Water on the Moon

*A Physician's Memoir of Service
from the Vietnam War
to Humanitarian Crises Worldwide*

FREDERICK M. BURKLE, JR., MD

Edited by Jan K. Herman *and* Megan Snair

Foreword by Arthur L. Kellermann, MD, MPH

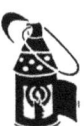

McFarland & Company, Inc., Publishers
Jefferson, North Carolina

ISBN (print) 978-1-4766-9664-5
ISBN (ebook) 978-1-4766-5435-5

LIBRARY OF CONGRESS AND BRITISH LIBRARY
CATALOGUING DATA ARE AVAILABLE

Library of Congress Control Number 2024046953

© 2025 Frederick M. Burkle, Jr., MD. All rights reserved

No part of this book may be reproduced or transmitted in any form or by any means, electronic or mechanical, including photocopying or recording, or by any information storage and retrieval system, without permission in writing from the publisher.

Front cover images: incoming Marine casualties (author's photo). The author beside a CH-46 Sea Knight helicopter. These helos were one means of transporting casualties to and from Al Khanjar (author's collection).

Printed in the United States of America

*McFarland & Company, Inc., Publishers
Box 611, Jefferson, North Carolina 28640
www.mcfarlandpub.com*

To
Philomena Klerx Dinnean Burkle
"Phyllis"
My darling wife of 63 years who has always been by my side—
even when we were thousands of miles apart.

To our loving children
Christopher, Jennifer, and Heidi

And to our family of Huskies and Golden Retrievers
we have loved and cherished
Anu, Emily Blossom, Tucker I, Oliver, Guinness, Finnegan,
Poochini, Sebastian, Pooh Bear, Chauncey, Okian, Tucker II,
Cashew, Bentley, Cooper, Willoughby, Peggy Sue, Benno,
Kipling, Henri, George Armstrong Custer

Contents

Acknowledgments	ix
Foreword by Arthur L. Kellermann, MD, MPH	1
Introduction	5

Part I: Planting the Seeds

1. Crossing the Street	9
2. Fulfilling a Dream: Frederick Martin Burkle, Jr., MD	19

Part II: In the Heart of War

3. How Did I Get to Vietnam? 1968–1969	33
4. A Moon for the Souls: 1969	53
5. Homecoming and Readjustment: 1969–1975	61
6. Operation Babylift: April 1975	66

Part III: Building a Humanitarian Career

7. Becoming a Global Health Professional: 1975–1990	85
8. Back to War—Iraq: December 1990–March 1991	103
9. Operation Provide Comfort: Spring 1991	119
10. On Call in Africa, Southeast Asia, and the Balkans: 1990s	134
11. The Center of Excellence: 1994–2000	150
12. Baghdad: April 2003	166
13. Sleuthing in Liberia: August 2003	183

Part IV: Bringing It All Home

14. A Wound Forever	199
15. Hard-Earned Lessons	209

Epilogue	221
Appendix 1: Tributes	223
Appendix 2: Four Perspectives on the World's Challenges and Concerns	233
A Physician in Peril	234
Sowing the Seeds of Global Autocracies	243
Politics and Public Health: An Explosive Combination	259
The Untold Cost of War on Civilians	266
Index	279

Acknowledgments

Writing and completing a book is not a one-person accomplishment. I would therefore like to express my deepest appreciation to those who kept prodding me to finish this memoir. Living in Hawaii, one of the most heartfelt Hawaiian words so often spoken is "mahalo," meaning "thank you." I therefore wish to say mahalo to the following extraordinary, make-it-happen contributors to this memoir—and to my life.

To Jan Herman, historian, film documentarian, author of many well-received books on military medicine, and a regular contributor to the *Journal of Health and Human Experience*. For 33 years, he was the Medical Historian of the Navy and Editor of *Navy Medicine* magazine, the journal of the Navy Medical Department.

And to Megan Snair, a first-rate journalist and editor. Megan is a science writer and an expert on public health subject matter, among many other health-related titles. She has supervised many scientific publications as Senior Program Officer and Study Director at the National Academies of Sciences, Engineering, and Medicine.

Jan and Megan were both determined to move this memoir along, and push they did to make this book come to light. Their names appear on the cover of this book—for good reason.

To my former civilian and military colleagues and humanitarian health care workers all over the world. You know who you are and you deserve my utmost appreciation and admiration. I have worked with professional teams in field hospitals, at Delta Med combat base in South Vietnam, and at Al Khanjar Navy-Marine Corps Trauma Center during the Persian Gulf War. I have had the privilege of being associated with expert health care teams during evacuee operations, as well as on worldwide inspection and assessment assignments to all continents. Hopefully, my professional and personal relationship with all of you made me a better physician—and perhaps a better person.

To physicians Dr. Albert Schweitzer and Dr. Tom Dooley whose humanitarian work inspired me at a very young and impressionable age to take the path I chose in life to the remotest parts of the world.

To Professor Zonghao Li, the former Director of Beijing Emergency Medical Center, whose friendship I have greatly treasured over the years.

To Brother Pierre at Notre Dame High School, who took a chance on me and paid my $25 application fee to Saint Michael's College.

To my Saint Michael's classmate, retired Senator Patrick Leahy, and to Bob Macpherson, Vietnam veteran, for their moving words that appear in the legacy section of Appendix 1, "Tributes." At this point in my life, those words of acknowledgment matter deeply.

To Arthur Kellermann, who wrote the Foreword to this book. He penned a glowing and highly complimentary tribute to my medical and humanitarian service. I thank him for his observations.

To Phyllis's parents, Neal and Margaret Dinnean, who encouraged me to pursue my dream of a career in medicine when my parents considered that profession a pipe dream.

To Luigi Boccherini, the 18th-century musician whose classical string quartet compositions got me through many of the proverbial writer's blocks and memory lapses. Grazie, Luigi!

To our two huskies and 19 golden retrievers, mainstays for our family over the years. We all shared their unconditional love and companionship.

To my three children, Christopher, Jennifer, and Heidi. I wish I could have spent more time with you in your childhood and adolescence. Thank you for your love for your mother and me.

Throughout the book, I have included some passages of Phyllis's remembrances of our life together and how my being away in war-torn lands touched her so personally. I went through many ordeals overseas, but Phyllis also went through many challenges during my long absences, the most important of which was raising three young children much of the time on her own. What affected me affected her. I strongly felt that some of her recollections should be included in this memoir because she was the other half of our enduring partnership in life. This is a love story.

Mahalo to all of you!

Perspective from the Other Half of This Love Story, from Phyllis D. Burkle

Skip and I are beginning our 64th year of marriage. If I were asked what it is about my husband that first attracted me to him and then saw my love continue to grow, the following words would be my answer: I met Skip at age 14 and knew even then that I wanted to spend as much time as possible with a warm, caring, and fun companion. When he realized his wish to be a physician, he faced many obstacles. But I knew he had the strength and determination to fight for what he believed was right.

During our early years of marriage when he was in medical school, his training required strength and determination. I had definitely married a man with unchallengeable convictions. During our married life, I witnessed many situations that required him to make difficult decisions—sometimes with uncomfortable results. I knew they were the right choices because he was true to his principles, and he lives true to them every day.

For much of our lives we were many miles apart, but there was never any mental distance between us. I always gave Skip my permission to do what he needed to do. All the major decisions were made as partners. We shared the sacrifices, joys, and disappointments, and our love was stronger because of it.

Skip is now battling a terminal illness. The time he has is spent motivating new humanitarians, giving advice, and encouraging their work. He is buoyed knowing that a cadre of humanitarians is increasing. They are continuing his work.

He insisted that this book be "our" book. I am proud to be married to this principled man. And yes, as Skip has already said, this book is a love story.

Foreword

BY ARTHUR L. KELLERMANN, MD, MPH

Memoirs and autobiographies, which are terms sometimes used interchangeably, typically fall into one of three categories. The first group of memoirs—and by far the largest—are works by individuals who are already famous for their past achievements or celebrity status—before they even sit down to write. Notable examples in this category are the autobiographies of Benjamin Franklin, Mark Twain, and Ulysses S. Grant, and, more recently, *Long Walk to Freedom* by Nelson Mandela and *Dreams from My Father: A Story of Race and Inheritance* by former President Barack Obama.

The second and much smaller classification of memoirs are those written by persons who are little known in their time, but whose works illuminate the era in which they lived or a cause they espoused. The best-known book of this genre is *The Diary of a Young Girl* by 13-year-old Anne Frank.

The third category consists of books by those people who are held in high esteem within a limited circle of colleagues, but not known by the general public. A prime example is *I, Rigoberta Menchú*, the story of a Guatemalan human rights activist who has dedicated her life to defending indigenous peoples in her country and, more recently, internationally. Nine years after the book was published, she was awarded the Nobel Peace Prize in 1992. Another book is *Witness to a Century: Encounters with the Noted, the Notorious, and Three SOBs* by George Seldes, a muckraking investigative journalist and foreign correspondent. Seldes wrote about some of the 20th century's most notable and disreputable figures, including Marshal Tito, Benito Mussolini, and Errol Flynn.

Water on the Moon: A Physician's Memoir of Service from the Vietnam War to Humanitarian Crises Worldwide fits firmly into this last category of memoirs. The author, Captain (Retired) Frederick "Skip" Burkle, Jr., Medical Corps, USNR, is little known by the public but revered by three generations of military medical officers and experts in humanitarian assistance medicine. During his extraordinary career, Skip not only witnessed some of the most pivotal moments in modern American history—he played a central role.

In 1968, for example, fresh out of his pediatrics residency, Skip was drafted into the U.S. Navy. Quickly deployed to Vietnam at a time when American military operations were at their peak, he was assigned to provide medical support to a Marine forward operating base near the DMZ. This area, barely south of the North Vietnamese border, was the site of the war's most intense fighting. Skip came of age in his late 20s while in Vietnam and discovered his true calling.

As the government of South Vietnam was collapsing in April 1975, he took leave from his graduate studies at the University of California, Berkeley to help an international relief group carry out Operation Babylift. This mission was one of the most audacious enterprises in the history of humanitarian medicine. His flight into Saigon, surrounded by North Vietnamese forces, and his venture into that strife-ridden city to find and rescue orphaned infants are tales for the ages.

In 1990, as a 50-year-old Navy Reservist, he was recalled to active duty and sent into the Arabian Desert near the Kuwait border in support of Operations Desert Shield and Desert Storm. Shortly before ground combat began, Skip was given the assignment as Senior Medical Officer of the Marine Corps' largest field hospital since World War II. With little time to spare, he swiftly brought his quarreling colleagues together and transformed them into high-performing team members who, in a brief amount of time, treated more than 450 severely wounded American and Coalition troops, as well as Iraqi prisoners of war.

In 2003, during the run-up to Operation Iraqi Freedom, Skip Burkle agreed to help the U.S. State Department prepare for post-conflict humanitarian assistance as head of the Disaster Assistance Response Team. He was repeatedly blocked by then–Defense Secretary Donald Rumsfeld and other DOD officials from taking the steps he knew were needed to prevent the health consequences that inevitably follow military conflicts. Skip nevertheless agreed to fly into Baghdad shortly after it fell in an attempt to stabilize Iraq's rapidly disintegrating health care system.

Once on the ground, he learned—through an Iraqi radio broadcast—that he had been named "Interim Minister of Health" for Iraq. During the next few hours, the dangers he faced eclipsed his most harrowing moments in Vietnam. What transpired in the days that followed will help readers understand why U.S. forces could not exit Iraq within weeks, as the American people had been promised, but instead remained for the next 18 years.

In addition to these and other riveting accounts, you will encounter a remarkable cast of characters, including Burkle's cold and imperious father, who concluded that his asthmatic and stuttering son would never amount to anything. His meek but loving mother finally stood up to her husband, however, to help Skip gain admission to a competitive high school. You will also meet dedicated military physicians, warriors, international relief workers, State Department officials, and intelligence agents. And you will come across both noteworthy and historical figures, such as Ambassador Wendy Chamberlin; General Jay Garner, who was Director of the U.S. Office for Reconstruction and Humanitarian Assistance for Iraq; Saddam Hussein; and Iraqi Shiite cleric Muqtada al–Sadr, who put a price on Burkle's head. Several pivotal chapters will offer fresh historical perspectives.

Historians should study this memoir for many new insights into the politics of humanitarian assistance. I also hope that many Americans will read it to understand that even in moments when elected or appointed officials act in foolish, arrogant, or shortsighted ways, military service members and other government officers, such as Dr. Skip Burkle, will put their lives on the line time and again to do what's right. In my experience, such selfless dedication has characterized America's military physicians since the early days of our republic.

Young people, who have to contend with disabilities or struggle to fit in, may find inspiration in reading the pages of this book, and realize that their physical or social difficulties need not define their lives. Dr. Burkle transcended his childhood stuttering and learning disability to become an outstanding scholar, quadruple board-certified specialist, international humanitarian, and an elected member of the National Academy of Medicine.

Finally, I hope that *Water on the Moon* motivates some number of high school, college, and health sciences students across the country to pursue careers of humanitarian service. In the book's first chapter, Dr. Burkle relates that, as a child, he was captivated by a 1949 *Time* magazine article about Dr. Albert Schweitzer. Thumbing through the photographs time and time again, he recalls, "I wanted so much to be like Dr. Schweitzer. He was my hero."

One day, perhaps, future humanitarians and health professionals will say the same about Skip Burkle.

Dr. Arthur L. Kellermann is one of our nation's healthcare thought leaders, and he has led, at various points, a city EMS system, a public health research center, and the Department of Emergency Medicine at Emory University. From 2013 to 2020, he served as dean of the School of Medicine at the Uniformed Services University. A longtime National Academy of Medicine member, he has published more than 400 scientific papers and public commentaries.

Introduction

"I learned this, at least, by my experiment; that if one advances confidently in the direction of his dreams, and endeavors to live the life which he has imagined, he will meet with a success unexpected in common hours."—Henry David Thoreau, *Walden*, 1854

When Thoreau wrote those words, he was talking to future generations, especially to me. Born less than a century later, I secretly embraced that confidence and the life I imagined, despite the limitations others initially placed on me. My dream was to practice humanitarian medicine wherever disasters unfolded. And it has been quite a journey.

Many obstacles stood in my way, not the least of which was a serious learning disability and an abusive father who saw no future for his seemingly indolent and difficult son. To put it mildly, I was not "college material" in my father's eyes.

Despite that inauspicious childhood, I created my own protective world and even my own juvenile language. But I also developed an insatiable thirst for learning. My first and most influential models were neither military heroes nor our Founding Fathers, but rather healers and humanitarians. Long before reaching my teens, Drs. Tom Dooley and Albert Schweitzer ignited my vision of practicing humanitarian medicine. Only after many years of education and experience, however, would that dream be fulfilled.

Looking back on the beginnings of my medical practice in the 1960s, and then my tour in South Vietnam, I find it incredible to see the trajectory my career took. The seeds of ethnic sensitivity, which were planted in that war-ravaged country, would set me on a path of enhanced cultural understanding for the rest of my career. When I left South Vietnam, the die had already been cast as to which direction my medical calling would take me. Just one year in Vietnam changed me forever.

Coming home, I wove a carefully crafted career in pediatrics and certifications in supplementary specialties, which eventually led me to teach other incoming professionals. I was getting ever so much closer to my dream of practicing humanitarian medicine in distant lands.

Eventually, that dream came true. I found myself back in South Vietnam rescuing infant orphans, deployed to the Persian Gulf War, and then a blur of responding to humanitarian crises in Kurdistan, the Balkans, and several African nations. I saw my share of war's aftermath in many places and witnessed what poverty and disease can inflict—even in the absence of conflict. Civilians are always the ones to suffer.

Practicing medicine globally meant dealing with power struggles and politics. I encountered sociopathic and narcissistic authoritarians, observing their gross lack of empathy for their respective nation's refugees. Following the Persian Gulf War, I negotiated with Saddam Hussein, as part of a small American Red Cross team, to provide relief for the beleaguered and struggling Kurds in northern Iraq. After that dictator's overthrow just 12 years later, I survived several coordinated attempts on my life while serving in Baghdad as Iraq's first Interim Health Minister. Yes, humanitarian medicine can be hazardous to your health.

Approaching my waning years, I cherished a Senior Fellow and Scientist position at the innovative Harvard Humanitarian Initiative, a Senior Scholar post at Johns Hopkins School of Public Health, and a Global Fellow post at the Woodrow Wilson International Center for Scholars in Washington, D.C., when I was in my 80s. Most appreciated was election by my peers to the prestigious National Academy of Medicine. Teaching, writing, and research were my focus to establish global public health as a recognized and harmonized multidisciplinary authority.

My life has gone in directions I never could have imagined—nor could Thoreau have pictured a career taking off in so many ways, always tied together by the need to think upstream and outside the box. Working in disaster preparedness and response, I quickly learned that a "next time" will always be on the horizon. It's just a matter of what that "next time" might look like and how it will appear.

But understanding who is most affected by disasters, as well as focusing more on the root causes and areas of breakdown, is the key perspective that I have always tried to address in my work. In addition, working across disciplines is certainly the only way we will ever be successful in solving some of these global problems. As these pages will reveal, confidence in my abilities, proficiencies which were built up across decades, played a key role. While at times both my wife and I paid a high price for this profession in the humanitarian field, both mentally and physically, we'd make that journey all over again. I hope you enjoy reading about the path our lives took.

Part I

Planting the Seeds

1

Crossing the Street

"I idolized Dr. Tom Dooley and other humanitarians for their altruistic deeds, and it was then that I had my first inkling that I wanted to be a doctor."

I heard it. We all heard it—the distant thrum of airplane engines, a noise that grew into a steady drone and then a roar. Sitting on the curb in front of my house, absent-mindedly poking bubbles in the hot asphalt, I looked up and saw them. Flying low over my Connecticut neighborhood were seemingly hundreds of bombers in formation, all heading southwest toward Long Island. This massive number of bombers darkening the sky was my first dramatic childhood remembrance. And these vestiges of war created a moment frozen in time that has stayed with me for the past eight decades.

To visibly take in this airborne phenomenon, everyone, mostly mothers and kids, ran to a flat area near the street where the trees didn't obscure the view. But then I suddenly found myself alone for the first time in my life—no mother, no father, no older sister to watch over me.

I was thrilled, of course, to witness this armada of aerial might, although something even more significant in my young life was also about to occur at that moment. With everyone preoccupied with the spectacle directly above and wildly clapping with excitement, I crossed the street to the forbidden side. I then turned around to view my house from a new perspective. This eye-opening event was every bit as significant as those planes passing in endless waves. The Second World War had just ended, but at age 5, I was now becoming aware of life beyond my small world on this street.

A War's Impact on a Child

I was born on April 29, 1940, in New Haven, Connecticut, to a typical lower middle-class New England family. Named for my father Frederick, I acquired the nickname "Skip" from early childhood. I was preceded by an older sister, Joan, and later a younger brother, Richard. Our house, built by my father, was a modest dwelling near the end of a dead-end street in the small town of Hamden, once noted for its apple orchards. The urban sprawl of New Haven has since gobbled up our old neighborhood, now under the jurisdiction of North Haven.

My father worked for the Southern New England Telephone Company as a drafter, and, on the side, was a tinkerer and an inventor. He contributed to the development of the original "walkie-talkie," which was used extensively in World War II. He even made one of those two-way radio transceivers for himself.

Reflections of the war impacted our daily lives. My parents taped maps to the wall so we could follow the far-off campaigns in Europe and the Pacific. And locally, we made family road outings around the neighborhood on Sundays in our old Plymouth sedan. My parents wanted to see which homes had their front windows displaying blue stars on small vertical Service Flags. A blue star indicated that someone, who had lived in that house, was serving in the military. A gold star on a Service Flag meant that a member of that family had been killed. We never lingered at those homes. Seeing those gold stars taught me about war and death at a very young age.

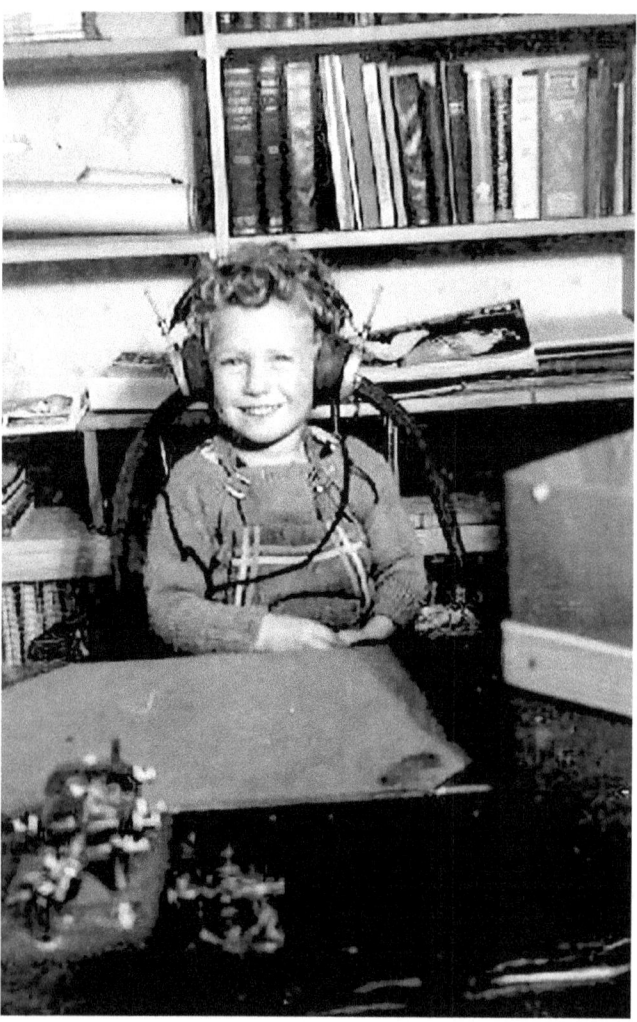

Skip commandeering his father's ham radio headset (author's collection).

My father was also a ham radio operator, broadcasting from our home at 97 Hartley Street, using the call sign "W10AS." He obtained the starter motor from a World War II Hellcat fighter engine and mounted the device in the attic. The motor turned a rod, which protruded through the roof. The motorized rod enabled him to rotate the huge antenna in any direction and receive and broadcast almost worldwide. He was very bright technical-wise, but too frequently he acted out his heritage as a cold Teutonic German.

As a psychiatrist, I am now aware that the influences in a child's first five years have much to do, consciously or unconsciously, with his or her direction in life. And World War II flavored every part of my daily childhood existence. I heard the term "rationing" but didn't understand what it meant at the time. War was different back then. Every person wanted to play a vital role in getting the job done. Rationing food and supplies in every home was among the many ways to support the men fighting overseas. Nowadays, even with U.S. troops deployed around the world, most Americans carry on with their own lives while being oblivious to the reality of war worlds away.

But the 1940s could not have been more different. It wasn't possible to read *Life*, *Look*, or *Time* magazines without seeing prominently displayed ads with patriotic themes. A helmeted GI grasping a candy bar appeared above the caption "He Comes First." Nestlé was presumably making this soldier's wartime experience more bearable with chocolate. The major automakers had ceased manufacturing cars for the civilian market and were now producing tanks and planes. General Motors and Ford reminded the reader that their new products, turned out by the thousands, would help defeat the Axis Powers. Even if I couldn't read yet, I certainly loved those advertisement pictures.

My playtime imitated reality. I wore helmets and shot toy guns. My friends and I pretended to be soldiers at war, even collecting and trading military patches. In the warm weather, we reconfigured the porch swing. Piled high with chairs, our overturned porch contraption resembled a plane's cockpit. Depending on the day, I was either a bomber pilot or a fighter pilot. As an adventurous 5-year-old kid with a wild imagination, I flew many missions—at least several hundred over Nazi Germany.

All my neighborhood friends collected model airplanes. My father would buy the plane kits but never let me build any of them. I had to watch in silence while he assembled the balsa wood parts and then painted the finished product. I hated not being allowed to help him. Nevertheless, I hung those airplanes from wires above my

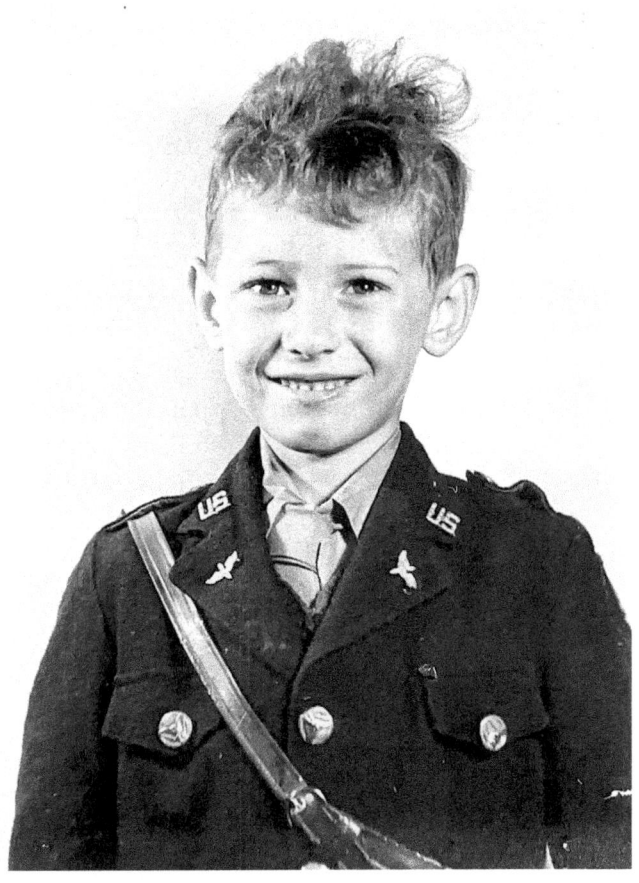

During the war years, a child's portrait meant donning a military uniform. At age 5, Skip posed as a "junior Army Air Forces officer" (author's collection).

bed and imagined what it would be like to fly one. I still have a few of those model planes my father had saved and stored in the attic. But they will never again see the light of day.

On some weekend summer days, my family drove to nearby Hammonasset Beach and looked for partially submerged enemy submarines that might be lurking in Long Island Sound. Living close to the water, German U-boats were on everyone's mind because one sub had already sneaked into New York Harbor in early 1942, and German subs were also torpedoing ships off the southern coast of the United States.

A Father's Scorn

Since we didn't talk much, my father's past was a mystery to me, and only later in life did I learn more about him. I found out that during World War II, he had served as a lieutenant in the Signal Corps of the Connecticut Army National Guard because of his talent with radios. With the formal Japanese surrender in September 1945, New Haven held a victory parade in which my father participated. I never saw him in uniform until the day he marched in that parade. With his eyes straight forward, he passed by me amid all the celebratory pageantry. I stood next to my mother in total disbelief. Even at a very young age, I never imagined my father marching in step, seemingly proud to have contributed to the war effort on the home front. He never glanced my way.

I discovered many years later that he had been accepted at and had attended West Point, but, for some unknown reason, he dropped out before he completed his first year. This well-hidden family secret remained buried until I was in my 20s, and nobody ever told me why he had left the Academy. While he was brilliant in math and science, it's clear, even in hindsight, that he didn't know how to raise a son, let alone a sensitive one. As with so many other young impressionable boys seeking their father's approval, I always sought my father's praise. I never got it.

Looking back, I really didn't know my father. He seldom said a word to me unless to bark an order. I grew up first afraid of him and then found myself despising him. I can't recall a single conversation with him on any subject. Information or orders—and there were many—were typically conveyed through my mother. When she alerted us that he was due to arrive home from work soon, we all went our separate ways and the house grew silent.

To add to my many childhood travails, I suffered from asthma. I was often up all night gasping for air and using the only home medication available, "Asthmador," a fine powder to be burned and the smoke inhaled. This nonprescription drug was later found to cause severe side effects and was eventually banned. But instead of concern for my asthma attacks, my father saw my illness as a personal affront, interfering with his sleep and other activities. I could often hear him yelling from his bedroom as my mother attempted to get my breathing under control. She would try to protect me from his wrath when my wheezing started, rushing me to my room and closing the door so my struggle to breathe would not disturb him.

Our family physician once cautioned my mother that I shouldn't be around smokers and asked if anyone in our house smoked. My father wasn't a cigarette smoker but he enjoyed cigars. When we returned home from that medical appointment, my mother told him about the doctor's warning. He angrily lit a cigar and blew the smoke in my face. When I didn't suffer any immediate breathing issues, he declared, "The doctor doesn't know what he's talking about. See, smoke doesn't cause any problem."

As I got older, I eventually realized my mother probably felt stifled and dominated during her marriage to a controlling, inflexible husband. Although relegated to the housewife role typical of that time, she had been among the first female graduate students at Yale in the early 1930s. In those days, Yale offered graduate degrees to women—although only in education and nursing. My mother received her master's degree in education in 1932, and two years later she wed Frederick Burkle. But because she was now married, she soon discovered that she was not permitted to teach grade school in the male-dominated teaching profession. Sadly, she never taught until the post-war years which produced teacher shortages. I was in her first class.

Early Obstacles

Elementary school was a real test for me. The birth rates were down, so there was room for kindergarten students to be placed in the first grade. To test our skills the school principal asked all to draw a horse. Most were simple stick figures but mine was a detailed trotting horse with a flowing mane. I was rushed from kindergarten to first grade, but being a year younger than my classmates was just the beginning of my dysfunctional childhood. Not only was I battling asthma and constantly falling ill, but I was also the shortest and skinniest kid in class. Making friends was a challenge, and, to top it off, I had three major obstacles to overcome. I stuttered, which made me a prime target for bullies. I had problems in both reading and math, a disability later to become known as "dyslexia." And I was left-handed in a right-handed world. My teachers were determined to "correct" my left-handedness, making my days even more difficult. Dealing with any one of these issues would have been hard enough, but I had to overcome all three every single day.

School continued to confuse me as I advanced from one grade to the next, and I struggled to fit in. Reading was very difficult and laborious. I could read but wasn't as fluent as my classmates in comprehension until I was in the fifth grade. I was jealous that other kids were learning more from books than I was absorbing. I often walked around with books in my hands to make myself look good, hoping to be accepted.

To cope with all these ongoing embarrassments, I invented my own world and developed my own selective way of acquiring knowledge that focused only on what

I felt was relevant to me. I constantly thumbed through books and magazines, concentrating on the illustrations. With my talent for creating pictures and drawings, I was able to make up stories to accompany the pictures. My fascination was with the world beyond, a captivation no doubt fueled by those wall maps of exotically named World War II campaigns. Those maps likely influenced my love of geography, a subject that I developed into a strength.

Being a loner, I even created my own written language in addition to my made-up world of pictures. I filled a notebook with pages of invented words and phrases. That treasured book was my alphabet and my dictionary. But when my parents found it, they were both equally confused as to what to do with me.

Their bewilderment led to an appointment—with my notebook in hand—for an assessment with a psychologist at Yale Medical School. I think my mother knew something was inexplicably wrong. The term "learning disability" wasn't even in the lexicon yet, though the psychologist said I was "very bright but lazy." I had some "sparks of intelligence," he added, but nothing my father could understand concretely. It didn't matter anyway. My father took in all he needed to hear from the psychologist who seemed to validate what he had been thinking all along about his son. In my father's eyes, I would never amount to anything. Hearing the word "lazy," he concluded that I was intentionally defying him. From that point on, I believe he stopped thinking of me as his son. I was only 9 years old.

My response, which I can now see being fairly predictable for a child my age, was to double down on fantasies about escaping from my home and small town to the countries whose names I had memorized. My daydreams went beyond running away, however, because I wanted to help people in need in those faraway mystical lands. I increasingly relied on photos or illustrations in books and popular magazines, such as *Life*, *Look*, or *National Geographic*, for my connections to the outside world. Those photographs may have been my salvation. I realized early on that something exciting awaited me on the outside, and a world existed beyond Hamden. At age 9, I still wasn't proficient at reading, but I knew what those magazine pictures were telling me. I needed to know what was out there.

What particularly intrigued me was a July 1949 issue of *Time* magazine with photos of Dr. Albert Schweitzer running a jungle hospital in French Equatorial Africa. For more than 50 years, he treated patients afflicted with every kind of tropical disease. I would study those pictures endlessly of this world-famous physician and humanitarian, as well as learn about the doctors and nurses working loyally by his side. I'd then make up a story of what I thought was going on in those remote, hot, and humid hospitals. I wanted so much to be like Dr. Schweitzer. He was my hero.

Defying the Odds at Notre Dame

Notre Dame, a Catholic high school for boys, was located about an hour away in West Haven, and several of my friends were planning to take the school's entrance exam. I also wanted to attend this prestigious high school so I talked my mother into letting me apply. My father had already said no. But without his knowledge, my mother arranged for me to take the tests on a day when he was away. Amazingly, I was accepted to Notre Dame High School.

My parents quarreled openly about whether or not I should enroll, with the focus on the annual tuition's prohibitive cost of $400. But my mother persevered. She rarely got her way when she tried to stand up to her domineering husband, but she firmly backed me up on this dispute. He eventually relented but stated flat out that he would not pay the tuition. She then had to ask her mother for the money.

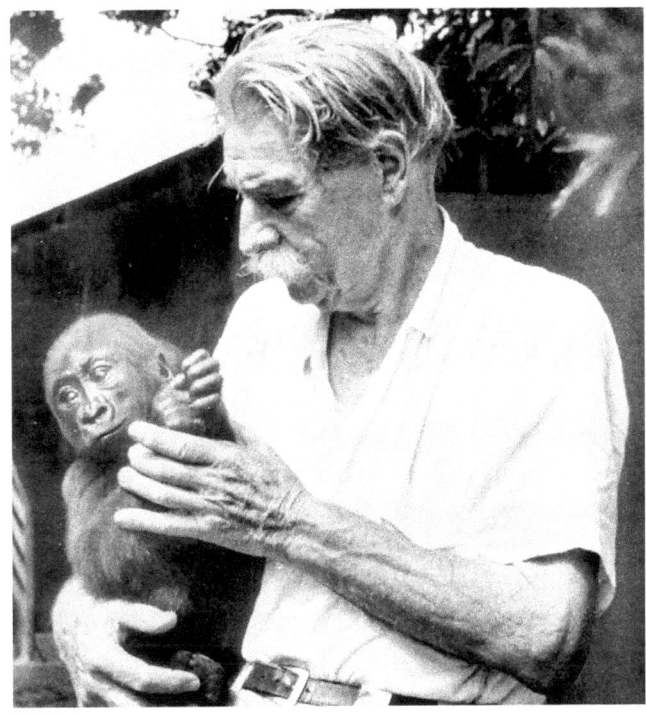

One of Skip Burkle's childhood ambitions was to become a physician-humanitarian like one of his heroes, Dr. Albert Schweitzer (National Library of Medicine).

I grew to love my time at Notre Dame. And though I enjoyed high school, I didn't understand the importance of studying other subjects that I found less interesting. I didn't see education in my future after graduation. I threw myself into history and science—but on my terms. I studied and learned in a unique way by listening rather than reading. I was a whiz at memorization. Slowly but surely, I taught myself to read but found I processed the words on the page in a different way than how others comprehended the meaning of the written word.

Once I finally overcame my reading disability, I became a voracious reader. If the books kids were reading in the 1950s were *Tom Swift and His Flying Lab* (1954) or the popular *Black Stallion* series (1940s), my fare was Tom Dooley's *Deliver Us from Evil* (1956) and *The Edge of Tomorrow* (1958). Tom Dooley was a physician who became another of my heroes because of the work he was doing healing the sick in Vietnam and Laos.

Through this extraordinary man, I learned about Southeast Asia and studied my cherished maps in more detail. I idolized Dr. Dooley and other humanitarians for their altruistic deeds, and it was then that I had my first inkling that I wanted to be a doctor. But I also had enough sense not to say anything to anyone at the time because I would have invited teasing and ridicule. I'm sure everybody in my immediate world thought I would be the last person who would ever become a physician. My father had already decided that I wasn't going to college—or anywhere else in life.

The First Day of the Rest of My Life

In the fall of 1954, I first set eyes on Phyllis—and my life changed. I was a sophomore at Notre Dame. At that point, I was the classic insecure, self-conscious teen with very little in the way of social life. When we first met, Phyllis was a freshman at a Catholic school for girls, visiting her classmate around the block from my house. I was on my bicycle and we made small talk. The conversation went smoothly, much to my surprise. But when it was time for me to return home, I picked up my bike and the front wheel fell off, leading to snide remarks from a group of kids nearby.

With great embarrassment and sneering laughter in the background, I said goodbye to Phyllis. I headed back to my house carrying the wheel in one hand and dragging the remains of my bike in the other. For many other teens, this mortifying bike incident would have made for a depressing day, but I found myself walking on air. I met Phyllis Dinnean.

Even though I had now found out where Phyllis lived, I didn't know anything else about her. My mission was clear: I wanted to talk to her again. Two days later, I found the name "Dinnean" in the phone book and nervously dialed her number. In the mid-1950s, we had a party line, which was a telephone line shared by others. If that party line was clear, I rationalized, then I was meant to call her. If the line wasn't free, then I would hang up and try again later. As luck would have it—or perhaps it was fate—the line was free and Phyllis answered. After some light conversation to break the ice, I told her I was going with "the guys" to the Whitneyville Theater that Friday near her house and asked if we could sit together. Much to my amazement, she said yes. This was one of the most exciting moments of my adolescent life.

On our first few encounters, we didn't talk much. She was shy. I was shy. But I was also afraid that if I didn't muster the nerve to speak with Phyllis at length, I'd lose the opportunity to get to know her better. Fortunately, my stuttering from a young age had abated significantly, and I prayed my stammering wouldn't rear its ugly head again when I was around her. My luck prevailed, thankfully. The stuttering seemed to have vanished into thin air!

I loved being around Phyllis during those high school years. As we became closer, I quickly realized that I also wanted to be a part of her nurturing family. I saw for the first time what a loving and caring home should look like. I paid close attention to their family interactions, making mental notes about their communication skills, which almost always resulted in warm and caring relationships. I observed their conversations during dinner and the way they supported one another throughout life's everyday challenges and unexpected turns. I also noted her parents' encouragement for their kids in school. Their family life was so different from the negatively charged environment I grew up in just a few miles away.

Unlocking Minds at Saint Michael's

Thankfully, Phyllis's home became my safe space during those high school years. I spent as much time as I could with her and her family. If her parents hadn't welcomed me into their family fold, I'm not sure what direction my life would have taken. As I inched my way toward high school graduation, my father made it clear, in no uncertain terms, that I was not going to college, and that I shouldn't even bother applying. But dealing with his hostile presence in our small town was never an option for me. Despite his discouraging words playing on a loop in my mind, I secretly defied my father, knowing that somehow I would apply to my college of choice, Saint Michael's, a Roman Catholic school in Colchester, Vermont. I was going to work out my academic future on my terms and conditions.

I had a job at a grocery store on weeknights and weekends, as well as a part-time position at Saint Raphael Hospital in New Haven learning how to draw blood and working in its blood bank. But I still didn't have enough money for the application fee. I pleaded with Brother Pierre at Notre Dame for a $25 loan, promising to pay him back. The next morning the requested check was waiting at the desk. The secretary wished me good luck when I picked it up. As if that check wasn't enough, Brother Pierre also wrote an encouraging letter of recommendation on my behalf. I couldn't believe it. The next chapter of my life was playing out right before my very eyes. I sent in my application and was fortunately accepted, but my joy was short-lived. When I told my father, he unwaveringly proclaimed, "You're not going!"

Refusing to speak to me for weeks, my father again blamed my mother. This highly emotional situation was ironic since she never knew I had applied for admission. But by this point in my life, I was done letting him dictate my future. I ignored his resentment and insults and followed through with the admissions process.

Knowing my father's strong disapproval of his college-bound son, Phyllis's parents once again came to the rescue and took me to Saint Michael's for registration in the fall of 1957. My mother thought it was a fine idea, but I suspected this trip created additional friction between my parents. Surprisingly, my father didn't object to another family taking me. I suppose he was happy for the weight of my defiance being removed from his shoulders. I was heading to college with unending gratitude to Phyllis, her parents, and a Brother of Holy Cross, all of whom had faith in me. I could not, and would not, disappoint my band of cheerleaders championing me all the way to college.

Leaving my toxic upbringing was the best decision I had made at that point in my life. I chose this small rural Vermont college based on strong recommendations for its pre-med program. But more importantly, I wanted to attend Saint Michael's because of its emphasis on the humanities. The college's courses were designed to teach students new ways to think and reason. The classes were so devised to convert our youthful concrete, black-and-white view of life to a more abstract way to see and deal with a complex world. My brain had matured enough that I was eager to grasp and analyze the more intangible concepts and arguments.

I excelled and broke all my previous scholastic records. I joined practically every club at Saint Michael's to learn and hopefully improve my stressful and weak social skills. In my junior year, 1959–1960, I even formed the Pre-Medical Honor Society. I was truly thriving.[1] And each summer, I continued to hone my medical skills by returning to Saint Raphael Hospital.

Later, I applied to an early acceptance program at the University of Vermont Medical College in Burlington and was admitted. For two years, the setup was experimental: The last year of college was combined with the first year of medical school. I was the only student from nearby Saint Michael's who was accepted into this program. But now that medical school was in sight, I spent many sleepless nights wondering how I would pay the tuition.

* * * *

By the time of my high school graduation from Notre Dame in 1957, I had overcome asthma, stuttering, dyslexia, and a father's contempt. I was accepted at a prestigious college and by 1960, I was entering medical school. I had "crossed the street" in ways that surprised even myself. But more important than any of these achievements against all odds, Phyllis Dinnean was now a part of my life. And whatever life would throw at me, I could deal with it because Phyllis would be there with me.

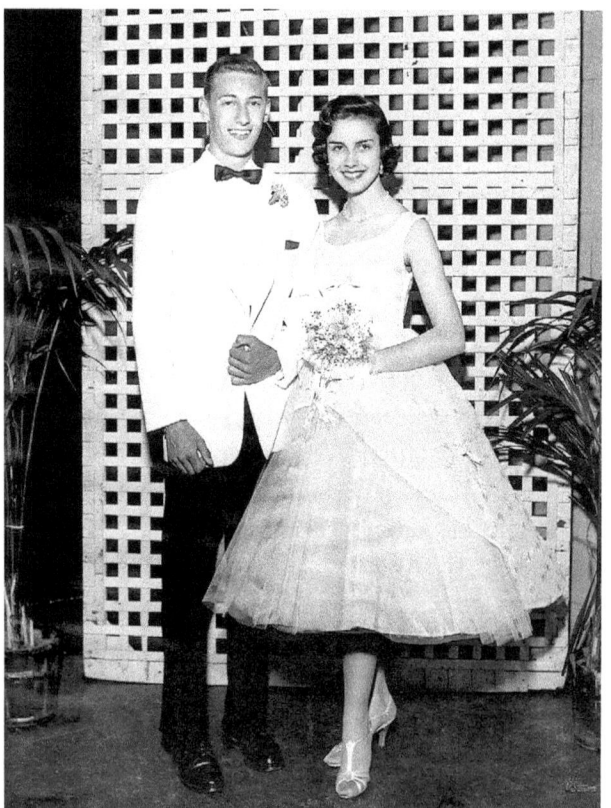

Skip and Phyllis dressed for the Notre Dame High School prom in 1957 (author's collection).

---

1. In 2016, I was honored to be invited back to Saint Michael's to give the commencement address to the Class of 2016. The text of my talk appears in the "Legacy" section of Appendix 1, "Tributes." This speech to my alma mater was recognized and placed in the *Congressional Record* on June 7, 2016 (pp. S3535–S3537) by one of my fellow college classmates, Patrick Leahy, senator from Vermont from 1975 to 2023. Available at https://www.govinfo.gov/content/pkg/CREC-2016-06-07/pdf/CREC-2016-06-07-senate.pdf.

2

Fulfilling a Dream

Frederick Martin Burkle, Jr., MD

> "At that point, a senior resident said matter-of-factly, 'Skip, you've been contaminated. We'll have to treat you.'"

Phyllis and I continued to date throughout college and planned to get married when I got into medical school. And I was now in my first year of med school at the University of Vermont in Burlington. Our wedding took place in a church in our hometown with a small formal ceremony on December 26, 1960. We were both 20 years old and ready to take on the world—together.

As newlyweds facing the beginning of that new med school program year from 1960 to 1961, we had to start off our marriage, much to our youthful regret, by leading separate lives. As Phyllis remembered, it wasn't the best way to begin a marriage since we couldn't be together, but it was worth it. She continued her classes several hours south of me at Southern Connecticut State College. We talked by phone only on weekends with the main topic being our critical lack of money.

But I had to find a way to pay for this medical school program because I couldn't let go of this opportunity. The Navy had created a scholarship program that paid for med school, which seemed to be a perfect solution for our ongoing financial dilemma. The program would include being commissioned a naval officer, and I would then go into a Navy residency program after I graduated from Saint Michael's in the spring of 1961. But my application for this Navy scholarship program was, unfortunately, rejected simply because I had a history of asthma. With that option off the table, the only alternative I could see was to pay for school with multiple student loans. I received a partial scholarship through the company that employed Phyllis's mother, and that money helped. But, as a result, I ended up with loans I never thought I would ever be able to pay off.

Phyllis started teaching kindergarten in Burlington, Vermont, after graduating from college in 1961, yet we struggled with finances through those trying, endless medical school years. But despite this demanding period in our lives, we both knew we wanted to have a family. We were thrilled to welcome our first child, Christopher, in 1963. As I was burning the midnight oil trying to make it through my courses, Phyllis was caring for our young son 24 hours a day. Neither of us got much sleep throughout the next several years which came with two more children, more debt, and my hospital residency. Phyllis never lamented our financial straits and my increased time away from the family.

In 1964, in my senior year at the University of Vermont Medical School, I applied for residency at Yale-New Haven Hospital. I anxiously waited to hear if Yale would grant an interview, the first step in the Matching Program for residencies.[2] Whether or not Yale ranked the applicant depended conditionally on the interview process, which was known to resemble an inquisition. The sessions were akin to hazing in which the interviewers made a sport of insulting the interviewees to see how they would react under stress. I knew this interrogation would be difficult, but had no idea what I was about to undergo. Yale, a teaching hospital, however, remained my first choice. If admitted into this program, Phyllis and I realized we would have to contend with additional economic hardship. The intern made $1,100 for the entire year and worked 24- to 72-hour shifts with eight hours off. A senior resident received $3,000 a year.

"Married to Yale"

Yale-New Haven Hospital had never accepted an intern who was married, not to mention married with children. But with a sigh of relief, I found out I was granted an interview at Yale. In a letter with a conditional and ominous overtone, the faculty wrote that they wanted to interview me—and they also needed to talk to Phyllis. Our son Christopher was 18 months old, and Phyllis was almost at full-term with her second pregnancy.

The setup included three interviews for me. The fourth interview was designated for Phyllis, which consisted of the three faculty members who had separately questioned me. They all sat behind a table in a long narrow utility room with just one gooseneck lamp shining on Phyllis's face, a very odd and intimidating room for an interview. Phyllis, who was quite nervous, had to sit in a chair about eight feet away. I sat in the back and was instructed not to speak.

One of the Yale faculty members, leaning forward and looking her straight in the eye, condescendingly stated, "We're interested in your husband. But you need to know that if we accept him, he won't be married to you. He will be married to Yale."

Then he sat back and waited for her response. Phyllis and I had never rehearsed any answers to probable questions, but being very insightful, she could tell this process was designed to be unnerving. After a few moments, she said she understood and added nothing else. The interviewers seemed satisfied with her simple reply. But I knew she didn't agree with the hospital's outdated regulations. Being

---

2. The National Resident Matching Program (NRMP) is a private, non-profit, non-governmental organization to put medical school students into residency programs in teaching hospitals throughout the United States.

ever optimistic, she thought we could somehow make ends meet and work out everything.

After those grueling interviews, I asked Phyllis what she was thinking when the interviewer made that provocative, seemingly smug statement about being "married to Yale." She responded simply and to the point. Having lived with me through medical school, she understood that I had to give just about 100 percent of my time to medicine, a commitment she supported.

I was accepted into the Yale-New Haven Hospital internship program, receiving that most welcoming news the day before I graduated from the University of Vermont Medical School. And somehow those exhausting years of "married to Yale" residency did work out though our financial circumstances seemed to always remain in the red.

We had two weeks before we had to travel to New Haven, but our second baby, about to be born, was oblivious to our schedule. Phyllis's due date was rapidly approaching while I tied up loose ends in Burlington and tried to prepare for our move back to Connecticut. Her Rh antibodies were increasing, which could be dangerous for the infant, so the obstetrician agreed to induce her. The delivery went well, but our new daughter, Jennifer, had to stay in the hospital to be monitored for possible anemia.

Much to our relief, Jennifer was discharged after three days in the hospital. But before her release, I had to settle the hospital charges at the Mary L. Fletcher Hospital.[3] Many married med students had babies during their time in school because they were not charged any hospital fees. I naïvely thought our situation would be the same, not wanting to add this large hospital charge to our ever-present financial burden.

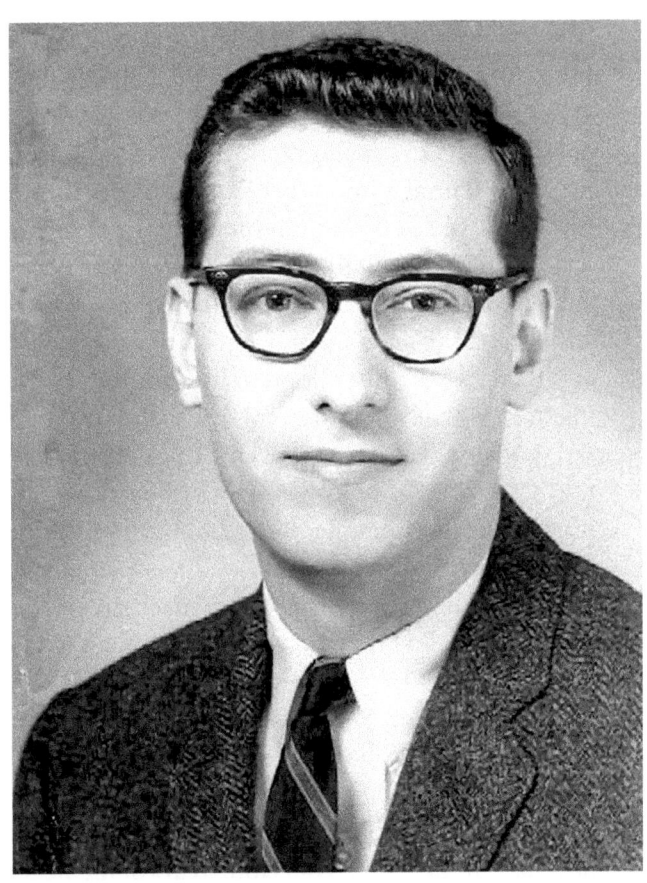

Skip as a Yale-New Haven Hospital intern (author's collection).

---

3. In 1967, Mary L. Fletcher Hospital became the Medical Center Hospital of Vermont.

My assumption was wrong. Our timing was just a bit late. Before the official discharge, the clerk at the hospital's front desk handed me a bill for nearly $400. I explained that I was exempt from any fees since I had just received my degree from medical school. He coldly responded that because I had graduated the week before, I was no longer allowed student coverage. My relief at our daughter's health improvement was suddenly replaced by sheer panic. I had just $13.83 in my pocket, enough gas money for the trip back to New Haven. I told the clerk that that was all the money I had.

The silence was deafening as he stared at me. Then he repeated, still unmoved, that he would not permit Jennifer to be released until the hospital bill was paid in full. I now had less than two weeks to move my family from Vermont to Connecticut to start another intensive phase of medical training. And here was this by-the-book clerk telling me he would not release our newborn daughter to us. My palms began to sweat as I scanned my brain for ways to come up with such a large sum of money on the spot.

My panicked, anguished deliberations, however, produced results. Amazingly, I forgot that I had a check in my pocket for $150, which had been presented to me at my recent graduation. The award was designated "for the greatest proficiency in obstetrics and gynecology." The irony of that "proficiency in obstetrics" wording was not lost on me as I stood there unable to pay for my daughter's release. I showed him the check. The clerk then disappeared through an office door.

The minutes felt like hours until he returned and conveyed that his superior had agreed to accept the check as full payment. I let out a huge sigh of relief and could start breathing once again. I signed the check over before he could change his mind and then took Jennifer home. We drove to New Haven the next day, fully appreciating the fact that we had never been so broke—or so lucky.

Looking back on this event, I can only love and admire my wife even more, if that's possible. I was consumed with ensuring Jennifer's health and safety, wrapping up my life from medical school, and thinking of the residency looming ahead. But Phyllis had just had a baby and was also caring for our young son at home. A few days after giving birth, she had to pack up everything that comprised our home—and our life—and then drive to Connecticut to start yet another of life's adventures together.

As I signed in for my first day as an intern at Yale-New Haven Hospital, I suddenly realized just how far I had come. At Saint Raphael Hospital where I had volunteered in high school, I had gone from being an orderly to working in the autopsy room, to drawing blood, to doing lab tests, and finally to working as an extern.[4] I now had all those skills plus four years of medical school behind me.

I was beginning the next phase of my training. I loved coming into the hospital

---

4. The "extern" classification refers to an unpaid medical student who wears the white hospital garb of an intern without an intern's privileges. An extern, for example, has no authority to write orders.

daily, inhaling all its associated smells, and dealing with the frenetic nature of a superior medical environment. I was happy and oddly felt at home here. Diseases increasingly fascinated me as my medical career advanced. And Tom Dooley, the humanitarian in Southeast Asia, remained my idol.

I decided to complete the three-year pediatric residency and become board certified in pediatrics before entering the surgery program. At that same time, in 1965, the war in Vietnam had intensified, so I thought the draft might require me to serve two years before I could apply for the surgical program. But I doubted the military would want me after being rejected from the Navy scholarship program, especially given my history of asthma.

At that time, we lived in a questionable New Haven neighborhood, but low-income apartments were the only rent we could afford on my paltry hospital stipend. I always worried about my family's safety and security during the longer shifts. But if I could struggle through the next three years of financial hardship, I was sure I could get a decent job, find better housing, and start paying back those ever-mounting bills. We had come so far and I could almost see the light at the end of the tunnel. I couldn't stop pursuing my dream now.

But before fulfilling that long-anticipated dream, Phyllis provided an accommodating routine for me during these stressful years of my residency—challenging years not only for me but for my entire family. Phyllis would have my dinner waiting, practically handing me the plate as I walked through the door. If the meal wasn't quite ready, I'd sit on the couch and the inevitable happened: I would crash. Unfortunately, with my demanding schedule and lack of sleep, we didn't have much of a married life. Phyllis never complained. My dream was her dream.

A Family's Worst Nightmare

On one fateful day in 1965, an event unfolded that permeated our lives for a very long time, something that had major family ramifications. The experience was both traumatic and terrifying, involving a closely held family secret from the distant past that had been hidden from me for decades. On this particular day, Phyllis was outside with several other mothers watching their young children play on our apartment's front lawn.

As Phyllis recalled, she heard baby Jennifer crying as she awoke from her nap upstairs in the apartment. She went into Jennifer's room to check on her. When Phyllis went back outside, she found that the mothers and their children had gone back inside, but Christopher was nowhere to be found. She hurriedly ran from door-to-door looking for him, assuming he had been taken into another apartment by one of the mothers.

Phyllis's mind was racing in trying to decide what to do next. Several minutes later, though seemingly like an eternity, Phyllis saw a patrol car driving to the apartment complex. Two policemen got out of their squad car, each one holding one of Christopher's little hands. Surprisingly, they knew to come to our address. One of the policemen said that an elderly man had flagged them down, pointed to our building, and then told the officers that he thought the child lived there. The older man said our little boy had wandered off on his own. The fact that this man knew where we lived was never explained to us. A highly distressed Phyllis phoned me at the hospital in tears, but full of relief that our son was safe.

Several weeks after this incident, I told Uncle Robert, my father's brother, about this alarming family episode. After a momentary silence, Robert then coolly related that he had already found out about this old man taking Christopher. I stood transfixed for a moment, trying to process how he could have found out. But to make this nightmare even more disturbing, Robert added that the elderly man was my grandfather, a man I had assumed was long dead. I was thunderstruck. Robert explained that my paternal grandfather and his family had engineered Christopher's capture. My emotions exploded. I was stunned and confused, not to mention speechless. But my overriding reaction was anger beyond belief.

Trying to take in this nightmarish scenario, Robert then conveyed a buried family story. This man, my grandfather, allegedly abused my father when he was a child. The parental offenses even included a claim that he had attempted to drown my father in a bathtub. I was now thrown into this depressing ancestral history. I suddenly viewed my father's internal struggle through a new lens.

"Baby Boy M"

The years I spent as a resident were a blur of constant cases, emergencies, and very little sleep. I became more proficient in diagnoses and skills. But medical incidents always arose that went beyond my scope of knowledge or practice, and new medical occurrences kept me humble. During the summer of 1966 and my first year of residency, I was called across the street to Grace-New Haven Hospital in the middle of the night to attend to a woman in labor. She hadn't received any prenatal care throughout her pregnancy. The baby was breech and small, so the obstetrician on duty wanted to have a pediatrician present in case any problems might occur with the delivery.

It was 2 a.m. when the baby boy was delivered, weighing just 4 pounds, 11 ounces. He gasped yet failed to take a deep breath. The obstetrician then handed the baby to me. At that moment, the infant's cardiac rate was getting slower and did not improve by "bagging"[5] him with oxygen. For newborns, we had short, soft rubber intubation tubes that went from the mouth to the trachea. Even with these kinds of specialized tubes, it is difficult to intubate a baby because its anatomy is so tiny.

---

5. Bagging is the artificial ventilation performed with a respirator bag, such as an Ambu (artificial manual breathing unit) or the reservoir bag on an anesthesia machine. The bag is squeezed to deliver air to the patient's lungs through a mask, an endotracheal tube, a laryngeal mask, or another breathing device.

I was finally able to get the tube into the baby's upper trachea. I placed my mouth on the outside tip of the short tube and breathed for the little boy. I was essentially doing mouth-to-mouth resuscitation. I felt immediate resistance, however, and the pulse rate increased only slightly. I repeated the intubation. But with each successful insertion, the obstruction occurred once again. I was able to get air only into the upper lungs. I couldn't do anything for the lower part of the lungs.

I told a staff member to quickly call my senior resident and she came immediately. We tried every breathing technique imaginable and continued for almost an hour to keep the baby alive. We were giving the infant enough oxygen to keep the pulse up to about 50 beats per minute, but this heart rate is much too low to sustain life. A healthy infant's pulse should be closer to 120 to 140. The heartbeat eventually failed and his little body gave up. We had to reluctantly declare the baby deceased. My senior resident and I had performed all the required resuscitation procedures in the delivery room, trying to keep this infant boy alive—but sadly to no avail.

With great regret and sorrow, I informed the mother, now back in her hospital room, that her baby had died. I told her we would perform an autopsy to determine the cause because we always need to consider the many reasons why infants have respiratory failure. The mother was heartbroken. But on the far side of the room, I noticed a stern-looking man dressed in a suit and tie standing against the wall. He was the father.

From my side of the room, I introduced myself and said, "Your baby just couldn't breathe. I'm very sorry. We tried to do everything to save him. We will learn much more with an autopsy."

But to my surprise, the man then charged across the room toward me. He grabbed my scrubs and lifted me off the floor before smashing my head against the wall. His malevolent eyes were fixed on mine.

"I want to know why my baby died!" he shouted. I pushed him away and yelled, "Back off! We need the results from the autopsy. It's the only way we can find out."

He and his wife had no problem signing the autopsy permit. But since she did not receive prenatal care from a hospital or clinic, we had no known medical history. The parents did not contribute any additional details. With a heavy heart, I filled out the paperwork for "Baby Boy M."

Contamination

A week later, I attended the mandatory monthly "black book conference," which convened in the basement housing the Pathology Department. These meetings were held to review the disease findings of children who had died or who were considered unusual cases in the hospital. A pathology resident was typically the only one who attended these meetings. But on that particular day, two faculty members were also present.

One of doctors asked, "Who had 'Baby Boy M?'" I responded that he had been my patient. I then began searching through my notebook for whatever history I had of the infant to share with those present.

Unfortunately, these two physicians hadn't heard a detailed account of the attempted resuscitation. The pathologists initially thought the delivery was a stillbirth. Reading from my notes, I reported the update: "This baby had presented without spontaneous breathing, attempted resuscitation, and worked on him for 50 minutes without success."

The faculty members looked at one other with raised eyebrows after I described the attempts at "tubing" the infant. I could tell they were growing concerned for some unknown reason.

I next heard the alarming words and I was petrified. The baby had died from syphilitic pneumonia—the first case in New Haven in 35 years. Pathology even obtained spirochetes, a form of bacteria, from the infant's mouth. I tried to digest this new and staggering information, recalling how close I'd been to him and how much air was exchanged as I tried to keep him alive.

At that point, a senior resident said matter-of-factly, "Skip, you've been contaminated. We'll have to treat you."

After this "black book conference," I was immediately taken to the ER and given mega doses of penicillin. I then knew what I had to do next and I dreaded it. But I worked up the courage to make that call to Phyllis about possibly being infected with syphilis. Although churning underneath, I calmly tried to explain the medical situation and the absolute need for penicillin injections for her and the kids since they were all exposed through me.

I was still on call that evening. Despite my exposure to syphilis, my immediate task was to perform an exchange transfusion on a newborn, a procedure that could take several hours. As a resident, Yale "owned" me and since I hadn't displayed any symptoms of syphilis, they had no qualms about my treating patients. I was not feeling well at this point, but I was already gowned and masked in a warm and crowded corner of the nursery. Halfway through this lengthy procedure, I suddenly began shaking with chills and fever. I asked a nurse to call my senior resident. When she arrived, I requested that she take over, insisting that I couldn't continue in my condition.

The senior resident sent me back to the ER. On arrival, I had a 105-degree fever, abdominal pain, and an enlarged spleen. I told the ER staff the history of my bizarre day and the devastating pathology report, adding that I had been given large doses of penicillin. The antibiotic had destroyed any spirochetes in my system, as intended. But when the spirochetes were killed, they released endotoxins in large numbers into my bloodstream, causing a detoxification condition known as a "Herxheimer reaction." My chills and fever spikes were symptoms very similar to severe malaria.

The ER doctor wanted to admit me but I refused. Then I called Phyllis to pick me up. After a fitful night of sleeping, I awoke the next morning exhausted, having sweated profusely during the night and soaked our bedsheets.

Trusting in my medical judgment, Phyllis and our kids got the penicillin injections the very next day and their test results indicated no signs of syphilitic pneumonia. And I never tested positive for syphilis. My relief knew no bounds.

Code Red

One unusually quiet night on the pediatric ward, I tried to get a few moments of much-needed sleep. But then the resident in the Pediatric Emergency Room brought me back to reality with a call for assistance. He had admitted a 6-year-old boy with meningitis to another pediatric ward. The mother had just arrived directly from Puerto Rico—with luggage in hand—at the Yale-New Haven ER. She also brought her younger son, a 4 year-old. Social Services had found a place for the mother to sleep but children were not allowed. The resident in charge decided to admit the younger brother to an empty bed, calling it a "social admission." His stay would be for one night only, he said, insisting this younger child was well and would be released in the morning.

When the 4-year-old arrived on my ward, I did a physical exam, got him to laugh, and tucked him in for the night. The nurses loved him immediately. I left the ward at about 1:30 a.m. Suddenly a "Code Red" alert for cardiac arrest was sounded throughout the hospital. I ran back to my ward wondering which child had caused this dreaded alarm. The nurses hurriedly brought in the resuscitation equipment to the room of this 4-year-old, who I had just made comfortable and had wished him good night. I rushed to the head of his bed and noted at once his dire condition. I ordered all the nurses, except one, to leave the room right away.

The little boy was covered from head to toe with large hemorrhagic lesions that were rapidly progressing before our eyes. With a massive, prolonged seizure, his body slumped and became lifeless. He died within minutes. I knew instantly that he had meningococcal septicemia, caused by an extremely virulent microorganism that rapidly invaded all his vascular organs.[6] Resuscitation was not an option because he was extremely contagious. I had studied this disease but could hardly believe how quickly it had destroyed this child's body.

The staff members on duty, as well as me, received prophylactic antibiotics. Everyone else, who had interacted with this little boy, was contacted immediately to get antibiotics. Ironically, his older brother, who had been admitted with meningitis, recovered well. But little did I know that I would soon be dealing with unfamiliar and infectious diseases in a far-off land—on an everyday basis.

---

6. Meningococcal septicemia, a highly contagious bacterial infection, allows bacteria to enter the bloodstream, multiplying and damaging the walls of the blood vessels. This bloodstream infection causes bleeding into the skin and organs.

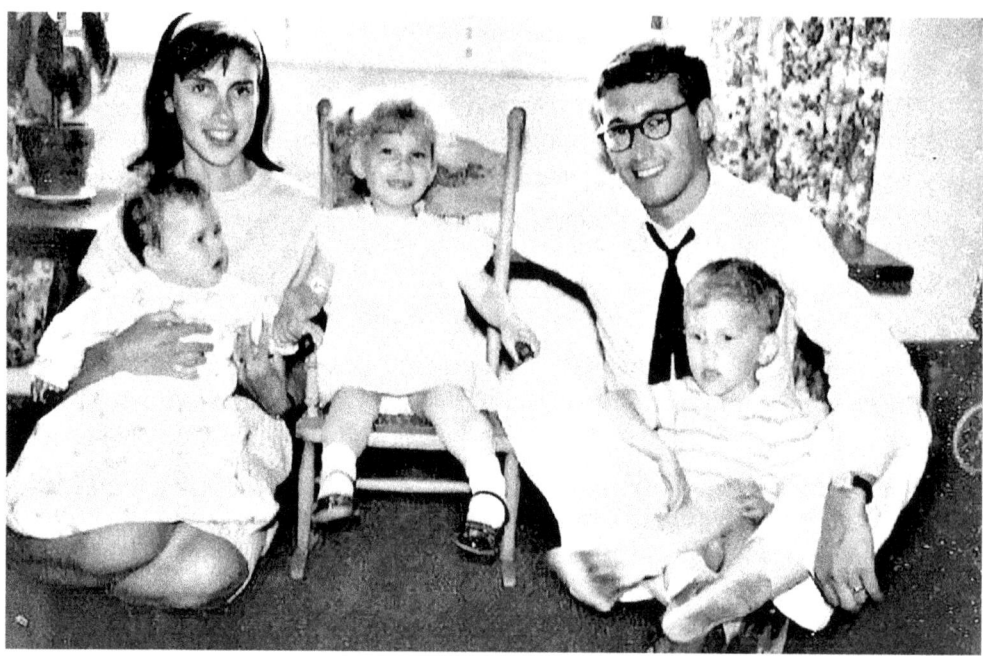

The growing Burkle family in late 1965: Phyllis holding Heidi, Jennifer (center), Skip holding Christopher (author's collection).

Vietnam Always Looming

Despite the hardships of these years, our family happily continued to grow. Our third child, Heidi, joined us in 1966. All three children were born in the very turbulent 1960s, a time that got more disruptive and tumultuous for Phyllis and me before it was over. The Vietnam War was escalating and racial disturbances had broken out into full-scale riots across the country. Yet during my medical training, I was sharply focused and had only one goal in mind: becoming a physician. I had almost no time to read newspapers or listen to news broadcasts. I barely had time to be a husband and father.

But according to Phyllis, she felt that she had a job holding down the fort, probably the most important job she would ever have. She was a mother and responsible for three wonderful, understanding children. She claimed that having that awesome responsibility kept her going, which enabled me to keep me going.

Being a resident was draining, grueling, and arduous. I also learned about the fragility of life and relationships in the very city I grew to love and admire. I barely understood the culture of those men, women, and children I lived and worked with in New Haven. Who knew that I would soon be sent to a country whose peoples' way of life was dramatically different from our culture. Ironically, it was a culture Tom Dooley had come to know and love. For some reason, I felt even closer to my lifelong dream. But those demanding years also altered my end goal of performing cleft lip plastic surgery and other medical techniques on children in need.

2. Fulfilling a Dream

* * * *

Time passed quickly and I graduated from the residency program, despite my father's hostility toward me throughout my childhood, adolescence, and early adulthood. I never let his resistance and intimidation get me down. Instead, I overcame every obstacle thrown in my path, including my father's ongoing conviction that I would never make anything of my life. I had at last earned my new title of Dr. Frederick Martin Burkle, Jr., MD, and nobody, not even my father, could take it away from me.

Part II

In the Heart of War

3

How Did I Get to Vietnam?
1968–1969

> *"One corpsman, using a common hose, washed pools of blood into two large drains in the triage floor. The drumming from the chopper faded away and a sudden quiet enveloped me—and this was just my first day at Delta Med. My inner voice finally broke that lingering silence and became loud and clear: I don't belong here. I'm useless at Delta Med."*

Suddenly a roar filled my ears, a sound I had never experienced before. Just outside the blast wall, all other clamor was drowned out by the loud and heavy "thwapping" sound of the helicopter blades, a noise that suppressed any possible chatter. We threw on our helmets and flak jackets, as ordered by the Chief Hospital Corpsman, and ran for the triage bunker. One section of the wall had not yet been built, allowing small rocks and dirt to be whipped through the small entrance to the hospital triage bay. We turned our backs to the chopper to avoid getting pelted.

Conspicuously uncomfortable, we stood and watched as small groups of teams were lined up against a far wall triaging and caring for this newest batch of Marine casualties from I Corps. The deafening helicopter noise made it difficult to talk and be understood, so three Navy corpsmen, who were bringing in casualties from the choppers, used hand signals to communicate. I looked to them to follow their lead. Not normally a religious man, I whispered, "God, please give me something I can handle."

Casualties were being offloaded with great efficiency and placed on the sawhorses closest to the triage entrance. Hospital corpsmen in combat gear rounded the single curtain barrier that separated each individual triage bay. The corpsmen then hurriedly slipped our casualty onto the awaiting sawhorses. I watched as three sets of talented hands, knowing exactly what they were doing, flew into action. Where a man's mouth had been was now just flattened bloody tissue with air bubbling up from the center. The only recognizable facial features were his eyes rapidly sweeping from one side to the other in anxious fright.

One corpsman placed a small surgical drape over the Marine's face, and the other corpsman, who was on the opposite side of the stretcher, immediately poured antiseptic fluid on his neck. Without hesitation, he performed the most beautiful tracheotomy I had ever witnessed. Simultaneously, a third corpsman cut down the side of the combat boot exposing the Marine's upper ankle, which was considered a relatively clean area. He deftly inserted a large-bore IV needle and the lifesaving fluids began to rush in.

More hand signals ensued. The casualty was whisked back outside to another chopper being loaded to take four newly resuscitated casualties to the Navy hospital ship 20 miles offshore in the South China Sea.[1] The corpsmen then routinely went back inside to perform their next tasks. One corpsman, using a common hose, washed pools of blood into two large drains in the triage floor. The drumming from the chopper faded away and a sudden quiet enveloped me—and this was just my first day at Delta Med. My inner voice finally broke that lingering silence and became loud and clear: I don't belong here. I'm useless at Delta Med.

How I Got There

The inevitable had happened. I received my draft notice in the fall of 1965, a few months after the start of my three-year pediatric residency at Yale-New Haven Hospital. After completing the residency, I was planning to enter the pediatric surgical program at Yale. But those dreams would now have to be put on hold. Vietnam happened. Luckily, I was able to get into the three-year Berry Plan, which was a Vietnam-era federal program that allowed physicians to defer obligatory military service until they completed their residency training. I therefore would not have to report for active duty until 1968—a much-welcome and necessary reprieve.

Those challenging, sleep-deprived, exhausting three years of my pediatric residency passed all too quickly. I received my orders in early 1968 assigning me to the 3rd Marine Division at San Diego. Great news! I called the base in San Diego to see about housing and moving my family. But the Marine on the other end of the phone broke the euphoric spell. He tersely stated, "You'll spend about six weeks training in San Diego and then you're going to Vietnam." Dead silence at my end. This moment of realization likely crystallized Phyllis's fears as well—that she would be on her own for a year or perhaps longer with young children. She would also have to deal with mounting debt, and a husband off to a war-ravaged country. We both just stood transfixed, trying to digest the Marine's parting words: "You're going to Vietnam."

With great sadness, I said goodbye to Phyllis and our three young children, the oldest being only 5 years old. Due to a lack of funds to move my family into an apartment during my year-long deployment, they had to move in with my parents and make the best of a situation that would have otherwise been intolerable. I was torn between my responsibility to my family and my medical obligation of going to Vietnam. Phyllis understood my dilemma, but, as she said, she knew that I wouldn't even

---

1. During this period, two Navy hospital ships, USS *Sanctuary* (AH-17) and USS *Repose* (AH-16), took turns taking aboard I Corps casualties.

consider finding a way not to go.

Into the Breach

Before I knew it, I was sitting on a United Airlines flight filled with physicians, whose numbers could make up the equivalent of three medical school classes. I wondered how it would play out in the press if our plane went down filled with dozens of much-needed doctors on their way to a war zone. Upon landing at the coastal air base of Da Nang, South Vietnam, we were surrounded by the overwhelming sound of silence. After the door was cranked open, the stifling heat and humidity entered our consciousness.

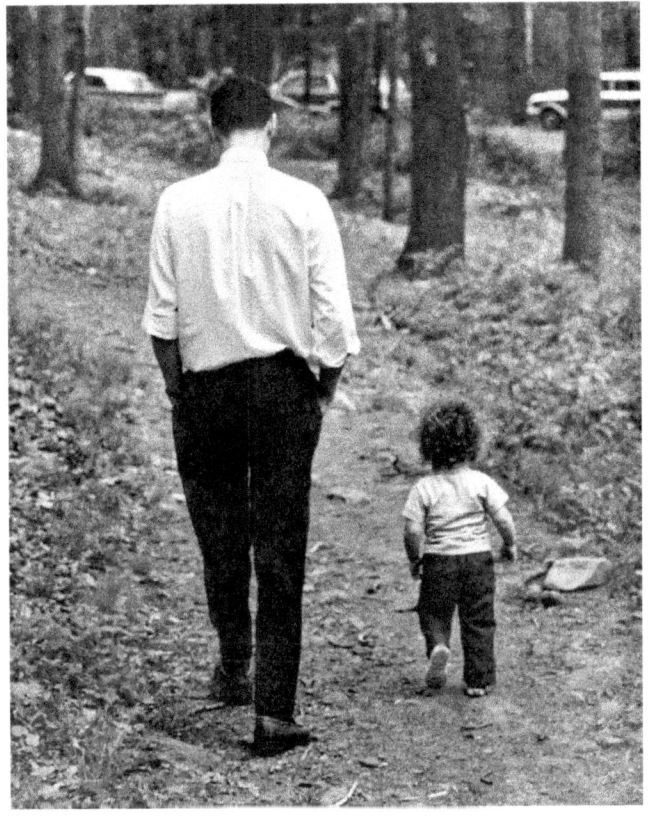

Before leaving for Vietnam, a contemplative father takes a walk with his youngest daughter (author's collection).

As we exited the plane, we saw Marine troops already lined up next to the plane's ramp, eagerly waiting to board for their trip home. As we walked past the men, whose uniforms would suggest they had just come from their last days in Vietnam hell, one Marine cried out, "You'll regret this!"

Another Marine yelled, "Get the hell back on that plane!" They were tanned and fit in disheveled uniforms that revealed they had just come from their last days in the nightmare called "Vietnam."

We were rushed to the north side of the airstrip where our group piled into a manmade network of wood and wire mesh only to wait four hours in the hot sun. Walking back and forth through this labyrinth, we heard Marine fighter jets taking off, an ear-piercing din that drowned out any chatter among us. This process seemed endless. All of us were lost in thought of what might occur once we reached the end of the line. Reality set in: Our lives were no longer in our control.

At the end of the maze, we were greeted by an impatient sergeant blurting out the names of those who were to immediately board a waiting C-130, parked only 10 yards away. I joined seven other guys on the four-engine C-130 military transport. Once in flight, against the constant roar of the engines, one of the crew shouted,

"We're going to be landing at Quang Tri.² When we hit the runway, the propellers are going to reverse. You'll be thrown forward so hold on. The back is going to open so move out quickly to the side of the runway to the foxholes and ditches. Dive into the closest one and keep your helmet on!"

As if landing at Da Nang and hearing the Marines' warnings wasn't enough to sufficiently frighten us all, suddenly and with a very steep descent, we touched down on a short airstrip. A deafening noise erupted as the propellers reversed. The rear ramp dropped down and everyone ran out looking for a foxhole. But instead of hearing bullets whizzing past my helmet, I caught the laughter of Marines. It was pretty clear that we, as rookies, were the butt of this joke.

Once the drama died down, we noticed the main highway, soon recognized as the infamous Route 1, or, as the French named it during the Indochina War, "La Rue Sans Joie"—"The Street Without Joy." The road ran along the coast from Saigon to Hanoi. Alpha Med³ and its imposingly large Red Cross flag were a stone's throw ahead.

So Alpha Med was to be my new home. Not bad at all. But my journey wasn't over yet. "Stand fast!" an officer yelled, as he called off the names of those who would continue north. "You four guys are going to Delta Med at Dong Ha," a place name I didn't want to hear. As he shouted out my name, I thought back to a Marine sergeant in San Diego who had cautioned us to stay away from the exact location where we were now headed.

It was almost nighttime when we left Alpha Med for our final destination. Several tanks were advancing up Route 1 to the demilitarized zone (DMZ),⁴ and they gladly took us "newbies" on their ride north. I'd never been on the back of a tank. Just figuring out how to get up on this metallic monster was an ordeal. I desperately searched for some toehold as I threw up my duffel, only to have it come tumbling back down. The tank's engine coughed loudly as it started to move. The six-hour journey to our destination was long and filled with many silent thoughts as we all tried to help each other maintain a stable foothold on the hot steel—our life support. The sky was darkening. The tank's engine was so loud we didn't bother trying to talk to each other.

I looked around at the passing villages, the poverty, and the destroyed thatched homes that defined the lives of the inhabitants. I was in a semi-dream state, my fingers numb from holding onto the tank's imposing metal protrusions that were our only safety net. As we abruptly turned left, the tank strained as the front lifted and

---

2. Quang Tri Combat Base near Quang Tri City was a major Marine logistics and aviation support base.
3. Alpha Med was west of Quang Tri City. Delta Med, about six miles north, straddled the village of Dong Ha on Route 1.
4. In 1954, at the end of the Indochina War, a military-political line, established by the Geneva Accords, ran approximately along the 17th Parallel in Vietnam from Laos east to the coast. The 17th Parallel essentially divided the country into North Vietnam and South Vietnam. During the Vietnam War, the line became the DMZ, or demilitarized zone, with several miles on either side to serve as an additional safeguard. With Vietnam officially reunified in July 1976, the military function of the DMZ was no longer necessary.

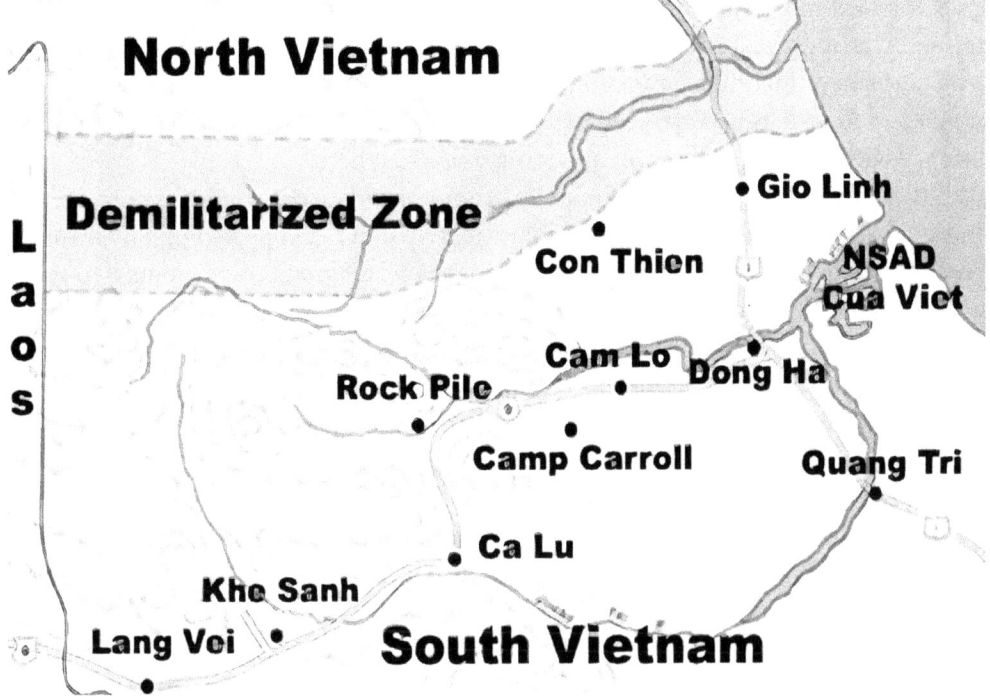

Theater of operations in South Vietnam (author's collection).

then sank onto what appeared to be a metal corrugated helicopter pad from which multiple choppers were rapidly landing and taking off.

"Dance of the Casualties"

Delta Med awaited us. The war awaited us. We slid down from the tank and stood at the edge of the pad until the last helicopter flew off. At that point, our little group headed into the apparent triage area through a narrow opening in the massive blast wall that appeared to surround the entire structure.

The Chief Hospital Corpsman approached us and defined the hand signals that the corpsmen used: "If you hear choppers or an announcement, someone will give the numbers of the casualties coming in. First number means how many are seriously injured. The second number means how many are walking wounded. The third number means how many are dead. That's it! Doesn't matter what time of day or night. Everybody responds. And always show up with helmets and flak jackets!"

This senior corpsman then read off our assigned triage bay numbers. I drew triage area number 7 which had 10 spaces on that side of the bay. Number 7 would hopefully be a lucky omen. He took us to our living quarters or "hooch," consisting of multiple cots lined up so close that we could barely stand in between them. The hooch had no lights and was oppressively hot and humid. All the smells were foreign and damp. I felt anxious and vulnerable.

The next morning, after another casualty experience in triage, we began orientation. At that point, I had already witnessed that incredible tracheotomy performed by a corpsman. I felt like an incompetent bystander, but I noticed only two rookies now when four of us had arrived the day before. "They were removed," I heard someone say within earshot. "They're not going to make it here."

If anyone wasn't going to make it, I thought for sure it would have to be me. But here I was near the DMZ. The remaining two of us then picked up our thinner, recently washed camouflage uniforms, all of which had previously belonged to casualties. They were covered in blood stains. I ripped off the name tag from the uniform and tried to clean this hand-me-down. No matter how hard I scrubbed, the multiple reddish blots stared back at me, becoming my daily reminders of death.

In the nearly 20-year-long war, almost 80 percent of major battles occurred in the northern half of Quang Tri Province. Delta Med, the northernmost Marine Corps Forward Casualty Field Hospital, was just five miles south of the DMZ. Because of its proximity, Delta Med was often a target of the North Vietnamese Army (NVA). The enemy had large artillery units just above the DMZ and could easily hit our base.

To protect against these attacks, Delta Med had a blast wall made from two layers of corrugated steel more than 20 feet high. Dirt was sandwiched in between the ribbed metal. Every structure on the premises was sandbagged and always caked in a thin layer of dust. Our entire world existed on our side of that blast wall. We knew little of what went on beyond that physical and cultural barrier.

The "dance of the casualties," or triage process, required a great deal of coordination. Due to the intensity of the fighting in that region, Delta Med received a huge number of injured, usually via helicopter. Those with head wounds typically couldn't be helped unless the patient could quickly be medevacked to the Navy hospital ship off the coast. The walking wounded would be moved to the side to wait. The chest and limb wounds and nearly severed appendages were the ones the medical staff would quickly act on to try to stop the bleeding, stabilize the patient, and get fluids going to save their lives. Ideally, these casualties would then be placed aboard a helicopter and sent to a hospital ship or to the Naval Support Activity Hospital in Da Nang, a better-equipped facility than what Delta Med had to offer.

Beyond the Blast Wall

But another world existed just outside Delta Med. The Chief Hospital Corpsman kept track of the pulse and needs of Dong Ha, which butted against us on the northern side of the base. He understood the village's political workings. On-site corpsmen and physicians would take trips to nearby villages to do basic health checks, today's version of a mobile health van. But being so close to the DMZ, we never knew if enemy soldiers were watching us, or if they were embedded among the local villagers.

My second day at Delta Med seemed to do its best to overshadow my first day. Because of my previous experience in the civilian world, I was asked to see a woman in the village who was having difficulty delivering her baby. The Chief Hospital Corpsman and two Marines with loaded M16s drove us by jeep to a community building on a dusty knoll in the village. This small, isolated structure was traditionally used by women to give birth. By the time we arrived, the mother had already given birth and was doing fine, lying on a primitive thatched table used for deliveries.

I was equally aware of the multiple smells—some oppressive, some pleasant—that were pervasive in this poorly ventilated structure. Scanning the room for the newborn, my gaze was drawn to two wriggling black mounds on a nearby table. As I approached the table, I couldn't believe my eyes. Upon closer inspection, I discovered the masses to be swarms of black flies, completely engulfing what I now realized were two babies. The flies covered every inch of the infants' faces, devouring the remnants of the placental membranes. They were also consuming the newborns' white, cheese-like protective coating, known as "vernix caseosa," found on a baby's skin. This coating protects them from heat loss, and it produces the characteristic smell of all newborns.

Though shocked, I couldn't help but admire the centuries-old symbiotic relationship between these villagers and the black flies, a tradition upheld in their birthing customs. I wasn't quite sure how to examine the infants, but they were both actively moving and crying, seemingly healthy. The mother and village attendants didn't expect me to do anything else, so I left the birthing house.

That day I realized the trajectory of my medical career had changed. I became much more aware of the Vietnamese character that surrounded me beyond the blast wall. This cultural sensitivity would set me on a path of enhanced understanding for the rest of my career. I recognized that this kind of insight into another society's traditions, such as this rural Vietnamese way of life, was a gift. I didn't have a name for this new type of perception but I knew that other people's thoughts and values should be based on their own culture. They were not to be judged by the criteria of our views.

I then started a new kind of double practice. One moment I was treating substantial wounds of Marine casualties, injuries that defined this war and its weaponry. But in another role, I was trying to take in the broader, socially driven life of the people who surrounded us. The Vietnamese culture always surprised and enchanted my consciousness. What I absorbed in this one short year would have taken me decades to learn anywhere else. I loved the prospect of discovering more about their beliefs and practices.

As my time continued in Vietnam, I increasingly realized the vital importance of understanding and valuing another country's customs and traditions. At one point, the higher levels of military leadership decided that we would build and staff a children's hospital to upgrade the existing forward casualty receiving facility. Then our eyes opened to what was happening all around us: the suffering of civilians. In the 1950s, more than 40,000 refugees had come down from the north and settled into camps and villages, all very close to the future location of Delta Med. These Vietnamese were the most vulnerable in this ongoing war. We opened the children's hospital in just two months, thanks to the expert execution and building by Marine engineers.

Because the ground war primarily went on at night, we had to perform double duty now. We spent most nights attending to the many Marine casualties, and during the day we were seeing long lines of sick children. Sleep was a luxury of the past, so unscheduled catnaps had to suffice. Once the hospital opened, the sick and diseased youth of all ages came in like a flood—more than 300 a day—and many with bizarre illnesses and injuries. Their medical cases were anything but simple.

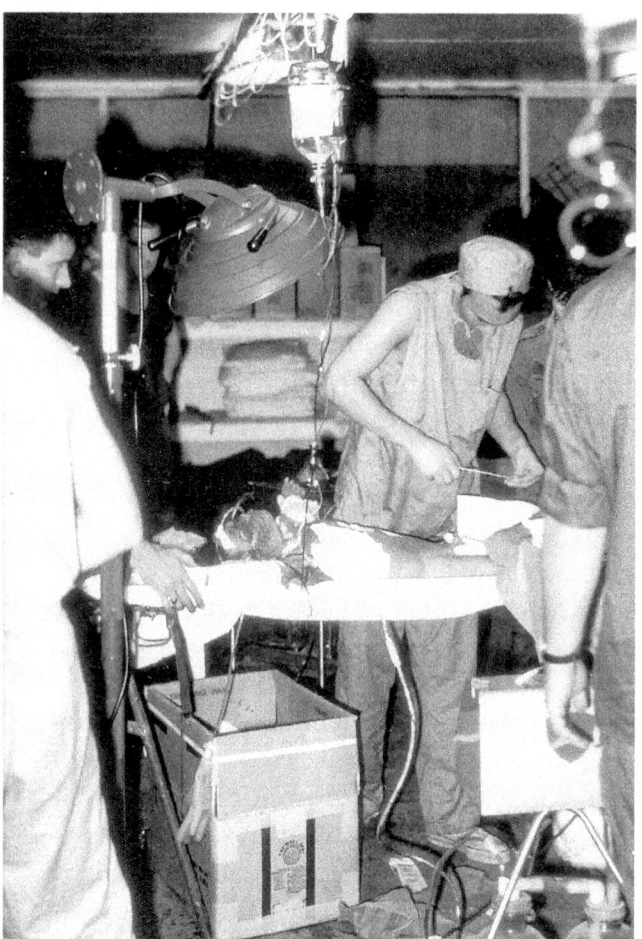

Surgery for a child at Delta Med (author's collection).

We had 100 beds to use for the Vietnamese, often with three or four patients in each bed. Multiple wounds, amputations, various kinds of pneumonia, bubonic plague,[5] blackwater fever, meningitis, scurvy, tuberculosis, and severe malnutrition cases pervaded the ward.

One of my staff members exclaimed, "And this has been going on around us?" We were so distracted by the war that we didn't see or recognize the local villagers' ailments, wounds, and diseases encircling us. The big blast wall was our symbolic perimeter and barrier in more ways than one. Ironically, this protection isolated us from the local outside world.

A new entrance to the large common triage management bay was created where the children were screened

---

5. Frederick M. Burkle, Jr., "Plague as Seen in South Vietnamese Children: A Chronicle of Observations and treatment Under Adverse Conditions," *Clinical Pediatrics*, 1973 May;12(5): 291–812. Available at https://journals.sagepub.com/doi/10.1177/000992287301200512.

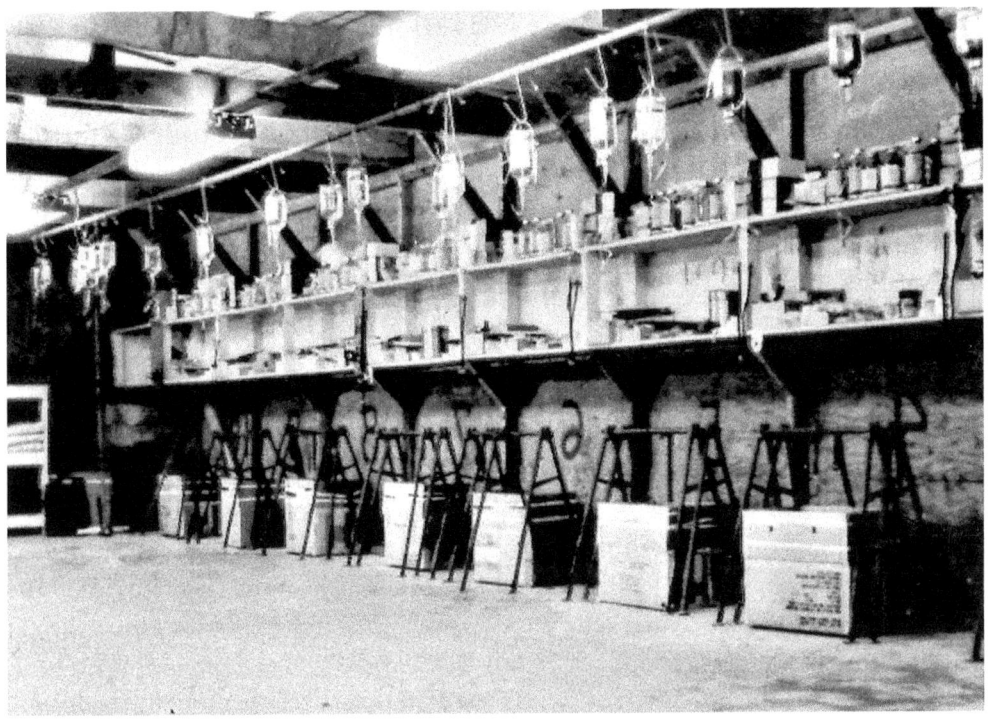

Triage bunker where treatment began (author's collection).

and the parent, always a female, had their belongings searched. One day a small commotion occurred about 15 feet away from me just inside the entrance. A little boy, about 2 years of age, stood alone looking at me with an innocent smile, trying to keep his balance. He had a loose jacket that was open, revealing two grenades attached to the straps holding up his overalls.

Everyone froze as two Marines gently removed the grenades before I took him in my arms and placed him in the care of a Vietnamese nurse. The woman accompanying the toddler appeared extremely old. She was defiant and resisted the Marine guards. The child did not seem ill. Hours later he was reunited with his tearful mother, the wife of a South Vietnamese soldier stationed at Dong Ha. From that point on, we all had to wear heavy, hot World War II-era flak jackets every day.

Being so close to the weaponry across the DMZ, Delta Med had the dubious recognition of being the medical facility most repeatedly hit during the war. We had several underground bunkers for the children and medical team. The corpsmen were often seen rushing from the wards to the bunker entrances with two to three children under each arm between bombardments. But even these bunkers were not totally safe. They were dark, damp, and, unfortunately, a gathering place for snakes.

It's still not clear how many Vietnamese died during the war. Some statistics show 500,000, but I believe that figure is wrong. In April 1995, 20 years after the war had ended, the Socialist Republic of Vietnam released official statistics reporting

2 million civilians had died in what was at that time both North and South Vietnam.[6] And we saw many of those civilian casualties.

Nevertheless, as someone especially interested in infectious diseases and critical care, I found the maladies endemic to that part of the world truly fascinating. With some illnesses, I had difficulty coming to a diagnosis. As for smallpox, I saw only one suspected case. An Army Special Forces captain, among several others from Special Forces, took me by helicopter to the Laotian border to see an alleged case of smallpox in a remote village. Special Forces needed verification immediately. Everyone was concerned about the dire consequences of a smallpox epidemic.

The air was eerily silent because the villagers had been evacuated for fear of contamination. Special Forces guarded the perimeter. I entered the thatched hut of a shy, healthy—appearing adolescent female shaking from fright. I tried to calm her by saying I was a doctor, using the Vietnamese term "bac si." Her torso was pox-covered and she also had the characteristic lymph nodes that distinguished her condition from that of smallpox. I told her she was fine and then reassured the nervous medic, saying, "No, it's the monkeypox virus, not smallpox, and it should not be a major problem. She might be an isolated case. She should be slightly ill for about two weeks." If smallpox cases existed, I didn't see them, but that doesn't mean those diseases weren't infiltrating rural Vietnam. Had this young girl had smallpox, it would have changed the course of the war with different military strategies.

A colleague once stated that the military medical system is always about 10 to 15 years behind, and I found this assertion to be completely accurate in Vietnam. Many of the medical provisions at Delta Med were from the Korean War era. For some reason, Army medical teams were better supplied. They even worked in air-conditioned buildings.

When I arrived in Dong Ha and opened my first surgical pack, I found sulfa powder, dating from battlefields in World War II and Korea, to treat infections. We didn't use sulfa powder because we usually had enough antibiotics if we used them sparingly. Physicians and corpsmen, however, were extremely meticulous in utilizing everything else in those surgical packs before unwrapping a new one. No supplies went to waste.

But even with this careful management, we were still always running out of supplies, especially antibiotics. I was constantly requesting them through military channels, but we could never get the needed supplies fast enough. So one day I tried a different resource: By mail, I asked the Yale-New Haven Hospital Pediatric Department to send these necessities. It was like Christmas every time that very distant hospital, which was almost 9,000 miles away, sent a big medical package to us!

---

6. Philip Shenon, "20 Years after Victory: Vietnamese Communists Ponder How to Celebrate," *The New York Times*, April 23, 1995, p. 12. Available at https://www.nytimes.com/1995/04/23/world/20-years-after-victory-vietnamese-communists-ponder-how-to-celebrate.html.

Dying at Attention

During my time at Delta Med, we saw an average of 50 to 70 Marines and almost 300 civilians every day. With triage being constant, we had to make life-and-death decisions on the spot and get creative with solutions. Options for chest wounds were limited. Ron Bohn, one of our senior corpsmen, along with his fellow corpsmen, opened a patient's chest. But they realized that a defibrillator, the standard equipment to restart a heart, was not available.

All eyes darted around the ward for a substitute. One of the team suggested stripping the wire from a lamp cord, wrapping the ends around two combat knives called "Ka-Bars," and plugging the electrical cord into the outlet. Another corpsman would next quickly yank the cord out of the power socket.

Someone then asked the inevitable question, "Who's going to hold the knives?" Everyone's attention landed on Bohn. "Me?" he exclaimed in disbelief.

A tactless response came from a corpsman. "You're the only one who's not married or has kids."

Swearing under his breath, he took each of the knives while the others threw down rubber mats and put everything else into place.

"You better revive me if this knocks me out!" Bohn cried out. A corpsman inserted the cord into the wall and then pulled it out, just long enough to send a jolt of electricity through the wire to the knives and the sinus node, the heart's so-called "natural pacemaker." Ron received a painful current of electricity through his body, but the patient's heart started beating again in perfect rhythm. He later swore that he was going to find a defibrillator even if he had to steal one from the U.S. Army.

Regrettably, neither Bohn nor any of his fellow corpsmen were able to beg, borrow, or steal a defibrillator from the Army. In a subsequent instance, one of our surgical patients went into cardiac arrest. With the assistance of the then–Commanding Officer (CO), surgeon Bob Rowe, I again attempted the "lamp cord trick." But this time that "trick" was not successful and the Marine died.

Part of the triage process includes making quick decisions. What was the patient's chance of survival? What evacuation options were open to us? How far away was the hospital ship? With triage, we had to manage all kinds of logistical situations, not just the casualty. We did a lot of "meatball surgery," that is, immediate amputations, chest tubes, and tracheotomies. Since most of the casualties who came in had multiple injuries, their best chance at survival was for us to immediately take care of the ones with severe bleeding, which often meant cutting off one or more limbs. The body could then focus its energy on the potential mortal wounds.

Though I believe we saved hundreds of lives during our time at Delta Med, many patients were not so lucky. The average age of death for the Marines in Vietnam was 19. Many Marines I treated in triage at Delta Med were just kids. They were physically mature and confident in their operational prowess. But once they were wounded or saw friends killed, the protective façade they had built up became vulnerable and began to crack. On one particularly bad day in triage, a young wounded Marine started to whimper and call out, "Mommy! Mommy!" His pleas were picked up by more injured Marines wailing for their mothers.

As committed physicians and corpsmen, we continued our work, dutifully trying to attend to everyone as best we could. We were living in a nightmare. But these Marines never complained. I didn't hear them yelling or crying out. They would follow orders to the letter, lying on the stretchers at attention, quietly and respectfully. They even died at attention.

An early lesson for all the medical staff was learning just how deadly the AK-47 and M16 bullets were to the body. These weapons of war were designed to kill. Once the bullet penetrated the body, the blast wave caused considerable widespread damage beyond the entrance wound. As triage officers, we had many Marine casualties. We had to decide who needed immediate surgery at Delta Med. We also had to select among the remaining casualties who, and in what order, would be sent to the hospital ship.

Bubonic Plague

Rats were also plentiful, some as big as cats. They ran between my legs at night as I trotted down the walkways to the wards where most of the sick children were housed. Aside from making us uncomfortable, these rodents were a major concern because they harbored fleas that carried bubonic plague. Children were the most endangered and they got the plague more frequently. Kids under the age of 6 typically didn't wear anything below the waist, and they spent most of their time with village rats. Both rodents and children would pick through garbage bins that bordered the bases.

I quickly learned that bubonic plague was not merely a disease of the Middle Ages. That kind of bacterial disease was endemic in war-torn Vietnam—and rats were the vector. During my tour at Delta Med, several hundred children and adults showed up with bubonic plague. On a daily basis, we saw many kids with large abscesses on their heads and covered with bites. Their hair came out in large clumps. This horrible situation was made worse by poverty and chronic filth. By examining the children closely, we could distinguish those pustules from the early buboes.[7] The inflamed lymph nodes were soft, hot, large, and painful.

I almost misdiagnosed my first case. A young girl with a large closed soft abscess under her left armpit was my first encounter with bubonic plague. I had seen many cases like hers so I just assumed it was of bacterial origin, and routine antibiotics would supposedly take care of it. My Vietnamese-Laotian interpreter tried to convince me that something else was going on with this young girl's condition.

---

7. A bubo is a swelling of a lymph node, especially of the armpit or groin, which is characteristic of bubonic plague.

His translation into English didn't make sense to me. He left and hurriedly returned with a Vietnamese-to-English dictionary. He squatted down next to the end of the stretcher, then tugged on my fatigues and called out the all-too-familiar name for "doctor." "Bac si! Bac si! Please look!" He pointed to a Vietnamese word in the dictionary that translated into "plague." He said he had seen this disease before.

I was silent for a moment then affirmed, "Yes, it could be bubonic plague." Using a syringe, I evacuated pus from the abscess and then placed a sample on a slide under a microscope in the lab. The slide was covered with rod-shaped bacteria that distinguished the plague. The bacteria looked like safety pins. I had all the lab techs and corpsmen line up to see the findings, commenting that what they were viewing was probably the beginning of an epidemic, one which came on frightfully fast. I immediately admitted the child and started her on sulfa antibiotics intravenously. The young girl was one of five cases of bubonic plague that day.

Later that afternoon, I examined a boy with similar symptoms and noted that he had onion flakes in his hair and on his forehead. I had learned earlier that the application of this substance was a village remedy to take the fever away. Intended to ward off evil spirits, a plaster cloth, which had been adhered to the boy's lower abdomen, contained Chinese characters. The Vietnamese believe the Chinese are the fathers of medicine.

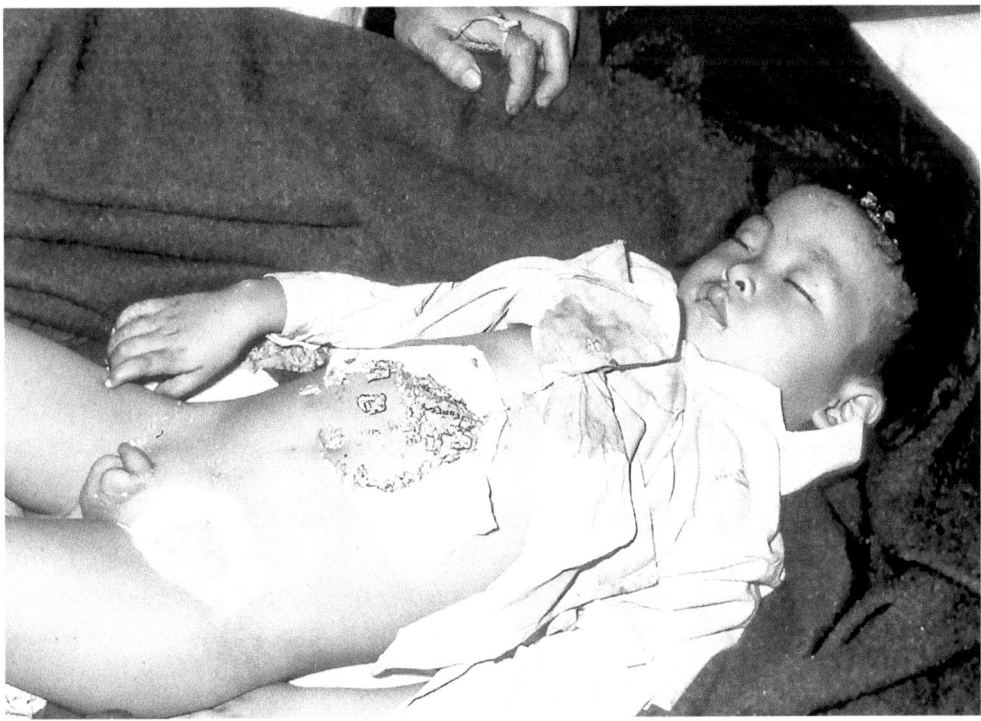

This comatose child had an enlarged lymph node (bubo) surrounded by a lime paste over the umbilicus. The Vietnamese believed this paste would prevent evil spirits from entering a child's body (author's collection).

The young boy was semi-comatose, toxic, and septic, that is, infected with harmful bacteria that had entered his bloodstream. The disease wasn't just limited to the groin. I grabbed my camera, realizing that I needed to get a photo of this condition. As the flash went off, the boy had a grand mal seizure. His whole body was convulsing. For the Vietnamese, a paroxysm meant those evil spirits were in the body. The mother thought the camera with a flash had instantly put evil spirits in her son. Panicking, she lifted her boy off the stretcher and fled the hospital.

Several hours later, a contingent of corpsmen and Marines found the child in a refugee camp and convinced the mother to return him to us. Her only condition was that the "bac si" would not go near her child. I did treat him but only from a distance and through the gentle corpsmen. I didn't dare impose our Western medical practices on their traditional cures, and I also did not want to ignore those village practices they trusted even more. The boy's mother never showed any civility toward me, and I didn't expect any courtesy after what had happened. I was learning cultural awareness day by day as I saw more of these patients. Every disease and each event came with traditional importance and challenges.

If a child's fever abated, often within 24 hours of the first antibiotic dose, the mother would frequently assume that her child was now well. She would then remove the IVs herself and escape with the child. A few days later, she would inevitably bring the infant or youth back, but this time the child would have to deal with an antibiotic-resistant plague. Unfortunately, this lesson still goes unlearned today by many in the Western world. Patients will stop a 10-day course of antibiotics on the second day once they start to feel better.

While treating these patients, I did not remove the onion flakes or the paste on the children's abdomens. The Vietnamese didn't understand "bacteria" or "viruses" or our Western explanations for disease. Those two words were not in their vocabulary. If they didn't see something tangible, then it didn't exist. If they were well, they had good spirits. If they were ill, they had bad spirits. I just added my medication to that particular boy's treatment and he did fine. I didn't want to dispel any Vietnamese beliefs, thereby insulting them. My complementary system seemingly worked. When offering my remedies, I would tell them, "This might help." Their concept of a "bac si" was that a doctor had better communication with the evil spirits that caused disease.

Dong Ha had a Catholic church that served as a tuberculosis hospital operated by the French-Vietnamese convent nuns. The priest was allegedly a double agent, working with NVA forces and the United States. He had to be a double agent to survive. One evening a Marine contingent came to Delta Med asking for me, explaining that one of the elderly nuns had the plague. The priest had requested I see her immediately so I contacted the Marines who knew his situation.

With flak jackets and medications, I followed the Marine convoy into the darkness of Dong Ha. U.S. troops controlled Dong Ha during the day, but the VC dominated it at night. We silently walked down totally blacked-out narrow streets and

3. How Did I Get to Vietnam?

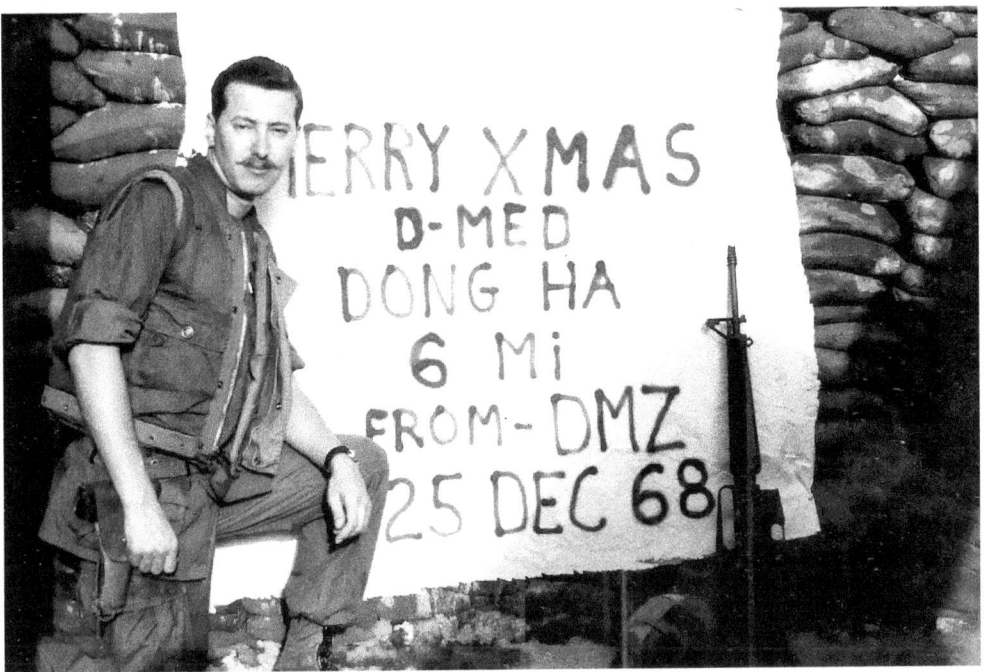

Nineteen sixty-eight Christmas card from Dong Ha, just a few miles south of the DMZ (author's collection).

alleys, with me holding onto the back of the Marine ahead of me. Their M16s were locked and loaded. Bent over so as not to be seen, this surreptitious trek through Dong Ha seemed endless.

We came to an ancient stone building, the tuberculosis hospital, and an entrance to the basement. In the distance, I could see candles illuminating a stone altar structure with a human figure lying on top. Elderly Vietnamese nurses moved aside as I approached. I slowly did my exam. The nun was hot and comatose but moved in apparent pain when I found a bubo in her right groin. I brought along Streptomycin glass syrettes, gave her a loading dose,[8] and then taught the nurses how to use these disposable syrettes.

As we left, I confided to the Marine lieutenant that I thought this older nun would die. Two busy days went by before that officer arrived to tell me that she was alive and the priest most grateful. Since news of this nun's recovery traveled fast, I thought maybe I'd see sick children earlier and therefore they would have a better chance at survival.

The height of the bubonic plague was in January 1969, about six months into my service at Dong Ha. With a one-year deployment, I was automatically given R&R, the military term for "rest and recuperation" or "rest and relaxation." I took advantage of it despite the plague taking on new life near our base—and I was in charge.

---

8. At the beginning of treatment, a loading dose of a drug is a higher initial dosage given to a patient to increase the drug's effectiveness.

The R&R meant flying 6,000 miles to Hawaii, compliments of the U.S. Navy, to rendezvous with Phyllis, who would have to fly 5,000 miles, considered an out-of-pocket flight expense on her part.

Phyllis understood my hesitation and reluctance to make this journey halfway across the Pacific at that point. But I took advantage of the situation and made the long flight to Oahu. We stayed at a resort for three days on the Big Island near Kona. As Phyllis recalled, she knew I was being pulled in two different directions: feeling the pressure to be at Delta Med since I was the go-to guy for the plague crisis, but also wanting to have much-needed time together. This R&R was to be a momentary escape from war and disease. After three days in paradise, we each went back to our different realities.

Losing It

Bubonic plague wasn't the only disease connected to our rat population. Rabies also entered the scene. Marines would often claim they had been bitten by rats as an excuse not to be sent into the field. This story was often used to get out of going on patrol. Marines came in every morning for the rabies vaccine: 14 days of seven shots up one side in the upper abdomen and seven shots down the other side in the upper abdomen.

A young black Marine walked into the triage area one day, claiming he had been bitten by a rat that morning. As the doctor on duty, I talked with him and took down his medical history. I assured him that I didn't doubt his word, but he would have to undergo the 14-day series of injections. He was very cooperative and displayed no signs of hostility. During the next two weeks, we developed a very congenial relationship. He was from New York and had been drafted into the Marines. At that time, the Marine Corps took draftees. He had been a student at a New York City college majoring in sociology, with aspirations and dreams for his future. I was pleasantly buoyed by the whole situation. I told him about my family and growing up in Connecticut.

This Marine was a short-timer and had just a few more weeks to serve before shipping out for home. He didn't have to go out on any more missions, but the Marine Corps higher-ups pushed their men up to the last minute. He left my office one final time, and I wished him luck with college and his career. This friendship offered me new insight into another world because I had never had a relationship with any blacks. African Americans were a rarity in rural Vermont where I had gone to college and medical school. The only blacks I had encountered were patients in Yale-New Haven Hospital.

A week later, I went to Graves Registration after a large number of body bags had recently arrived. During my year in Vietnam, the Graves Registration staff discovered three "deceased" casualties still breathing in body bags. After they were rushed to triage, all sadly succumbed despite attempted resuscitation.

As physicians, one of our lamentable duties was trying to identify the dead's matching body parts. I would see piles of heads, half a head, torsos without limbs, torsos without heads, and many severed limbs. Atop a pile of torsos was an exposed upper body with black skin. I immediately spotted an area on the upper abdomen where rabies shots had been administered very recently. I recalled my newfound friend, the black Marine, but didn't make a connection. Then I saw another pile of stacked heads. They were separated from the torsos at various angles. But one head caught my attention. The eyes were shut and the face was on its side. The attached shoulder seemed to go with what was missing from the torso. First recognition, then disbelief. These body parts belonged to my former patient, my friend.

I stood silently in that room, sudden grief overwhelming me. A few minutes later, after pulling myself together, I approached one of the Marines on duty and said very soberly, "That head and shoulder go with the top torso in the pile over there."

He never asked me how I knew. He just said, "Thanks, Doc." As I walked across the helipad to the triage entrance, I cried. I waited on the pad and wept more, not wanting anyone to see me in that demoralized state. Even today, I can still see my friend's face.

Becoming a Casualty of War

On the first day of November 1968, I became a casualty—just three months after my arrival in Vietnam. I was working on a Marine with a chest wound and getting him ready for a helicopter medevac when suddenly incoming enemy rounds began landing nearby. I had just inserted a chest tube into my patient lying on the floor on a stretcher. But when the corpsmen picked up the stretcher, one of them inadvertently stepped on the chest tube, and it flew out of the Marine's chest and across the cement floor like a long whip. I shouted, "Give me another chest tube!"

The corpsman looked around and said, "Don't have any chest tubes. They're all in surgery."

I didn't have any choice but to wipe off the tube on my fatigues and then put it back into the Marine's chest. While he was still lying on the floor of the triage area, I rapidly took some thick silk sutures and tied them very tightly to secure the chest tube. With the chest tube now in, the patient was breathing fine. Then we gave the hand signals. The corpsmen picked him up and ran him out to the awaiting chopper. The pilot was angry because he had been on the ground too long between bombardments. All medical personnel escaped to their own protected bunkers because a new set of rounds from the north was expected at any moment.

I ran toward the entrance of the secondary triage bunker but stopped to grab my helmet from my adjacent hooch. I then stepped off the back steps facing one of the entrances to the triage bunker a mere 10 feet away. Both entrances were L-shaped, making an abrupt right-hand turn to limit any blast from entering from the outside.

Not aware of any detonation in real time, I was lifted and thrown forward, my helmet blowing off and hitting the outside wall of the bunker. I don't even remember hitting the ground from the explosion. I then saw what is best described as a "reverse tornado," somewhat like a funnel with a wide base circling upward toward my face and taking my breath away. The impact was as if I had been hit by a large heavy metal object.

To my right and back, the projectile struck the corrugated roof of the hooch next to mine. I crawled the rest of the way into the triage entrance. Everybody was busy and harried but efficiently taking care of casualties. I slowly stood up. All I could hear was an overwhelming hollow whooshing sound. My head felt like it weighed 50 pounds. I was pale and had profound nausea. People were talking but I couldn't hear anything. I wondered, "What's going on?"

On the wall nearby were shelves containing IV bottles and other medical supplies. A corpsman pointed toward the shelf, obviously wanting me to grab an IV bottle. Stunned as I was, I grasped the bottle but then instantly froze. Behind the bottle was a large, thick black snake with narrow white stripes. The banded krait slowly undulated across the back of the shelf.

A corpsman finally turned me around and took the IV bottle from my hand. He realized something was wrong and helped me to sit down in the nearby corner of the bunker. I spent the rest of that time in a haze, observing the usual professionalism of the triage teams. I was finally taken to my rack where I fell into a very deep sleep.

When I awoke almost 20 hours later, I slowly made my way to triage. Dr. Bob Farkas examined me and found blood behind my right eardrum. I couldn't hear and the high-pitched ringing tinnitus was remarkably strong with that characteristic whooshing noise throughout my head. Although the right ear was noticeably worse, I had hearing loss in both ears. The Commanding Officer said he would evacuate me with the next group of casualties to the hospital ship to see an ear, nose, and throat specialist. I refused because it would have been too difficult to find my way back without first going 100 miles south to Da Nang.

Combat veterans experience hearing loss because the cochlea is right at the outside of the skull, making it vulnerable to every blast. What concerned me more than the loss of hearing was that the roof of my mouth was extremely painful and that aching lasted for another two weeks. I also felt soreness in all my teeth, and two days later five fillings fell out. I would learn years later that blast waves go through normal tooth structure at a different rate than amalgam fillings, causing the fillings to loosen.

My hearing eventually returned to my left ear, but the hearing has always been diminished in my right ear. Unfortunately, some blood accumulated in my left eye that has remained to this day as a small clump of cells closely grouped. The result is impaired vision. More than 50 years later, in my left eye, I see as though I am looking through an uneven gray-black veil. Regrettably, this "veil" has chronically affected my reading ability. I had no idea then that I would be habitually reliving what was eventually called a "traumatic brain injury" (TBI), which has stayed with me for decades after that long ago day in Vietnam. While I had survived my closest call at Delta Med, I would have even closer brushes with death in the years to come.

A Dark Side of War

War is a complex, dynamic, and multifaceted concern. In Vietnam, the war, not surprisingly, was politically complicated. The Viet Cong had been decimated by the time I had arrived in 1968. The hardcore North Vietnamese Army was therefore replacing the Viet Cong, largely taking over the ground war in the south. I treated NVA soldiers, now referred to as "POWs," several times during my stretch at Delta Med. They came in with rashes and various chronic and acute infectious diseases acquired from being in the jungle. The 17th Parallel wasn't a dividing line for disease and death. The North Vietnamese troops suffered just as much as the troops south of the DMZ.

Many North Vietnamese soldiers were tall, muscular, committed, and well-fed. They were impressive soldiers. They stood at attention and made eye contact in an intimidating manner. The NVA soldiers were always kept under guard. However, after being brought back to our base, one wounded soldier bit down on a cyanide pill before we could grasp what was happening. He died a minute later, and everyone began speculating where he had concealed the lethal pill. I thought he might have hidden it in his cheek or a hollow tooth.

On another occasion, when we were receiving incoming rounds, two NVA casualties were brought into the secondary triage bunker. The CO was on leave so I temporarily held that post. One casualty had a bullet wound in his right upper chest, just under his collarbone. He held his eyes shut and never once winced in pain. A corpsman had prepared a chest tube as I checked for other injuries. Minutes into the procedure, three Marines, in full combat gear with blackened faces, appeared at the triage entrance with their M16s aimed at us. "Get out!" they screamed.

Another doc and corpsman, who had been tending to the second prisoner, immediately left. I stood still and shouted, "Wait! What are you talking about? These are wounded soldiers. Under the Geneva Conventions, we are required to treat everyone." In legal terms, "wounded" means a soldier is "out of combat." The Marines maintained their angry demeanor and again ordered us out. For emphasis, they wielded their M16s just inches from my chest. With arms held high, we turned and left the triage area. Everyone else had evacuated to the underground bunkers. But I found a few physicians and advised them of the situation, questioning why we were ordered out. We all agreed this action was a possible Geneva Conventions violation. "It's too quiet," I thought. "I'm going back in."

The triage bunker was long, narrow, and dark with only two single hanging light bulbs. All the stretchers and surroundings blended into a characteristic military brown and green. My casualty was about 20 feet away. The Marines were busy doing something at the head of the stretcher. Even from that distance, I was struck by seeing a fresh, brilliant white cloth hung over the head of the casualty. That snow-white cloth stood in stark contrast to the surrounding drab colors of the bunker. The Marines were pouring normal saline IV solutions over the white cloth. The NVA soldier was struggling and kicking.

The Marines saw me and yelled again to get out. I stood motionless because I wanted to see what they were doing. But once I understood what was taking place, I quickly left the triage bunker. I told the other doctors what was going on and then ran directly to the administrative hooch, which had a radio connection to base headquarters.

"This is Delta Med!" I screamed into the radio. "I want to talk to someone in charge!" I was immediately connected to a colonel. "This is Lieutenant Commander Burkle. Your Marines are preventing us from treating wounded NVA soldiers and are actively torturing my patient right now. This is a violation of the Geneva Conventions and must stop!" All I heard in response was a soft click as the Marine colonel hung up.

I went back a second time to the triage bunker where I found the two NVA patients—but no Marines. My patient was dead and the other was barely alive. We later learned that these two enemy soldiers were forward observers, and they had been shot trying to cross the base's barbed wire perimeter. Both NVA soldiers had gotten very close to our blast wall.

* * * *

We eventually learned that we had witnessed the act of "waterboarding." No one talked about it. The incident allegedly never occurred, and we never heard anything from the base's Marine colonel. Weary, we continued our duties that day, but I never forgot what had happened right before my eyes.

4

A Moon for the Souls
1969

> *"For the Vietnamese, as my interpreter had earlier explained, their luminous sphere could not be dismissed so cavalierly. Instead, the moon was a destination for the soul."*

Though my cultural curiosity had been piqued since my second day with the black flies covering the babies, I often recognized that I still had much to learn, not only about our own military culture but also about Vietnamese ethnicity. On one excessively hot, humid day, I left a ward and headed toward the back entrance of the north-facing compound. I saw a gathering nearby of Vietnamese nurses and my interpreter, who was pointing up to a perfectly round, massive cloud drifting slowly from the north. This visual phenomenon seemed as if someone had blown a huge smoke ring. One of the nurses said this cloud indicated that Ho Chi Minh[1] had died—the third such claim of Ho's death while I was in Vietnam. Moments later, several anxious nurses scurried past me and rushed back home.

To the right of the cloud formation was a particularly large and low hanging moon, clearly revealing its markings more prominently than I had ever witnessed. I asked my interpreter, who had stayed behind, "Do the Vietnamese believe they have anything like a soul that leaves the body of the deceased?"

"Yes! The soul goes to the moon," he exclaimed. When pressed for more details, he declared that a soul needs water, and the dark parts of the moon, which we see as craters, were large tracts of water. "Water on the moon" seemed a strange concept to a Westerner but quite acceptable to the Vietnamese. I certainly did not argue that the shadowy areas were large lunar craters.

Coincidentally, around this same time, NASA's Apollo program was in full swing. The December 1968 launch of Apollo 8 became the first manned spacecraft to leave Earth's orbit, circle the moon, and return. Every American was proud of this accomplishment. Before long, however, the news filtered down to the Vietnamese working at Delta Med, many of whom were furious and offended by what they perceived as propaganda.

---

1. Ho Chi Minh (1890–1969), president of the Democratic Republic of Vietnam (North Vietnam), died on September 2, 1969.

The December 21 launch date was the first time the moon came alive for me. The moon had always been what my science classes confirmed: a rocky leftover from the solar system's creation, a distant world for man to conquer.

For the Vietnamese, as my interpreter had earlier explained, their luminous sphere could not be dismissed so cavalierly. Instead, the moon was a destination for the soul. And now, as the blindingly bright disk barely kissed the tropical horizon, the optical illusion made it appear even grander and more mystical. Earth's satellite had a presence that consumed all of us, Asians and Westerners alike.

I then understood why the Vietnamese were insulted by the claim that Americans had sent men to the place where the soul eventually resided. To the Vietnamese, moon exploration was blasphemous. But to me, with the Apollo 8 launch, I stood and gazed upon the moon as never before. The lunar marvel, now shimmering in the tropical heat, spoke to me as it had done for centuries for the Vietnamese.

And another conviction permeated the ranks of the South Vietnamese troops, who were often positioned to protect American flanks. The Marines distrusted these troops' willingness to fight. Digging deeper, I learned the cultural reasons for Vietnamese hesitancy. Many South Vietnamese troops were not from the Dong Ha area or the surrounding region. Many were from villages much farther south and closer to Saigon. These soldiers were afraid of dying up north because, according to their beliefs, if they were killed and buried far from home, they would never make it to a beautiful afterlife. The Vietnamese admittedly thought life on this earth was hell's equivalent, but hoped that a worthy life on Earth would earn them a good place in the hereafter. Witnessing their country and their lives torn apart by war, I couldn't argue with their logic.

Transfusions of Life

One day, a corpsman brought in a 5-day-old baby. The decaying umbilical cord was still attached. The infant was hot with fever and experiencing apneic spells, so his erratic breathing required resuscitation. The baby was obviously at the edge of death which, initially, could have been caused by pneumonia. The chest x-ray didn't reveal anything unusual. The problem, most likely, was sepsis or bacteria invading the bloodstream. I administered fluids and gave the newborn large doses of IV antibiotics. Despite this aggressive treatment, the infant was not improving, leaving me unsure what to do next. I wondered what other procedure I could perform.

Before antibiotics were discovered in the 1930s, physicians occasionally performed exchange transfusions for desperate cases. I didn't know the success rate of those transfusions but I was running out of options. The purpose of the exchange transfusions was that someone else's healthy blood, which contained globulins and good white blood cells, might help fight the infection along with the antibiotics.

I asked the Chief Hospital Corpsman to call for some Marines who had the

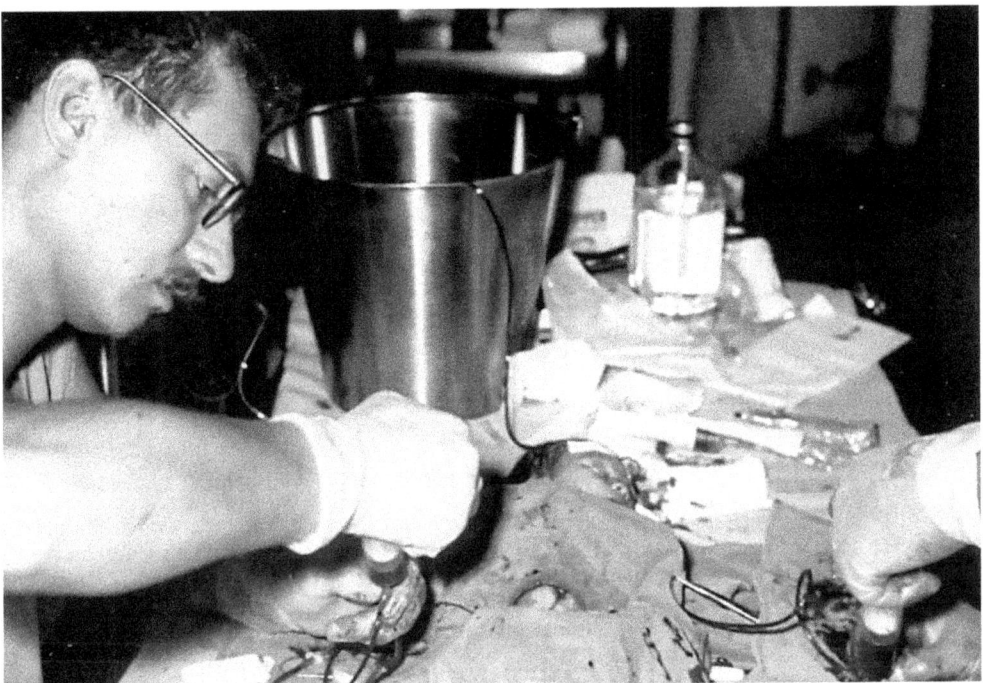

Dr. Burkle performs two volume blood exchange transfusions to save a critically ill infant at Delta Med (author's collection).

same blood type, and I would confirm compatibility with a cross-match. The baby's blood was A-positive so that blood type would be easy to obtain. Within minutes, we had several young, healthy Marine volunteers, but I needed only two to serve as donors. We drew their blood right next to where I would do the baby's exchange transfusion.

Their blood went into a sterile tube, which then entered and curled around in an aluminum bucket filled with warm water. I next cut the decaying umbilical cord and exposed the small vessel that led up into the liver. I didn't have the equipment I had used at Yale-New Haven Hospital, but we located a small urinary catheter that I improvised. I fed it up into the liver and then, over several hours, completed a two-volume exchange. I replaced the baby's blood volume twice with that of two U.S. Marines.

All the while I was calculating what the infant's blood volume would be at that moment. In between these blood exchanges, I gave pushes of IV antibiotics so the drugs would circulate. I did one total volume exchange and, so far, the infant was in stable condition. I then proceeded with the second exchange. Interestingly, about three-quarters of the way through the procedure, the baby was no longer having apneic breathing spells. He was clinically doing better; the heart rate was good and strong. I finished the exchange procedure just as the sun was coming up.

The infant's mother arrived at the hospital. I had never seen the mother. She had just passed her baby over the wire gate the evening before. The guards let her in early. She had brought a small gray-white wooden coffin, clearly expecting that her infant had died. Upon seeing her baby breathing again and moving on the table, she ran over and dropped to her knees. She threw her arms around my legs and cried. To this day, I can remember that moment. Though we couldn't communicate well, her gratitude was crystal clear because she gave me a huge smile later when I walked into the ward. She was the wife of an enlisted South Vietnamese soldier and had followed him north to Dong Ha.

With the success of the infant's transfusion, I was hoping now that the local villagers would realize that I needed to get to these kids early to effectively treat them. For the blood exchange baby and family, this story had a happy ending. But that transfusion was responsible for further complicating a situation for me and for my fellow physicians. During the next several days, the lines of patients waiting at the children's hospital became much longer. We were now to the point of seeing even more children than the usual 300 per day.

With the surge in patients, our supplies took a hit, and we had to ration everything we used, especially antibiotics. Everyone in the line watched us take care of patients as though we were being examined under a microscope. The line crawled forward and the hours ticked by. We were so exhausted that even the days of the week seemed to blur together.

Soon after the incident with the septic infant, the early morning long line of patients unexpectedly parted like the Red Sea. An older Vietnamese man, clearly an honored village elder with a chin tuft of long facial hair, entered the compound with an entourage of other males. The villagers immediately showed their veneration. He didn't speak but others spoke for him, directing their pleas to me. My interpreter told me the old man was a village chief who demanded that I take out all his blood and replace it with new blood. He raised his garment and pointed to his umbilicus.

I then gathered that the account about my transfusing the baby had spread widely around Quang Tri Province. This man was obviously important and well revered. I assumed he must have had some kind of chronic illness based on his aches and pains. But I was definitely not going to do a total blood transfusion.

Through my interpreter, we went back and forth about this procedure. No matter what I said, I couldn't clinically explain my decision to refuse him without attacking his dignity. "I'm sorry," I finally said. "I cannot do it. It is impossible. I can only do this procedure with infants." He was visibly angry. My interpreter and the village chief exchanged words, but the elder never spoke directly to me. I could see from the looks on the faces of his followers as they departed that I had offended their esteemed chief. Small groups of mothers and their sick children also left.

During the next few days, the number of villagers waiting in line diminished noticeably. But they eventually came back. I learned a good lesson that I have since been trying to teach students and other young humanitarian professionals: Never perform a procedure that cannot be reproduced by local medical workers in their culture and in their own facilities. This mistake is still made by humanitarians the world over.

Sensitivity, Camaraderie, Connection

As difficult as the job was at Delta Med, I felt this wartime experience was a gift. For the first time I began to understand the culture of the Vietnamese as the villagers arrived to be treated. Throughout my one year in in this war-ravaged country, I came to value and appreciate their customs and beliefs. In every humanitarian mission in which I had participated since serving in Vietnam, my priority has been to be sensitive to the native people's culture and to respect them and their traditions through our personal interactions. That comprehension has been critical in achieving some measure of global success.

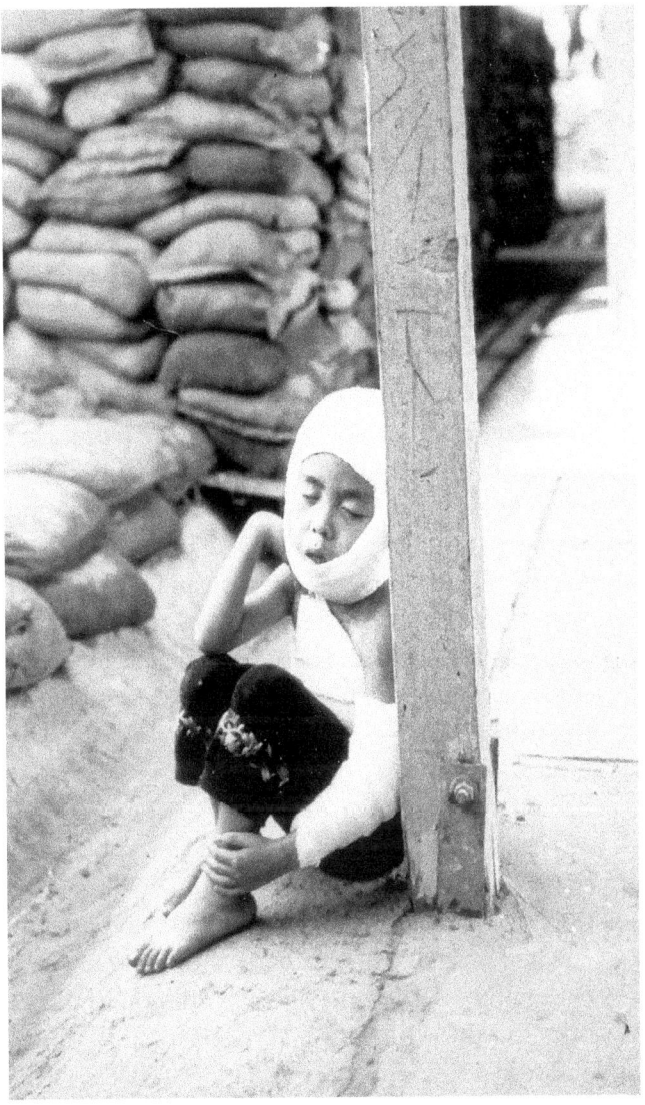

A little girl—the last remaining survivor of a family whose home was destroyed in an air raid. The child was mute and refused to be held or receive care in the hospital wards (author's photo).

After months of nonstop 24-hour triage, surgeries, disease, and death, coupled with little sleep and little communication from back home, I wondered if I could handle much more of the mental burden. Thoughts of my family consumed me. For four months, I had received no letters from home. I finally wrote to Phyllis that I understood if she had found someone else and wanted a divorce. My letters desperately asked about the three kids. They were mine, too, and I hated missing so much of their formative years.

One fateful morning, I traveled six miles south with several corpsmen to pick up urgently needed antibiotic supplies at Alpha Med. We stopped briefly at the main office where the Marine behind the desk asked for our names. On this errand outside of the base, we had, of course, removed all identification from our uniforms. When I gave him my name, he turned and retrieved a packet of letters from a shelf. The bundle had been tied and covered with dust and dirt. Not knowing my rank and figuring I had to be a newbie, he chastised me for not informing the command where I was posted. I was astonished but thought the charge comical.

I eyed the large packet of letters, grabbed them, and turned away. For months, they had been sitting on that shelf while I pined away at remote Delta Med. The desk Marine emphasized that I was lucky because he planned to burn the lot that very day. I read the last of the letters to assure myself that I was still happily married. To this day, I admit that I read only that final letter, not the earlier ones.

Phyllis later related that because Dong Ha was frequently mentioned in the press, her anxiety only increased knowing that I was stationed there. She watched Walter Cronkite's "CBS Evening News" program every night, as did the rest of the country. Casualty figures played a big role in his news program. Cronkite brought the distant war into every American living room.

At one point she heard on the radio about an attack on Delta Med with several medical personnel being killed. She got the run-around from the Navy and the Marines about which branch was responsible for giving names of any deceased in this attack. After three days, Phyllis learned that I was alive. But those were probably the longest three days of her life. If I was working in a living hell on a daily basis, Phyllis was suffering from uncertainty on an hourly basis.

Medically, my year in Vietnam was very rewarding. I learned so much about myself, especially realizing that I could be calm under pressure and that my education at Yale-New Haven Hospital had prepared me well. Pediatrics at that time was equated mainly with the care of infectious diseases because inoculating for most childhood diseases was not yet common in the late 1960s. We had only four antibiotics to work with, and every week we had admissions for meningitis, pneumonia, and sepsis.

Because the physician I had replaced from the outset was an internist who disliked dealing with contagious diseases, I quickly had become the go-to guy who treated transmittable diseases. With a big smile, he handed over that responsibility to me on the very first day I was in Vietnam. I was therefore consulted on a host of infectious diseases in both the military and the local population.

As a medical team, we were all quite different regarding our religions, prejudices, politics, and other social norms. But each one of us at Delta Med had been through our individual challenges and yet drew closer despite our many contrasts. The bonds that developed among my new colleagues were camaraderie and connection, which, I believe, everyone strives for in life. For the most part, we all had the highest levels of respect and admiration for each other.

Even now, more than five decades later, I frequently think of my comrades and try to keep in touch. Veterans often talk about the brotherhood formed during wars, but comradeship is truly difficult to replicate in our everyday lives in more peaceful, developed countries. Those of us who have experienced that feeling of shared wartime experience know it well, and we cherish the memories despite the hardship and trauma we all endured together.

A Departure of a Different Kind

As my tour in Vietnam wound down in mid–July 1969, events took a peculiar turn. Earlier in the year, Bob Rowe, our surgeon, had successfully corrected a patient's ductus defect. This condition is a persistent opening between the two major blood vessels leading from the heart that should have closed before birth. The patient was a 10-year-old boy. No complications occurred.

Around the same time, I had diagnosed three children with correctable heart disease. But each of these children had a more complex heart issue, a problem way beyond what we could handle at Delta Med. With surgery, their disease could be reversed. I learned that several international non-governmental organizations (NGOs) were located in Da Nang, and I sent them information on these three children. Before long, representatives of these NGOs responded that all three qualified for treatment at a major hospital in San Francisco where they all finally ended up.

As the months passed, I almost forgot about those children and what had become of them back in the States. In June 1969, news of my pending departure filtered through the local population, mainly from the Vietnamese nurses we employed. My time finally came in July, 365 days after my arrival at Delta Med.

I was scheduled to leave the base in three weeks, but close to that time, Bob Rowe called me to triage. He somberly stated that some Marines had warned him that the local population had planned a demonstration the next day outside the hospital on Route 1. The villagers demanded that I remain a "technical hostage" until those three children were returned. One mother had come to the hospital several weeks before, claiming the Viet Cong had told her I had sent the children to the U.S. to be my "slaves and servants." I also learned that I had had a $125 price on my head—insultingly low, I thought—because of these three children being taken to the U.S. for life-saving surgery. That bounty had gone up by the end of my tour.

Bob then told me that the higher-ups had made a judgment call to fly me to Da Nang on a helicopter at 5 a.m. the next morning. I was not to mention this to anyone, especially the Vietnamese. I was quite taken aback by this decision. After all I had hoped to accomplish, this kind of discharge was not how I wanted my service in Vietnam to end. I had planned many farewells and expressions of thanks and admiration that now would not occur.

Back in my hooch, I reflected on what had just transpired. I wanted to put some meaning into my year of caring for Marines, soldiers, and Vietnamese alike. Initially, I couldn't quite believe I was going home, but the anticipation was tempered by mixed feelings. For the first time, I understood the kind of physician I wanted to be. The diseases and diagnostic challenges I encountered that year were intriguing, and I now realized I loved this kind of specialized medicine.

I sat down on the edge of my cot in the dim light. Less than three feet away was a solid wall of sandbags, lit by only a single bulb hanging in the center of the room. I then sensed a movement on the floor next to me and felt an odd weight atop my right boot. I looked down and saw a big, black, thick-bodied snake with white markings. It slithered by and entered a hole between the sandbags. The banded krait had been slinking around for some time. We had unknowingly been long-time neighbors.

Watching helplessly, the slow-moving krait invaded my depression, but I was so tired that I didn't have enough energy to be afraid. Thankfully, the krait had little interest in me. Despite the flooding thoughts of what would come next, I eventually fell asleep. At 5 a.m., I boarded the helicopter to fly to Da Nang, the first leg of my journey out of Vietnam and back to Connecticut.

I returned home a few days before Neil Armstrong first set foot on the lunar surface. But on that most historic night, July 20, 1969, I looked up at Earth's imposing satellite and stood transfixed, reflecting on my extraordinary experiences in that war-torn country. I also thought about crossing that cultural threshold to try to understand and appreciate other people's beliefs. Maybe there is water on the moon after all.

* * * *

More than fifty years later, thankfully, I've never suffered the torturous flashbacks of many veterans who have served in time of war. Phyllis put it so well when she told me that Vietnam would be with me forever. And her insightful remark reflects that I can still clearly recall every detail of those Marines and Vietnamese children I was not able to save. Strangely, in my dreams, they all survive.

5

Homecoming and Readjustment
1969–1975

"I hosed off the Dong Ha mud from my boots in the backyard, mud which instantly evoked memories of a war I could never forget."

Following my chaotic departure from Dong Ha in July 1969, I slowly made my way back to American soil with several stops along the way. Needless to say, I was apprehensive about my homecoming on many levels.

During the Vietnam War, service members returning from Vietnam in uniform were often harassed in public places, including airports. One of our surgeons at Dong Ha had to return home on emergency leave. He arrived at the airport in Los Angeles and was immediately confronted by a group of rowdy young men playing drums and singing anti-war songs. Calling this surgeon a "baby killer," these protesters grabbed his hat and grew increasingly confrontational. Unlike today, many airports had no security. No one at the airport, including terminal personnel, came to his aid. He was the only one in uniform—grubby camouflage fatigues that shouted out where he had been serving. Nobody knew he was a doctor who had been saving lives—not taking them.

Thinking of that incident as I made my way back home, I worried about how my own family would greet me. Would my two older kids even recognize their father after a year of separation? What would my relationship with Phyllis be like? Would it be the same as before I left? My year-long medical tour in Vietnam was both an education and an ordeal, but my actual homecoming was even more difficult.

All this distress weighed on me when we landed in Alaska, and then I had to anxiously wait for the next military flight to Dover Air Force Base in Delaware. I was exhausted, sleepless, and sick with a respiratory infection I was trying to conceal. I knew I had few options for getting to Connecticut. I was unshaven and still in my dirty camouflage uniform with muddy boots. I had little money in my pocket, most of it being South Vietnamese currency. Hitchhiking was my only option.

Upon landing in Alaska, I called Phyllis who was overjoyed that I was back on U.S. soil. "Don't worry," she lovingly reassured me. "We'll get there to pick you up." Phyllis contacted a friend, Bob McDonald, who, without hesitation, agreed to make the 250-mile trek down to Dover to get me.

In ordinary circumstances, this proposal would be seen as very generous. But predictably, my father did not view kind offers well. For some reason, however, Bob's proposal came as an affront to his pride. When he found out about Bob McDonald's intention to drive to Dover, he became inexplicably infuriated, yelling, "I'm picking him up!"

My father borrowed Uncle Robert's station wagon, and with my mother, Phyllis, and three kids crammed inside, they headed south to Delaware. Despite his insistence on personally picking me up, I later learned my father had angrily complained about this unwelcomed chore during the entire five-hour drive to Dover.

When I exited the terminal after days of interminable travel, I saw Phyllis standing beside the station wagon, searching for me with great anticipation. And, as in a typically romantic Hollywood movie, we rushed toward each other and embraced. After a few moments, my mother and the kids ran up to me. My father never got out of the car. For the next five hours on the trip back to Connecticut, he did not speak a single word to me. Heidi, our 3-year-old, didn't remember me at all because she was born shortly before I left. Chris, now age 6, didn't say much. Jennifer, age 4, clung to me all the way back home.

I was disoriented by an 11-hour time zone difference and drained from an all-consuming respiratory tract infection. I then callously reacted to these makeshift living conditions, along with my father's reproachful behavior. I took out my pent-up anger on Phyllis, saying, "I wish I was back in Vietnam."

Even as the words left my lips, I realized the pain I had just inflicted on this incredibly supportive woman. I had endured living in a war zone for a year but Phyllis had to accept living in cramped quarters with three young children for that same length of time. She had to deal with a father-in-law who, most likely, hated my family's imposition into his personal living space and intrusion into his life. I did not doubt that he made his feelings known daily. I immediately regretted—and long afterward—those heartless remarks to Phyllis.

The following morning, I had my first real shower in months. I hosed off the Dong Ha mud from my boots in the backyard, mud which instantly evoked memories of war I could never forget. Later that day, holding Heidi's tiny hand, I walked up the street to visit old neighbors. I had known this senior couple for years and wanted to say hello, perhaps just to experience a warm welcoming outside of close relatives. At the same time, I was very eager to leave my parents' house and begin a normal family life once again.

Trying to get back to a "normal" routine, though, didn't quite work. And Phyllis saw right through me. She understood that I just couldn't get back into a normal world after spending a year in a war zone, seeing death every day, and having a near-death experience. This attempt at readjustment was a trying time for us all. Phyllis realized that during this period I didn't quite have what was needed to feel like I was there for her and the kids. I was forcing myself to make them think that my period of readjustment was going smoothly. But sometimes I just wanted to be left alone.

5. Homecoming and Readjustment

This reacclimation was sometimes beyond my ability. As Phyllis said, Vietnam was still in me and nobody was willing to listen. Friends and family could acknowledge what I went through, but they couldn't understand unless they had lived through it themselves. And some people, she shrewdly remarked, didn't want to know. But I had to talk about it because, as she said, some people wanted to know.

After several weeks of bouncing back and forth between my parents' home and visiting Phyllis's parents, we needed to leave. I was due to report to my new duty station. Being a Vietnam veteran, I was able to pick the Naval Hospital at Newport, Rhode Island, as my first choice. The pediatric clinic needed a physician, so I gratefully accepted that duty. My first day was awkward and a bit trying. My handlebar mustache, not strictly within "military specs," was met with laughter. I wasn't familiar with the Navy's so-called "mustache length rule."

Shortly after beginning my post, I had an argument with a young patient's mother who insisted I give her son an antibiotic for his alleged viral infection. A duty nurse asked me to see a young child needing attention. Before any words were exchanged, the mother quickly declared that her child had strep and she wanted antibiotics to be given to him immediately. I didn't want to give him any drugs needlessly and cautioned her on the dangers of unnecessary antibiotics.

After asking if her son had any symptoms, I examined the boy. He didn't have a fever or any swollen lymph nodes, or even a red throat. I tactfully said that I needed to get a culture to determine if he really had this bacterial infection.

I reached for a sterile cotton swab in a glass container. But before I could remove the cotton stick to swab his throat, the mother slapped my hand and the container fell to the floor and broke. She then snatched her son and ran out the door, declaring, "You'll hear about this!"

I was shortly summoned to the CO's office concerning this encounter. I told the CO what had occurred and then angrily stated, "Maybe you should just send me back to Vietnam. I am not going to practice bad medicine."

Being an astute commander, he could see right through me, just as Phyllis could. He channeled my early duty frustrations into something substantial by assigning me to give medical presentations both at the hospital and in Newport about my Vietnam service. Talking about Vietnam to the medical world, as well as one-on-one with the CO, was psychologically very beneficial for me. The commanding officer and I chatted many times about my Delta Med experience, which he found genuinely interesting.

Every physician had to do shifts in the Naval Hospital ER, regardless of rank. During my first night pulling duty in the ER, I came across an unfortunate encounter between a corpsman and a nurse. As I watched him mop the floor, the nurse screamed demeaning names at him. Then I suddenly realized that I knew this corpsman. We had both been at Delta Med and had shared many wartime urgencies almost daily. He was that corpsman who performed that amazing tracheotomy on my very first casualty. He had carried out that lifesaving procedure yet now he found himself washing floors and being berated for some alleged minor infraction. I later told the nurse about this corpsman's background in Vietnam and his superb medical skills. She was unimpressed and said nothing. As I spent more time in military culture at home, the disparaging hierarchy mentality became clearer. Thankfully, I had not encountered anything like this in Vietnam, but Rhode Island was not Vietnam.

Toward the end of my two-year military obligation in 1970, the Navy wanted me to make a career in the Medical Corps. I said no. I had concluded that being in the Medical Corps was not the path I wanted to take. In Vietnam, I had taken care of young Marines in their late teens and early 20s. I had treated Vietnamese children, and I had developed a strong interest in adolescent and young adult medicine.

At this point in 1970, I learned about a fellowship offered in adolescent medicine at Harvard Medical School. I applied for it and was accepted. During the one-year fellowship at Harvard, I moonlighted in a few pediatric practices and in emergency rooms around Boston to make some money. In the early 1970s, I was in serious financial straits, and the expectation was that I would go into private practice. Although my dream to practice global medicine was still in the back of mind, I put that hope aside, realizing that I had to be a responsible husband and parent.

When my fellowship ended, I was offered a job as a co-pediatrician in a practice in Old Saybrook, Connecticut. I worked my tail off for four years, and sometimes even slept in the office, but I barely made it on my $20,000 salary my first two years.

Our practice did face some medical challenges, however. In 1973, my partner and I began seeing children who came in with strange symptoms resembling arthritis and certain indicators of rheumatic fever. Each child exhibited a red rash, painful joints, and a low-grade fever. My colleague and I had never seen an illness such as this one, and we had no idea what was causing these unusual symptoms.

Ticks were commonplace in southern Connecticut, just part of the natural environment. Ironically, our practice in Old Saybrook was barely five miles from Old Lyme, just across the Connecticut River Bridge. None of our young patients mentioned getting a tick bite, and we, as physicians, never considered ticks as a cause of these symptoms. Moreover, the physical manifestations may have developed many months after the children had been bitten.

At a loss to understand what was transpiring in our little medical community, we sent the children to the rheumatology experts at Yale-New Haven Hospital. The staff infectious disease specialists finally made a definitive diagnosis five years after we had seen our first cases. They had classified a new illness: Lyme disease.

The last year in that pediatrics practice I made $63,000. Even so, we just weren't making it financially. I wanted to use my more specialized medical skills, mostly relating to emergency medicine and infectious diseases.

Phyllis also wasn't happy in this small community. She had few friends in Old Saybrook society and didn't seem to connect with anyone else in this small historic town in southern Connecticut. According to Phyllis, we were living in a different world in this posh community and unwilling to keep up with these upper strata of society. She and I both agreed that living in Old Saybrook wasn't the life we wanted. And, as always with great insight, Phyllis saw that my medical practice, despite the hands-on aspect of being in a practice, was becoming a business and too routine. She knew that when medicine becomes a business, it was not medicine.

So we decided to follow my ongoing dream of applying my medical skills and aspirations to the global health arena and see where that goal would take us. In 1974, I applied to the UC Berkeley School of Public Health for a master's degree in public health. I knew by then that if I wanted to make my mark in global health, I needed the prerequisite academic public health credentials.

I was accepted into the one-year Berkeley program and informed my pediatric partner that I was leaving. We packed our Jeep Cherokee and drove across the country to Berkeley. In nearby Walnut Creek, we rented an apartment and once again I had to moonlight. Phyllis got a job at a Sears Auto Center and the kids attended local schools. We all made sacrifices. The apartment was small and crowded, but these tight living circumstances brought us closer as a family. Even though I had completed my military commitment on active duty, I remained in the Navy Reserves so I was obligated to attend periodic drills and other military activities once a month.

The master's program at Berkeley was my entrance into global health. If I planned to practice global medicine, I had to be qualified in public health and epidemiology that dealt with rapidly spreading contagious diseases. Berkeley was one of the very few institutions teaching those subjects in the early 1970s.

Once I had completed my coursework for a master's degree in public health, I was certain that some organization would hire me, perhaps the World Health Organization, a non-governmental organization, or even the American Red Cross. That latter agency enabled me to do my first humanitarian work with the villagers outside the Delta Med compound.

* * * *

I received my public health degree in the summer of 1975. But that spring during my studies in the Berkeley program in April, I could never have imagined that I would shortly be back in Vietnam under extraordinary circumstances.

From 1968 to 1969—just one short year, Vietnam changed my life forever. Now that far-off world would once again touch and alter my professional life.

6

Operation Babylift

April 1975

"We were in the heart of darkness—a world gone crazy. Chaos reigned in Saigon, a city in its death throes, and everybody seemed to be looking at us with some suspicion—or so I thought."

I certainly was not expecting to return to South Vietnam in April 1975 in equally dangerous circumstances as those I experienced in 1969. I was currently finishing up my master's degree in public health at UC Berkeley. A month before I headed back to Saigon, the North Vietnamese had precipitated a full-scale invasion of South Vietnam, overrunning every village, city, and province in its path toward the capital. To the dismay of all of us who had fought and served in this battle-scarred country, South Vietnam's collapse now seemed inevitable. My connection to Vietnam hadn't stopped in July 1969 when my Navy medical service ended. So once more into the breach.

In an event much less remembered than the Vietnam War itself, "Operation Babylift" began on April 3, 1975—the first of several missions following President Gerald Ford's order: Military Airlift Command to evacuate orphans from Saigon aboard C-5A Galaxy and C-141 Starlifter cargo aircraft. Many of the so-called "orphans" who would be whisked from Saigon weren't really orphans. They were children of poor Vietnamese who could not support them. As a result, their parents were forced to place their children in orphanages. American officials promised some families that their infants and young children would be reunited with their parents once conditions stabilized.[1] Several non-governmental organizations (NGOs) also weighed in by chartering aircraft to move out orphans and bring them to the United

---

1. Other children caught up in the chaos and confusion of war became separated from their parents and were simply classified as "orphans." Many of these orphans were the offspring of American GIs and Vietnamese women. The future of thousands of these Amerasian children remaining in Vietnam was in jeopardy, especially under the inevitable communist rule on the near horizon. These "alien" children, tainted with American blood and referred to as "half-breeds," would not be adoptable by Vietnamese families. Many of those who remained behind were ostracized because of their mixed race, and so they became street beggars with very uncertain futures. In 1989, 14 years after Operation Babylift, my wife Phyllis and I traveled to Vietnam. In Ho Chi Minh City, formerly Saigon, we encountered many Amerasian beggars, especially in the parks where they congregated. They were now all grown up, looking like American teenagers. They spoke only Vietnamese, were uneducated, totally destitute, and lived as gangs in parks. We gave them what Vietnamese money we had in our pockets.

States. Time was quickly running out to evacuate many of these children before the enemy captured the city.

A Fateful Pause

At that point in April 1975, while at UC Berkeley, I received an unforgettable phone call. A dentist from outside San Francisco contacted me saying that he had been asked by World Airways and the federal government to send in a team to take out as many orphans as possible from Saigon. I don't know how he obtained my name, but he unassumingly asked, "You were there?"

I responded, "Yes, I ran a children's hospital near the DMZ from 1968 to 1969 and can speak some of the language."

He quickly came to the point. "Would you be my medical director?"

I agreed and then informed my department professor at Berkeley. But I was instructed not to tell anybody else—except my wife—where I was going. This fateful pause in my master's program lasted for about 10 days.

Phyllis's response was very supportive and reassuring. She said she realized Operation Babylift was a humanitarian effort and that I was needed. She understood that this assignment would be daunting and dangerous, given that South Vietnam, barely a country at this point, was now almost nonexistent and in absolute turmoil. But my wife of 15 years knew me well and knew I had to go.

We took off from Oakland on a World Airways 747. The plan involved landing in Saigon and taking out a large group of orphans. The strategy was simply to get the orphans to the U.S. where many families had already volunteered to adopt these children. When I stepped aboard, I looked around to see what other medical personnel I was going to direct. I noted 13 nurses, 13 doctors, and 26 flight attendants, most of whom were nurses or who had nursing experience from World Airways. Due to space, I immediately decided that we would reconfigure the first-class section to be the intensive care unit for the sickest children. With the number of village children I had observed and treated at Delta Med, I knew many acutely ill children would need specialized care on this trip. Since the seats were still in place, we needed to put babies in boxes on top of those seats.

About two hours outside of Saigon, the pilot announced we were not being permitted to land. The North Vietnamese had advanced and the president of South Vietnam, Nguyen Van Thieu, had said he was unwilling to let any more children over the age of 6 out of the country. He also affirmed that the South Vietnamese were going to fight to the last person. Saigon was now surrounded and no more commercial flights were being allowed to land at Tan Son Nhut Airport, located four miles east of Saigon. The plane then turned around and flew northeast, setting down three hours later at Clark AFB in the Philippines. All the passengers got off totally exhausted. On the tarmac, I was introduced to two men who were associated with a Scandinavian humanitarian group, an international NGO.

Another plane, a Flying Tigers[2] 727 aircraft, had just landed, transporting about 30 infants and toddlers out of South Vietnam. They were in the back of the aircraft lying on thick padding material used to protect cargo. The children were unaccompanied, and none had name tags or any other form of identification. The pilots of this 727 said they were planning to return to Cambodia, but this time on a larger DC-8.

Ed Daly, president of World Airways, was also on the tarmac. He had just arrived from Saigon after his chaotic rescue flight from Da Nang Airport. Daly was aware of many orphans still in need of evacuation, and he arranged for the DC-8 to try to land at Saigon's airport before going on to Cambodia. He asked if I was willing to go along and support the effort.

From Bribes to Promissory Notes

As if my assignment to find and rescue children in South Vietnam didn't put me in harm's way, the NGO representative on the tarmac asked me to accept an additional task: tracking down and delivering four packets, each containing "good faith" funding. This financial backing included $3,000 cash and also promissory notes totaling thousands of dollars. The envelopes held the lists of people who were to be evacuated from Saigon, and the cash was to facilitate their departures, including payments to boat operators. Unfortunately, money previously sent to Saigon, which was to be used as bribes to get families out, simply "disappeared." Many were then left stranded at the boat docks. The potential evacuees were told to show up at the harbor at a certain time and boats would be waiting for them. In the end, no boats arrived. So the bribe money stopped and the promissory note system was substituted.

The representative from that NGO explained this next role in great detail. I had to make contact with the people in Saigon whose names were on the packets. I also had to let them know the conditions in order to receive the promissory notes. If the people on the list made it out of Saigon, including those who worked the evacuation exchange and who were then able to get to the U.S. themselves, then the promissory notes would be honored. They would also collect the additional cash that would be life-changing for them.

Once it was decided that I would go back on that DC-8, I gave orders to remove all the seats in the first-class area of the World Airways 747 while I was away. I had requested supplies but emphasized no milk provisions. I needed infant feeding bottles with electrolyte solutions for dehydration, saline IV bottles, Ringer's lactate, and other necessary medical supplies.

From my experience running a children's hospital for a year in Vietnam, I was

---

2. Flying Tiger Line, named after the 1st American Volunteer Group (AVG) of the Chinese Air Force (1941–1942), was dubbed the "Flying Tigers." As a U.S. cargo airline, it was a major military charter company during the Cold War. In 1988, Federal Express purchased the Flying Tiger Line.

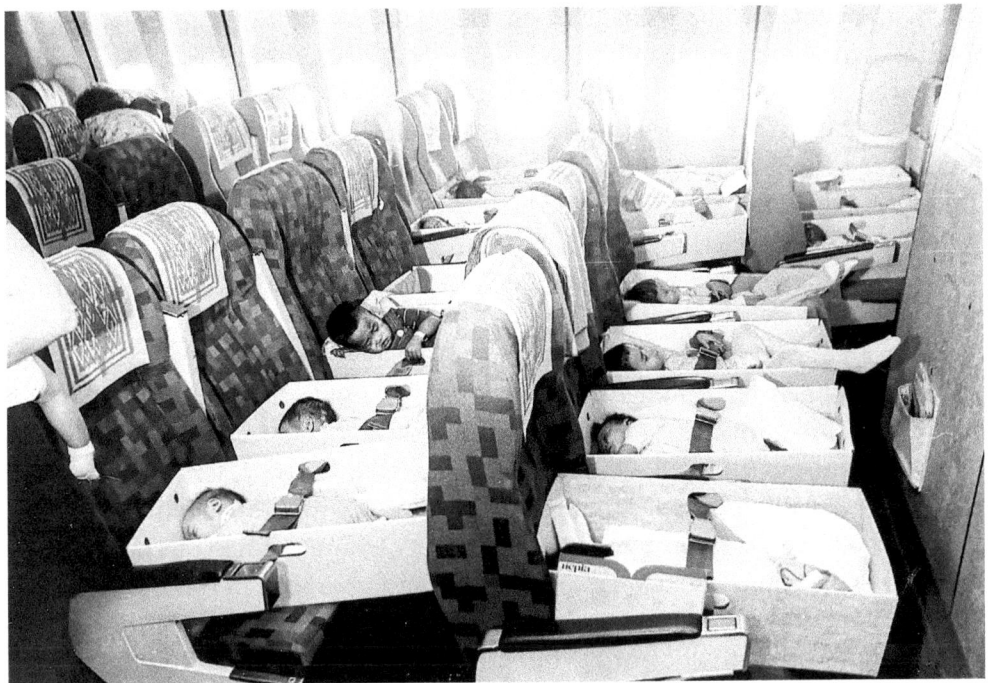

Strapped-in rescued orphans on their way to a new life in America (photograph by the late Robert Stinnett, used with permission).

aware that many Asian kids do not tolerate milk protein because it produces almost instant, severe diarrhea. This condition can lead to added dehydration. I specifically asked for clear electrolyte fluids that children often receive in hospitals worldwide. I assumed stocks of these fluids would be available at the U.S. military hospital tied to Clark AFB.

I sat in the cockpit facing forward right behind the pilot. The seasoned flight crew, all of whom had white hair, had flown in China during the Second World War with the original famed "Flying Tigers." Accompanying us was David, a young African American who was a new CBS cameraman based in San Francisco. David had broad shoulders and had played professional football. Once in the cockpit, we introduced ourselves and discussed our chances of being able to land in Saigon. The pilots said they would chance it, and if not successful, they would fly farther west into Cambodia because they were aware of some orphans who needed to be evacuated from that war-torn country as well.

G-Forces to Remember

As we flew over Tan Son Nhut at 20,000 feet, the crew requested permission to land. We could hear the control tower personnel but they could not hear us. Suddenly, the Tan Son Nhut control tower crackled through. The back-and-forth discussion alternated between "No, you can't land" and "Yes, you can land." We finally received permission to land but were warned that North Vietnamese troops were near the city and had surface-to-air missiles (SAMs). The tower personnel emphasized the real danger if we were to touch down. The pilots did a 360-degree diving turn to come down around 2,000 feet, hoping to line up with the runway. Those were the only moments in my life I ever felt G-forces, and I would be very happy to never again feel the power of those formidable gravitational forces. Sitting right behind the pilot, I was pushed up against the bulkhead. It was a diving turn to remember.

We came around and when descending to 2,000 feet, the pilots realized we had come too far and were definitely in range of not only SAMs but a lot of other heavy artillery. I could immediately tell these experienced pilots were scared. I had several of my close calls in 1968 and 1969, just a few miles south of the DMZ. I now thought that this upcoming perilous landing was an odd way to die. My mind drifted to Phyllis who knew I was heading for Vietnam but certainly couldn't be aware of the operation's dangerous particulars—and this landing was one of those particulars. The co-pilot stood up to look outside his side window, reassuringly calling out that he could not see any missile trails in our direction.

Metal Carcasses

We did another quick 360 degrees and made a very "hot" landing, that is, coming in very fast, at Tan Son Nhut. As soon as we hit the runway, I was overwhelmed by the shocking sight of the grassy areas between the runways. Small spotter planes, helicopters, and mid-sized planes littered the medians. Pilots had flown their aircraft in from bases all over South Vietnam, landing on this runway during these past several days before Saigon's impending downfall. Those South Vietnamese pilots had tried, in desperation, to escape the advancing North Vietnamese. The people aboard quickly emptied those aircraft and ran for their lives. Hundreds of planes and choppers were bulldozed into these grassy zones. The haphazardly stacked aircraft, all one on top of the other, looked like piled-up Mattel toys. These metal carcasses were once worth millions, and now they were just scrap lying on their sides and upside-down. The massive heap extended for hundreds of feet.

Our plane stopped just outside the Flying Tiger Line terminal, which that airline shared with World Airways. Once inside, I was introduced to a soft-spoken, middle-aged Vietnamese man who was shredding documents. He was the station manager for the Flying Tiger Line. I told him about my medical mission and showed him the addresses on the packets. He listened intently and promised to help, also agreeing to take David and me into Saigon to find the orphanages on my list.

David, our guide, and I tried to leave the chaotic confines of Tan Son Nhut on foot, but we were questioned several times by both the American and South

Vietnamese military who asked our purpose for being in Saigon. We walked through a small driveway where Vietnamese guards operated gate bars to be raised and lowered for vehicles. As soon as we got through the gate, the situation was totally different. It was estimated that at least 100,000 refugees were already in Saigon, many of them just roaming the streets. Some joined us as we walked toward the city.

It was April 11. I had four sealed packets with three Vietnamese names and addresses on each one. The instructions I received from the Scandinavians at Clark were to verify the identity of one of the three names on each packet before handing it over to that person. Each envelope, which contained that $3,000 and promissory notes, included assurances for more money—if those people on the promissory list were able to get out of Saigon.

At the same time, my major duty was trying to find orphans in several small orphanages that the Flying Tiger Line's office manager agreed to help me find. But those orphanages were small compared to the number of orphans, as I was informed, who were still present in Saigon. So my task was to find other orphanages, which were not run by Americans, to get those babies out. Under President Thieu's order, we could only evacuate orphan children under the age of 6 years.

"Black Holes of Calcutta"

My Vietnamese tour guide brought me to these so called "institutions," and each one could have been likened to the "Black Hole of Calcutta." These structures were old and decrepit. Located in poverty-ridden areas, these buildings didn't look appropriate for orphanages. The first one I entered had no lighting. I tripped almost immediately over an infant who was stuck to the floor in his own feces. I just looked at all these babies in disbelief. About 15 or 20 infants were in bassinets, maybe two to three in each one. They were orphans with no names and no stories.

I said matter-of-factly, "I'll take them all."

But how was I going to transport them to the airport several miles away? Through our guide, I gave instructions to the Vietnamese in charge of the orphanage about where to show up the next morning with these babies. We went to two more small orphanages, giving the same directives.

Those in charge of these "homes" were on their own to find a way to get their precious cargo to the airport. They were told which entrance to use at Tan Son Nhut. All the attendants at the orphanages were grateful and relieved, happily arranging for airport transportation.

My guide was able to find two people whose names were on the list but they talked rapidly back and forth—too fast for me to comprehend with my limited Vietnamese vocabulary. They then looked to me to acknowledge the details. These two named persons on the packet acted suspiciously but confirmed that they had made separate plans to leave for the United States.

A Dilemma

We eventually made the second packet transfer in a small but crowded circle, probably 40 feet in diameter, where several minor streets converged. The transaction took place and we were ready to move on when my Vietnamese guide quietly introduced me to his wife and two sons. They had been standing in the background. With a weathered face, she looked much older than her husband and was on edge about this encounter with me. He had somehow connected with her while we made our way around the city, arranging for them to meet me in this circle of humanity where it was difficult to hear and be heard. Their sons were probably 11 to 13 years of age. They were wearing identical white shirts, brick-red trousers, and matching brick-red ties. Their heads were bowed. I could not make any eye contact with them. They just stood nervously by their parents.

My guide explained their situation with the impending North Vietnamese Army takeover of Saigon. Since he and his wife worked for the Americans, they were no doubt going to be killed. They wanted me to take their sons out of the country to keep them alive. He then added, "They will be your companions and serve you for the rest of your life."

I didn't expect this kind of dilemma. With this obvious prearrangement to forcibly be introduced to his family, I had to emphasize that my only responsibility was to evacuate orphans. I could not take out anybody else, especially older children. I reminded him that President Thieu had declared that only orphans under the age of 6 were allowed to leave. I suggested that he find a boat on the Saigon River that led to the ocean. I asked if the Flying Tiger Line was making arrangements for their employees. He somberly said he did not know. I told him to take his family to his office and wait, knowing I would never see him again.[3]

In a brief moment of reflection, I thought this situation was insane. We were in the heart of darkness—a world gone crazy. Chaos reigned in Saigon, a city in its death throes, and everybody seemed to be looking at us with some suspicion—or so I thought. And here I am tracking down people on a list handed down from some unknown source, and promising money for their safe evacuation. Some of them had resources and had already arranged to leave on their own. Other orphans and families, who were not on my list, were stuck in the hell of Saigon without any solutions. Phyllis is often the voice of reason in my head, and I tried to think of what she might say or suggest if I was able to describe the situation. But I had no time for such deep thoughts.

My guide spoke to his wife in Vietnamese. I was no more than two feet from both of them when the woman screamed, then lunged at me and pounded my chest with her fists.

After attacking me, she fell to the ground crying. I backed away but this

---

3. Many years later, I learned that my guide/station manager and his family eventually made it out of Vietnam and settled in California.

noticeable commotion drew unwanted attention. People gathered around, curious about this strange, ongoing street event.

About 20 feet away, I saw a North Vietnamese soldier wearing a pith helmet, black shirt, and khaki trousers with an AK-47 slung across his chest. Our eyes locked on each other. He didn't change his expression. He was staring at this scene but made no motion to respond. We knew some North Vietnamese troops were in Saigon, but many officials hoped the NVA soldiers would leave the Americans alone to make an "honorable evacuation."

David, my cameraman, had been standing back, watching this incident unfold. I told him to get out of there—and fast. I started running, too, and then I realized he was now behind me hauling his heavy TV camera. I was certain we were going to be shot in the back. For about 100 yards, we both sprinted and dodged people standing in our way. The buildings were all tightly spaced next to each other. Thankfully, no shots rang out. We finally darted into a small alleyway between two buildings, our chests heaving and our minds racing. We sat down on our haunches to catch our breath. Thoroughly winded, I whispered, "Let's wait here." David and I were now on our own. The Vietnamese Flying Tigers guide leading us through town had disappeared so now we had to find our way back to Tan Son Nhut Airport ourselves.

On the roads into the city, I kept looking for landmarks so if I had to find my way out if the situation had changed, I could see prominent sites along the way. One spot across a small street from where we were sitting looked familiar so I knew we were going in the right direction. We waited for a while until it seemed safe, then headed back toward the airport.

We found our way to the original airport gate where we had started, and no one stopped us from entering. About 40 feet from the checkpoint was a white building with Air Force emblems and other American markings. The military personnel knew about me and my mission so they said we could stay and offered us some food and drink. But I still had two more undelivered packets.

After a few hours, a tall, handsome, well-dressed Vietnamese man came into the office asking for me, saying a nun was waiting outside. Her name was on one of the packets.

"Well, tell her to come in," I responded. "That's wonderful!"

With some authority, he stated, "No, you please come outside."

I went with him and he told me rather bluntly, "You follow my instructions. Go down the walkway," which was on the opposite side of the checkpoint's narrow entrance. "You will see Sister coming. And you do exactly what she says."

I swallowed hard and simply acknowledged, "Okay."

I walked down toward the gate, but before I got to the entry point's crossbar, I saw the woman. She was Caucasian, short, and slightly stocky with cropped black hair, wearing a white blouse and black trousers. She started moving toward me smiling and waving as if we were old friends. Somewhat relieved, I smiled in return. When we both got to the checkpoint gate, the charade abruptly ended, her demeanor instantly changing.

She sternly looked at me and cried out, "Give it to me!" So I gave her the packet and she immediately turned around and left the way she came. When I returned to the office building, the well-attired Vietnamese man had already left. Somebody later told me the nun was running an orphanage. I never saw her again. But I learned that she had come to that same checkpoint early the next morning in a jeep with infants under the seats. She smashed through the gate when the guards wouldn't let her through. That night I slept on a couch in the building. I never delivered the fourth packet.

The next morning, I was taken to where two Air Force C-141s were parked. They had just flown in and the crews were huddled under the wings. I was escorted onto what was supposed to be the lead plane. David was on the other C-141. I was introduced to the pilots, the two flight engineers, and the other Air Force crew. The side entrance to the cargo area was adjacent to the bulkhead that had a ladder to the flight deck. I saw a sizeable area where the children and infants could be placed. Most of the space was taken up by coffins, which, I would learn, contained the bodies of American personnel killed in the C-5A crash on April 4.[4]

As I was setting up, a crew member noticed some disturbance at the gates. Many of these infants were now showing up, but they were not being allowed to come out to the planes until a fee was paid for each child. An American, sporting a Hawaiian shirt, approached and asked me to identify myself. He spoke excellent Vietnamese and was in charge of some adults already on the plane. I assumed he was with the embassy. He told me that South Vietnamese officials were now demanding money as ransom for each infant and child who came through the gates, and that money had to be sent from the embassy. This appalling situation of making money off the evacuation of children was causing the delay.

Human Cargo in File Boxes

Then someone yelled, "They're showing up! They're showing up!" Blue Air Force buses filled with infants began approaching the planes. We assumed that the embassy had complied and sent the money. Each baby was in a file box that had hand openings on both sides so the handler could easily pick up the containers. I talked to the crew about how to secure these boxes holding the babies. Web seats lined both sides of the plane's belly with probably seven seats still vacant on each side. I stood at the door and could see the blue buses parked under the wings. Air Force personnel began grabbing the file boxes. The four engines were running, their deafening noise

---

4. The Air Force C-5A Galaxy had departed Tan Son Nhut Airport shortly after 4 p.m. on April 4, the first Operation Babylift mission. Twelve minutes after takeoff, an explosion tore through the lower rear fuselage, resulting in a rapid decompression of the aircraft. The crew, struggling to keep the plane in the air, attempted to return to the airport but the aircraft crashed into a rice paddy. The casualties numbered 138 killed, including 78 children, 35 Defense Attaché Office Saigon personnel, some embassy wives who offered to assist on the flight, and other volunteers.

almost drowning out every sound on the tarmac. At this point, I didn't know which children were going to make it onto the plane.

These smallest infant refugees were now being loaded on board. We put straps, which stretched from the rear of the plane forward, through the hand openings on the boxes holding this human cargo. We had four rows with the straps. Some infants were not in boxes and I said to put two or three kids in each web seat with straps firmly around them. Several of those children were ill and all were scared to death. Many vomited so we tried laying them down. Even though they had put the infants on their backs in the file boxes, I told the handlers to change their positions and place them on their sides. If they vomited on the flight, they wouldn't aspirate while lying in this position.

Everyone offered to assist, including the flight engineers. We had already loaded many of the file boxes from the rear of the plane to the front so we were getting close to the bulkhead. A small lavatory door in the bulkhead faced forward underneath the cockpit area. One of the flight engineers opened the lavatory door to get some paper towels to clean up a sick child's vomit. A few feet away in front of the bulkhead, I was straddling one of the boxes holding an infant.

The Bomb

At that point, I heard a commotion to my right. Out from this very thin lavatory door came one of the Vietnamese bus drivers. He was struggling with the flight engineer, who was then able to push the driver up against the bulkhead near me, threatening him with his .45 pistol. A purple felt pouch with a gold braid fell to the deck. The familiar-looking bag was a Seagram's 7 pouch that the company used to package their whiskey bottles.

The bag was bulky and everyone immediately realized it was a bomb. One of the crew instantly seized it and just as quickly removed it from the plane. Air Force security police came aboard and dragged the bus driver off the plane. During the chaos, I had been triaging the infants. In the confusion and noise of loading the babies, the bus driver had grabbed a file box from his bus and placed the satchel charge in the Seagram's bag under the infant's blanket. He entered the long line leading to the plane, handed the file box to me, secretly grabbed the Seagram's bag, and then slipped past everyone unnoticed. He had opened the door to the narrow lavatory and was attempting to lodge the pouch between some of the plane's avionics, but was fortuitously surprised by the flight engineer.

Right after the saboteur altercation, everything came to a halt. No more kids could come aboard the plane. The Air Force personnel stopped the entire process of loading these orphans. I could see that the other C-141 was filling up. But the Air Force security police on our plane started to search every space for other possible planted bombs. When they were satisfied it was safe for the plane to depart, the pilot was given clearance for takeoff.

About 10 minutes later, more infants in boxes started to arrive. I now surmised that the American in the Aloha shirt was probably CIA. He looked around and then turned to me, exclaiming, "Good luck, Doc! I don't know how you can do this." It was apparent that all the children were now sick. The plane's door finally shut.

Then one of the crew told me I had to go up on the flight deck during takeoff. I was hesitant because I wanted to be with the children. He said I had no choice, adding that as soon as we got to altitude I could return to my station. I climbed a ladder through a small door into the cockpit. I looked forward at the pilot, co-pilot, flight engineers, and all the instruments on each side. One seat was vacant at the back of the flight deck.

The two C-141s had been waiting for hours on the tarmac in blistering heat with the engines running. They had prepared for immediate takeoff if the airport was attacked. When the engines suddenly began revving up even faster, we heard a big explosion under the right wing. I was astounded to witness the rapid coordinated response when the flight engineers instantly shut down all the engines. Everyone thought a bomb had exploded, but it wasn't an explosive after all. One of the four turbofan engines had simply overheated.

Our crew then had to repeat the entire checklist procedure so the other nearby C-141 took off first. I looked at the pilot and noticed that his head was bent down between his legs. The co-pilot turned around and beckoned me to come forward. I gave him a puzzled look.

The co-pilot, reading my thoughts, asked, "Could you check the pilot? He's sick."

I kneeled in a space between the pilot and co-pilot and asked him about his condition.

The pilot reluctantly responded, "I just can't stand seeing sick kids." He was pale, nauseated, and perspiring profusely.

Lost for words, I desperately asked, "Can you fly this thing?"

He quickly replied, "Oh yeah, I'm okay," and offered a weak smile. I then turned and nodded to one of the flight engineers that everything was all right, even though I didn't have much evidence other than what the pilot had told me.

The turbofan engine that had overheated now seemed to be functioning. We sped down the runway, lifted off, then went into an extreme vertical takeoff. As we climbed, the engines were straining to the hilt.

I kept my eyes on the back of the pilot, willing myself to take slow, deep breaths, but soon he looked like he had recovered from his nausea. It appeared as though our climb approached about 85 degrees, and the ascent seemed to go on for the longest time. But at that point, the entire outside layer of cockpit glass suddenly cracked into a fine jigsaw pattern appearing like small geometric pieces. The pilots were unfazed because only the outside windshield had shattered so no breach had occurred in the integrity of the cockpit. I assumed the fragmenting happened from the rapid acceleration to a higher altitude. Everyone in the cockpit looked at each other, smiled, and shrugged. To relieve the tension after the plane had leveled off, people were half-jokingly asking, "Can anything else go wrong?" I did not want to know the answer.

After flying out of Vietnamese airspace, the crew clapped and cheered. The pilots soon let me go back to check on Vietnam's tiniest evacuees. The infants were all fine. I didn't go back up to the flight deck for the landing at Clark, a touchdown that drew an additional big hurrah from the Air Force crew. Our plane and the one that departed just before us were the last two Air Force flights out of Vietnam.

The World Airways 747 that I had left at Clark AFB was still sitting on the tarmac with all the medical staff and crew who had earlier accompanied me. When we landed, the 747 crew were already piling in the kids—those who were sick or who had been in the hospital at Clark, having arrived on previous flights. The base personnel were also loading children who were on that other C-141 that had landed 20 minutes earlier. When I got off the C-141, the 747 was not very far away. I climbed the ladder to greet my colleagues, all wanting to know what had happened. I gave them a brief report and then told them that we had a lot of sick children who needed immediate attention.

Diarrhea in the Extreme

I was standing in the first-class area with no seats. Several Air Force wives were also in that area, but I noted one who was definitely in charge. She was quite confident in her decisions and delegation of authority, clearly comfortable ordering everyone else around. Small pallets of infant formula had already been loaded on the plane. She was telling her staff to give the kids the formula, asserting they were all malnourished.

I quickly interrupted her and shouted, "No! No!"

She insultingly responded, "You don't know what you're doing." I was tired and had slept very little for the past several days. Believing she would follow my adamant directive, I backed away and walked down the aisles to assess the situation and hoped the doors would shut fairly soon. Maybe she was a nurse or the wife of one of the officers at Clark AFB. She considered herself in charge. Much to my relief, we were finally airborne.

By the time we reached altitude, the babies had had the infant formula and the damage was done. But within a few hours, even the ones who had started in stable condition came down with severe diarrhea. The milk formula was coming out undigested. These cases were so acute that halfway through that flight to California, the toilets were plugged up and nonfunctional. The stench in the cabin was horrific.

In no uncertain terms, I told that woman, who had appointed herself in charge, "I hope you've learned your lesson. You don't give Asian infants milk formula. You have to introduce milk slowly into their diets, allowing them to adjust to Western milk products over time." No response from her.

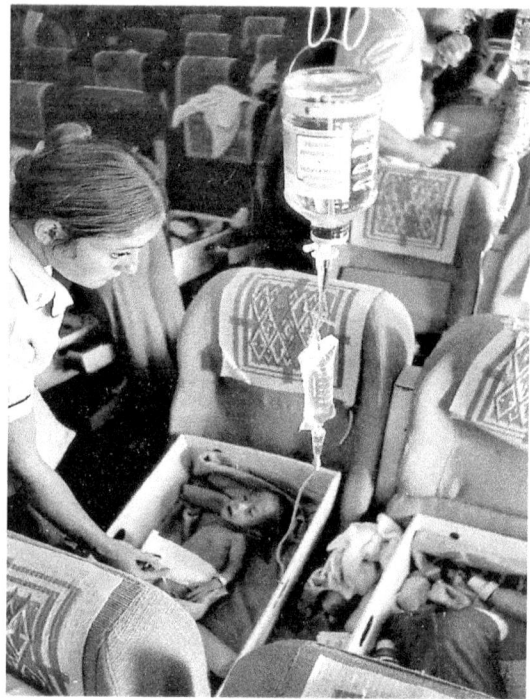 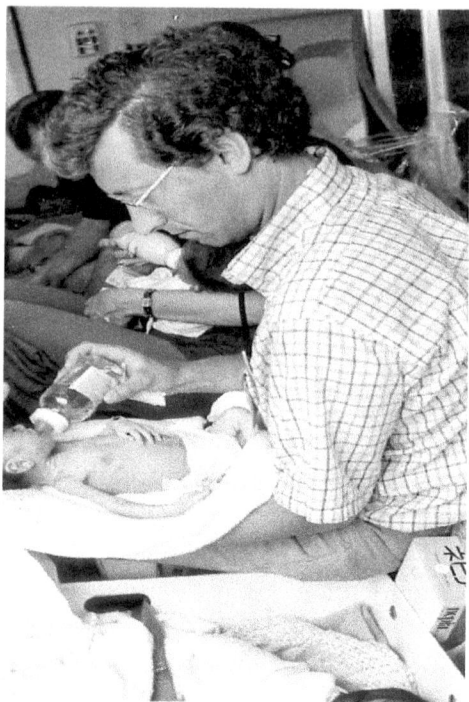

Left: Malnourished and dehydrated infants required IV solutions. Infants were placed in these cardboard file boxes with their handles secured by the aircraft's seatbelts. *Right:* Dr. Burkle feeds a severely dehydrated and malnourished infant aboard the 747 (both photographs by the late Robert Stinnett, used with permission).

To counter the babies' dehydration caused by diarrhea, we had to start placing IVs into these babies and very young children. The many cases of diarrhea were our biggest problem; otherwise, the trip was uneventful across the Pacific.

We were supposed to land in San Francisco, but authorities had agreed to accept only infants and children who were already registered in the adoption process. So we found ourselves diverted to Los Angeles, giving LAX only a three-hour notice.

We had many extremely sick children in the first-class section. One child's condition was tenuous from the outset and, sadly, he died on the flight. The LAX authorities asked if any kids on board were sick, and I gave an outline of six or seven who were critically ill. But the tower was more concerned about infectious diseases, especially since one child had already died.

As a result, the authorities automatically quarantined the flight before we had even arrived at 8:30 a.m. I warned the medical staff that confinement to the plane was a possibility, so they needed to prepare themselves by providing their personal medical history. We then attempted to take some children off the plane and onto the tarmac. But we, as the medical staff, were all ordered back onto the plane because we had not gone through immigration or quarantine ourselves.

Medical personnel on the ground were very irritated because they had had such a short warning prior to our arrival. The LAX authorities were infuriated with

6. Operation Babylift

World Airways showing up because we were the only flight that came to LAX from Saigon, via Clark AFB, and LAX wasn't prepared for our cargo of ill children. Fortunately, we were finally permitted to take the rest of these poor, displaced infants and young children off the plane.

I then took a quiet yet foul-smelling trip back to Oakland. Soon after landing, I had to attend a required briefing about this operation. I was the only medical person from that flight to be present at that meeting. The other doctors had quickly left. We were told to keep quiet about our participation in Operation Babylift. But a real political controversy arose about this entire mission that occupied the press for weeks. I didn't realize that the State Department had contacted Phyllis and told her not to talk to anybody about the flight due to the dispute flaring up among the State Department, the U.S. military, and Ed Daly of World Airways. The federal government was trying to prevent Daly's airline from making any more humanitarian flights in and out of Vietnam, and he was also being threatened with lawsuits. I didn't know the legal details, but the entire World Airways episode was kept secret for a long time.

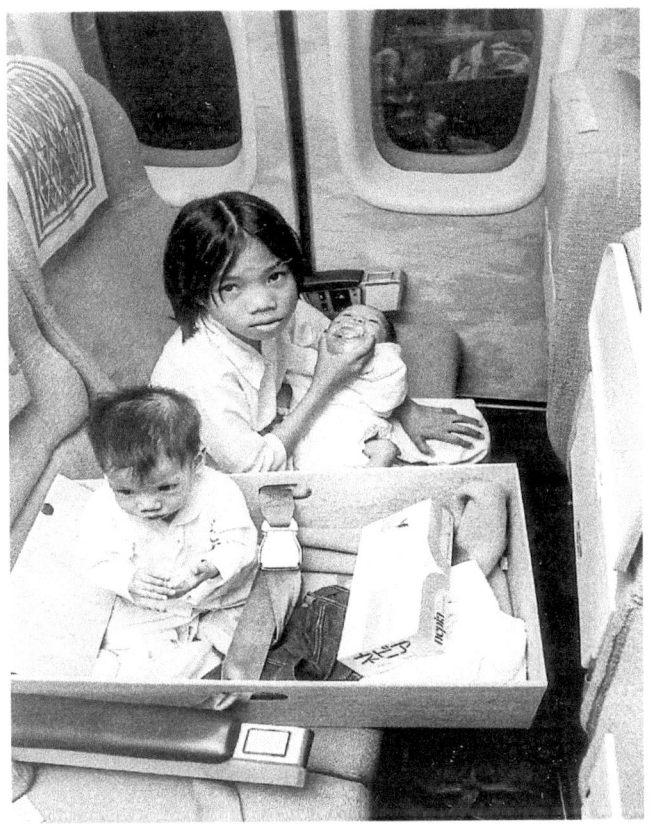

The not much "older" children helping the younger (photograph by the late Robert Stinnett, used with permission).

I was never contacted to offer information about this lifesaving rescue operation other than that informational session in Oakland soon after my arrival. The next day I went back to Berkeley. My colleagues thought I had come down with the flu. They had no idea that I had been almost 8,000 miles away in Vietnam. But an *Oakland Tribune* photographer, Robert Stinnett, had been on the plane and took those photos that documented that last flight out of Vietnam.[5]

Of the two C-141s, 133 orphans were on my flight and 120 on the other plane.

---

5. Robert Stinnett served during World War II as a U.S. Navy photographer in the Pacific. After the war, he worked as a journalist and photographer for the *Oakland Tribune*.

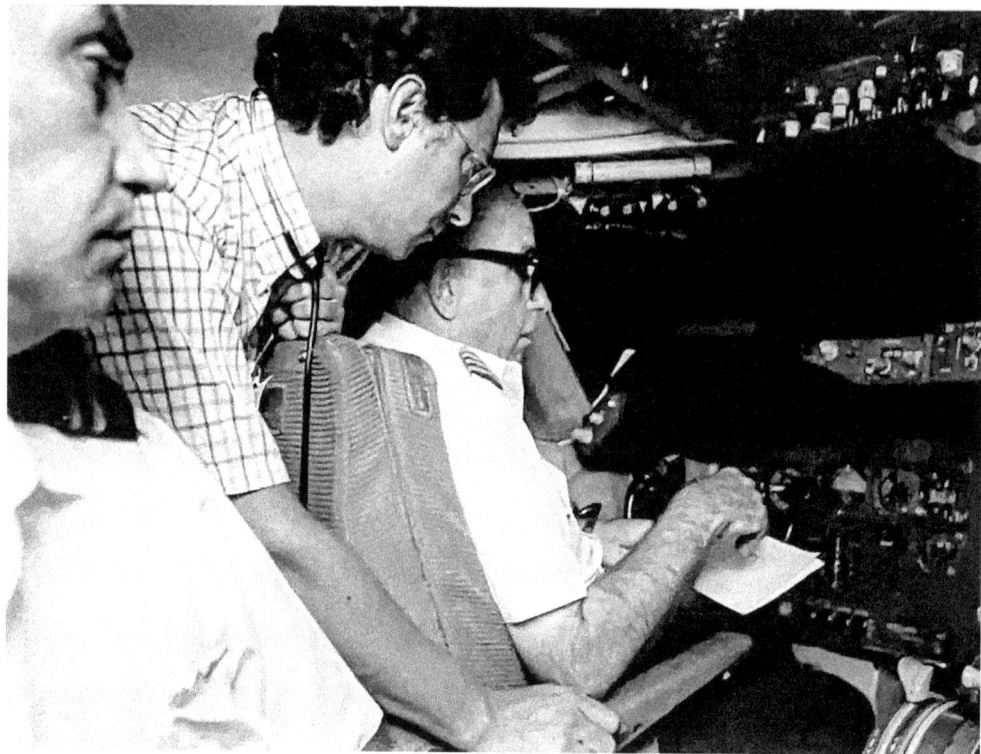

The return flight to the U.S. had been diverted from San Francisco to Los Angeles. In the cockpit, Skip Burkle clarifies medical information with pilot Ken Healy to transmit to paramedics on the ground (photograph by the late Robert Stinnett, used with permission).

The World Airways airlift to LAX carried 330 orphans, including 22 orphans who were intended to go to Norway and 52 Cambodian children to some unknown destination.

* * * *

As medical director of the last orphan airlift out of Saigon in 1975, I was secretly slipped into Saigon, which was already surrounded by the North Vietnamese Army. The city was in peril and packed with more than 100,000 frantic and desperate refugees. During the city's last gasps, I had to find abandoned and ill infants, many whom were alone and starving in dank and dirty orphanages. Operation Babylift had airlifted 330 nameless infants in file boxes from Saigon to California.[6]

After returning to Berkeley, I told Phyllis about the planted Viet Cong bomb aboard our flight out of Saigon. She thought I lived a blessed life. Knowing my perseverance and determination amid chaos, she astutely realized that my staff and I

---

6. Operation Babylift evacuated 2,547 orphans. Of this number rescued in these airlift missions, 602 were sent to other countries. Total adoptions in the U.S. numbered 1,945. Operation Babylift Report, Emergency Movement of Vietnamese and Cambodian Orphans for Intercountry Adoption—April–June 1975: Agency for International Development, undated, p. 1. Available at https://pages.uoregon.edu/adoption/archive/AIDOBR.htm.

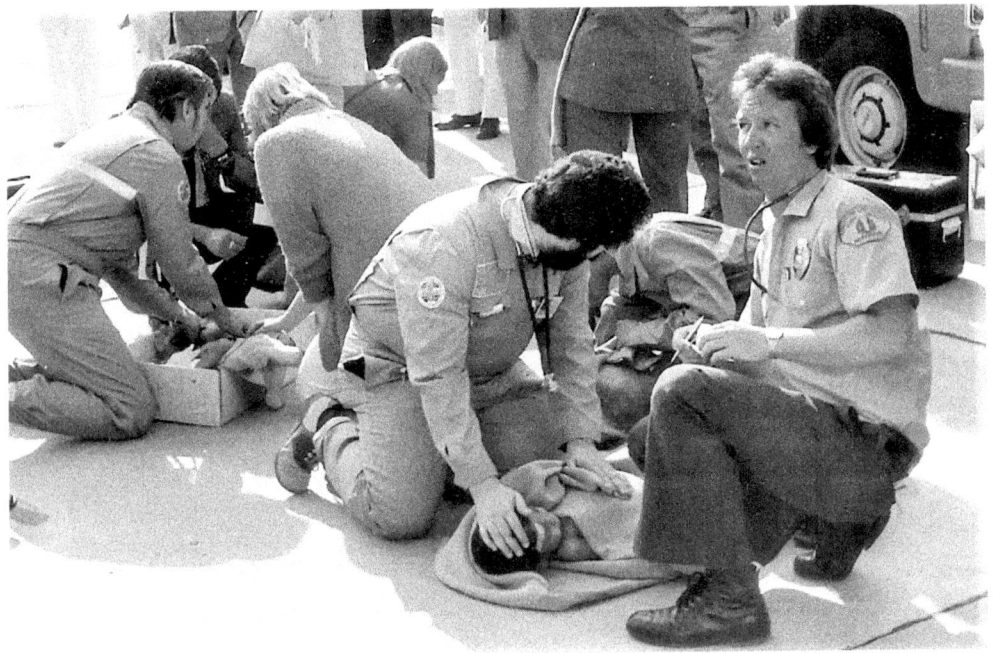

Awaiting paramedics treat several just-arrived sick infants on the tarmac at LAX (photograph by the late Robert Stinnett, used with permission).

would just keep doing what we were trained to do despite the terrifying circumstances. She added that she was sure none of the medical staff took more than a second of thinking about what might have happened if they hadn't found the bomb aboard that aircraft. And she was right.

By chance, 20 years later in a Honolulu restaurant, I met an attractive, ebullient Asian woman, the valedictorian of her college class and now a graduate student. She had been one of the infants I had rescued and had been on that World Airways 747 that had landed at LAX on April 12, 1975. Life had come full circle. Meeting this beautiful young woman on that consequential day in 1995 was a very good day for me.

Operation Babylift transformed the future of those infant refugees. Rescuing those children transformed me.

Part III

Building a Humanitarian Career

7

Becoming a Global Health Professional

1975–1990

"Standing in Tiananmen Square, one of the largest public squares in the world, all we had before us was an uncomfortably empty silence and hundreds of armed Chinese soldiers guarding our singular presence."

In 1975, I reached another significant milestone in my career: I earned a master's degree in public health at UC Berkeley. This degree and discipline were critically necessary for specializing in global public health, a developing arm of medical science at this point. Although the number of professional advocates and practitioners was increasing, this new branch of medicine didn't even have an official name. I had been trained in emergency medicine, pediatrics, adolescent medicine, and now public health, but I nevertheless felt I needed one more credential: psychiatry. Despite this essential medical field remaining the one specialty we know the least about, psychiatry would hopefully enhance my skills for the kind of global health medicine I wished to concentrate on.

During my tour of duty in Vietnam from 1968 to 1969, I quickly appreciated psychiatry's relevance in a war zone. Those 12 months of service in time of war always managed to influence my future medical career. I directly witnessed what strain and anxiety could do to the mind after treating grievously wounded Marines day after day. My commanding officer was even evacuated from Delta Med after "breaking down." A fellow physician was also medevacked from the base after he lapsed into a fugue state, freezing into a fixed position and losing his power of speech. This also occurred in one Vietnamese nurse and represents a sudden paralyzing attempt to withdraw and abolish an emotionally painful experience such as a traumatic war event.

The gravity and intensity of what the mind can do never left me. I was extremely curious to know more about these mental conditions. I'm sure my direct Vietnam experience with these scenarios was part of the reason I was driven to become more proficient in psychiatry.

While in Vietnam, I also realized that untreated mental illnesses are a major component of global health. Many psychiatrists can go through an entire career without encountering fugue states, an incredibly rare disorder. Serving in Vietnam for just one year, however, I observed several patients suffering from this intensely difficult takeover of the mind. Dealing with the suicides of two Marines in Vietnam also focused my attention on mental illness. These Marines, some as young as 18 years old, had to mentally escape unbearable apprehension and the pressure of unending conflict and threats. We should never forget the mental trauma of war's cruelty.

Honing Psychological Tools at Dartmouth

I also later discovered that when people learned that I was a psychiatrist, especially in refugee camps, I had instant credibility. Shortly after getting my master's degree at Berkeley, I was accepted for a psychiatry residency at Dartmouth Medical School[1] in 1975. Once again, Phyllis and I packed up the family and headed back east to Hanover, New Hampshire. As always, I admired Phyllis for her fortitude during these taxing and exhausting moving upheavals—relocating across the country, finding schools for our children, and creating a new and warm home environment.

I found the psychiatry residency at Dartmouth's teaching hospital, Mary Hitchcock Memorial Hospital,[2] more difficult than anything else I had previously encountered in my medical training. The patients I saw in this program illustrated the complexities of mental illness I had never really comprehended. However, most cases were biologically or genetically induced, conditions that played to my stronger diagnostic skills. I was also intrigued by the powerful control that manic-depressive disorders and postpartum psychoses have on an individual's life.

I dealt with many psychiatric cases, but I vividly recall two instances from decades ago. While I was unable to see the full picture in time to save these patients in need, I have since used them as teaching examples to prevent anyone else from having to go through the same stressful incidents with tragic outcomes.

One early evening while on night duty, a senior resident called from the outpatient clinic saying he was admitting a young, long-term patient with a major psychiatric condition. She was in a raging psychotic state and on a tricyclic drug, a standard antidepressant medication. The resident thoroughly examined her, administered an additional tricyclic dose, and then sent her up to the ward.

When I approached, I noticed the woman was extremely agitated with her back against the wall screaming and lashing out at the nurses who were trying to help her. She was scared to death, cowering and hissing in a corner. The nurses told me to

---

1. In 2012, Dartmouth Medical School, the fourth oldest medical school in the U.S. (1797), was renamed the "Audrey and Theodor Geisel School of Medicine." Theodor Seuss Geisel, who attended Dartmouth in the early 1920s, wrote and illustrated the classic children's books under the name "Dr. Seuss."
2. Built in 1893, Mary Hitchcock Memorial Hospital in Hanover was torn down in 1995. A new hospital was built in nearby Lebanon in 1991 called "Dartmouth-Hitchcock Medical Center."

return once the tricyclic medication had calmed her down. I had other admissions to see so I told them I would return later.

I was gone no more than 10 minutes when I heard the code alert. Rushing to her bedside, I observed that she was already in cardiac arrest. We tried to resuscitate her but our efforts were to no avail. The psychiatry resident did not realize she had recently taken a large dose of tricyclic drugs on her own, and being unaware of that fact, he had given her another dose. In such cases, other drugs can be given to flush the tricyclics from the system, but once we realized her situation, she was too far gone.

Although I was the physician who had responded to the code, and my care was limited to her attempted resuscitation, I had to present her case at the hospital's grand rounds. That

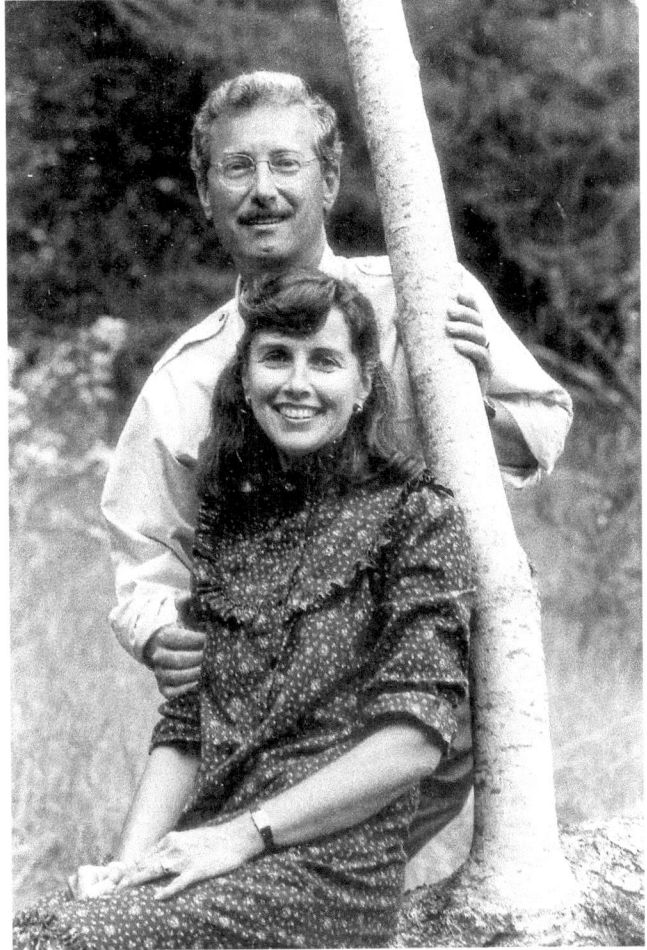

Skip and Phyllis grab a rare leisure moment between frequent international trips (author's collection).

discussion centered on the powerful effects of these medications, as well as the limited knowledge we had of major psychiatric disorders.

Another patient around that time was under my care for depression. After treatment, he seemed to be doing well and said he wanted to go home for the weekend. He was cheerful, smiling, and lucid. I did a thorough check on his condition, and then discharged him that afternoon to spend the weekend with his family. The next morning his wife called, obviously in great distress, to say that he had just shot himself in the head. That shocking event had a very sobering effect on me. Unfortunately, I didn't see the signs or consider that he had a condition called "smiling depression," always considered as an anguished state.

Most psychiatrists characterize "depression" as a condition that results in lethargic, sad, and apathetic behavior. But someone experiencing "smiling depression" often appears happy on the outside, displaying a seemingly conventional social life. This split between how a person is seen externally and how he feels internally still complicates a diagnosis to this day.

These two examples demonstrated to me how little I knew about psychiatry and these multifaceted mental illnesses. Yet despite my initial resistance while in med school to this medical specialty, I gradually honed both my diagnostic and counseling skills. By habit, I began to look at every case to find any potential mental health factors because they would influence the physical health outcomes. All these skills would prove crucial in the future when I inspected or assessed Nigerian and Somali refugee camps where no psychiatrists had ever set foot. Most mental health care at these sites had been performed by indigenous nurses who used medications that had not been administered in the West for years.

The Dartmouth psychiatry residency was demanding, rigorous, and didn't pay very much. To make ends meet, I again moonlighted every available free weekend in emergency departments in New Hampshire and Vermont. That old familiar pattern of minimal family life, as I dedicated myself to my work, had once again become somewhat "normal."

Maui: Hawaii's Valley Isle

In 1977, after a difficult two years, the Dartmouth residency ended. I now had a degree in another medical specialty under my belt. I was eager to carry out what I had just learned. Aside from the short stint in Berkeley, we had spent many years on the East Coast and were ready for something new. Hawaii beckoned with an opening at the Maui Community Mental Health Center in Wailuku, just west of Kahului, the island's largest city. But the job opportunity and island breezes weren't the only reasons I had my eye on the Aloha State. I still longed to practice global health in Asia, and living in Hawaii would make that prospect seem more like a reality—and also put me several thousand miles closer to the world's biggest and most populous continent.

After settling into our new home in Kula, about 14 miles southeast of Kahului, I began as a staff psychiatrist and Director of Community Consultation and Education at Maui Community Mental Health Center. The Center was part of Maui Memorial Hospital. Shortly after arriving, I was asked to evaluate a young adult male patient who had just arrived at the hospital's ER before he was to be placed in the mental health ward. His thinking was bizarre but he also had inexplicable drowsiness, weakness, and retching.

Yet something else wasn't quite right regarding this male's condition. Before transporting him to the mental health unit, I kept him in the ER and began my evaluation. After obtaining blood levels and doing a spinal tap, the results indicated that the patient had a condition called "water intoxication," or water poisoning, caused by drinking an excessive amount of water. This grave state of health occurs when a huge influx of water in the body upsets the balance of electrolytes and dangerously decreases sodium levels. Drinking too much water can lead to confusion, nausea, and vomiting as the body tries to expel the water and return to what is called "homeostasis" or the body's equilibrium. Following this diagnosis, we admitted the patient to the critical care unit first and the mental health ward later.

Maui Memorial Hospital was just beginning to staff its emergency room with trained ER doctors. Most of these physicians practicing this new field of emergency medicine were part-time staff. They came from family practice, internal medicine, and other medical disciplines, as was the case in many other hospitals around the country back then.

As this field continued to grow, I spoke at conferences addressing future physicians in emergency medicine. Some of my talks focused on triage and were based on my cases in Vietnam. My love and fascination with this developing realm of care also increased as my experience in that branch of medicine matured. Having an interest in this medical specialty was also due in part to the exhausting 24- and 48-hour weekend shifts in an ER several months after starting my new job at Maui Memorial Hospital.

While this position on Maui was the start of building a long life in Hawaii, I had several stints that interrupted my time on the Valley Isle. From 1984 to 1986, I served as Residency Director at Madigan Army Medical Center in Tacoma, Washington. I considered this job a great career move. Madigan advanced my prospects for becoming a global health specialist and gave me more leeway to pick up and go where I was needed in a global health crisis. But this academic post came with a challenge. I was hired because Madigan's residency program at that time was rated second from the bottom in the Army medical system. I had my work cut out for me.

I first had to surmount a procedural hurdle, however. The Madigan job was a military position. Since I was in the Navy Reserve, I thought the Navy could simply recall me to active duty and then detail or "loan" me to the Army. But, of course, the Army wouldn't agree to that simple arrangement. I would first have to transfer to the Army. Even though I had mixed feelings about this type of reassignment. I agreed and was brought aboard as an Army colonel.

My main task at Madigan was overseeing the residents' training. I guided them through their rotations and ensured they were getting the required education. When I left two years later in 1986, the program had risen in the ranks to be rated second from the top.

When I returned home, I rejoined the Navy Reserve. During my college days at Saint Michael's, I had been enrolled in the Air Force ROTC program, so within two decades, I had already been attached to four military services: Air Force ROTC—while in college; Navy—as a physician in Vietnam; Marines—when I was assigned to a forward Marine base in Vietnam; and Army—at Madigan Army Medical Center!

Back in Hawaii, I resumed my post at Maui Memorial Hospital for a reprise of my service in the ER. However, this time I was also given two new titles, first as Medical Director and then as Administrator of the hospital.

As the previous director had moved up in the Hawaii state hospital system, which was managed by the Hawaii Department of Health, one of my first projects was developing a survey to evaluate organization and staffing needs. When I took over as Medical Director, I was bombarded by many recommendations. My staff-directed survey was critical in receiving feedback from all those employees who were doing the work day in and day out under my supervision.

On one otherwise quiet day, two male strangers from California showed up at Maui Memorial. They first talked to the Business Director to claim office space, insinuating they were sent to Maui Memorial by the State of Hawaii to oversee the hospital's budgeting process. The Office Manager then insisted that I let him know what I had arranged. I faced the two men and asserted my role as Medical Director, demanding, "Excuse me, but who the hell are you?"

They thought I had already been informed by "their people" in Honolulu to expect them. I was infuriated by not having been notified they were coming and also offended by their insistent attitude. In no uncertain terms, I told them to leave my office. I then went to the hospital's accounting office and convinced the staff that I had no idea what was happening on our turf. We were all in the dark.

Acting on my anger of not being notified of these major changes and also in my capacity as Medical Director, I called the State of Hawaii Department of Health in Honolulu. I learned that this mysterious California group was determined to take over the budgets not only of Maui Memorial Hospital but also the state-run hospitals on Molokai, Lanai, and the Big Island (the island named "Hawaii" to the southeast). My superiors stated that those men were not authorized to come to the hospital, affirming that we needed to keep this entire disturbing incident quiet. I soon came to realize that this was all about politics, an area that was infiltrating the medical world.

Later that same week, the Head Nurse, who was about to retire, came to my office accompanied by another nurse whom I had previously met. Although I didn't realize it at the time, the senior nurse wanted her friend to replace her in the Head Nurse position. But I had no intention of making any staff changes until the survey was completed and analyzed. The results of this survey were going to be the backbone of my decision-making. I had a big job and needed more time.

A few days later, the State Senator from Maui sent one of his "aides" to take me out to lunch. He arrived alone in a large tail-finned black Cadillac. We headed to a small restaurant in the Iao Valley west of the hospital where we made small talk while we ate. But during that entire hour, I kept wondering about the purpose of the lunch.

Driving back to the hospital, my luncheon companion suddenly pulled the car over and ominously stated, "We know what time you go to work and when you return. And we also know the roads you take through the sugarcane fields and cattle ranch to Kula. It would be a shame if your wife learned that they found your body in the sugarcane fields."

I stared at him in utter disbelief. The State Senator, through his henchman, made it upsettingly clear that I had to designate that younger nurse for the Head Nurse position about to open up. I later found out she was the State Senator's niece.

The intent of the lunch and threat on my life had now become quite evident. I took the long way home that evening and told Phyllis what had happened. Tearfully, she pleaded with me to resign, adding that this confrontation was probably the first of many political demands. Even though I might have chosen that woman as the new Head Nurse, I resigned from the hospital that same day without any notice or explanation.

News of my hasty departure as Medical Director of Maui Memorial Hospital made the local island newspaper, *The Maui News*. I refused any interviews. Except for Phyllis, no one else knew at that time what had transpired. Both of us agreed that I couldn't take the chance of remaining at the hospital with that kind of surveillance, forced influence, and the constant risk of deadly violence.

Even before I left, I learned that the State Senator's cronies were also involved in trying to take control of the entire Hawaii state hospital system on the neighboring islands. With the combination of the Head Nurse episode, the lunch with the State Senator's so-called "representative," and physical intimidation, I was extremely glad to have left Maui Memorial Hospital at that point. I did not want to become a main character—or victim—in this strange evolving intrigue.

As an alternative medical employment, I decided to quietly practice psychiatry out of our home in Kula. Our three kids were all grown and in college, and Phyllis and I decided it was best to stay out of politics. At the time, I was also the Director of the Emergency Medical Services (EMS) system for the outer islands—Maui, Molokai, and Lanai, a job that gave me great satisfaction. Even with this peaceful retreat from my career, I was always vigilant, making sure I knew that Phyllis was safe. Feeling threatened on a daily basis was not a good way to go through life. But I thought if I just remained silent, nobody would harm us—and nobody did. I never drove through those possibly lethal sugarcane fields and that cactus-laden cattle ranch, a landscape we had dearly loved.

Paying It Forward on Oahu

In 1988, during my years of having a private psychiatry practice at my home, the head of the EMS in Honolulu called to ask if I would be interested in a position at Kapiolani Medical Center for Women and Children on Oahu. It would mean commuting by air, but I happily accepted the offer and started working in the emergency department, which also came with a professorship at the University of Hawaii at Manoa School of Medicine.

For the next four years, I made the commute between Kahului and Honolulu. This island-hopping travel comes with living in the Hawaiian Islands. Aloha Airlines at that time had two early morning flights filled with Maui residents who worked in Honolulu.

My shifts were 12 hours at the Medical Center, and when off duty, I slept on a sofa bed in my office. I would work three to four days and then fly back to Maui. But Phyllis and I eventually grew tired of this long-distance routine. Being away for such long stretches at a time was too reminiscent of my earlier years in med school, and neither of us was interested in returning to that disconnected phase of life. We rented our house in Maui and moved to Honolulu to live in a small apartment close to the hospital.

When not occupied with hospital duties at Kapiolani, I was at the School of Medicine teaching pediatrics, public health, and emergency medicine, a role I truly valued. Educating the next generation was a way I could pay it forward. I could also confidently add to the school's medical arsenal some important lessons in the prevention, diagnosis, and treatment of disease that I had learned along the way.

I enjoyed practicing urgent care medicine and teaching. I also loved to travel, giving talks on disaster medicine and humanitarian assistance plus seeing similar training programs being established throughout North America. I was now knee-deep in professional commitments and was frequently contacted to speak at conferences throughout the U.S., as well as in Japan, China, Indonesia, and Europe. I was invited to give lectures at medical schools that were developing curricula in disaster medicine and national and global health programs. I tried to take advantage of every opportunity to advance and bolster their coursework and research programs.

Improving the health of populations on a worldwide basis was becoming critically important. I was gratified to see this new area of medicine grow and to be a part of it. I wanted to ensure that those entering this field were given the right education, training, and tools needed to solve some of these complex and multifaceted global health problems.

Nigeria: Low-Tech Primary Health Care— October 1988

Late-night phone calls are never good. But I received one in October 1988 from the Naval Reserve Personnel Center in New Orleans. The official asked me to be a speaker at the WHO Collaborating Center Hospital Meeting in Lagos, Nigeria—in just five days. I was taken aback at the short notice. Making that trip from Hawaii is not easy; in fact, making any trip from the most remote islands in the world has never been easy. Nevertheless, the caller assured me that the request was of great importance to the U.S. Ambassador in Lagos, Princeton Lyman. The coordinator of this meeting had already taken it upon himself to give my talk a title: "Care of the Critically Ill." I felt well-versed on that subject so I agreed to go.

When I landed in Lagos a few days later, authorities took me aside to conduct a hand search. I was subsequently interrogated by security personnel as to the nature of my visit, followed by being sequestered in an airport office for several hours. A senior Nigerian representative finally arrived and quickly whisked me away in a U.S. Embassy car. We took a cutoff that brought us below the highway at which point we stopped, awaiting an opportunity to enter traffic. The driver, quiet until now, casually said, "This is where the other speaker was assassinated."

Quite taken aback, I asked, "What speaker?"

Thinking I must have known about the incident, he added, "Yes, the man who was to speak at the conference was assassinated right at this highway stop 10 days ago. You are to take his place."

The only words I could stammer were: "Well, it's the first I've heard about it." Silence followed but I needed to know more about this tragic event.

When I arrived at the U.S. Embassy, I met Alvin Crawford, head of orthopedic surgery at the Cincinnati Children's Hospital Medical Center. He, too, was a Navy Reserve captain and was also recently recruited to give a lecture at this upcoming gathering. Both of us were representing the United States and the U.S. military at this conference. Crawford's topic was to be "Care of the Traumatized Patient." He knew nothing about the recent murder of a speaker. He was eager, though, to talk about his arrival at the airport and then being detained in a narrow one-man cell for more than an hour. His hurried trek to Africa and being placed in airport confinement, similar to mine, didn't bode well.

Later that evening, we were briefed about our upcoming lectures and given a brochure for the National Orthopaedic Hospital "Multidisciplinary Workshop." The official stated that contrary to the printed schedule, Dr. Crawford would speak first followed by my presentation. He provided no further details.

The following morning, Alvin and I were driven to the lecture setting, a narrow one-story hall in which many young, eager physicians stood about curiously eyeing our white Navy captain uniforms. Alvin gave an impressive practical speech. Although he described several procedures that were beyond the capability of Nigerian medicine, orthopedics is fairly concrete—bones are bones. His listeners could certainly understand his talk's content.

Alvin's informative discourse gave me pause to rethink my lecture. I always tried to gauge the level of expertise and ability of my audiences and make sure my words were culturally sensitive. I could not fathom how my "Care of the Critically Ill" topic entered the picture. But I was certain that the latest technology in critical care equipment did not apply in this specific instance. In addition, having access to this kind of specialized equipment was beyond the reach of these physicians' professional knowledge. Primary care had to be their priority.

I decided at the last moment to ditch my prepared talk and PowerPoint slides and instead focus on primary care. My real emphasis was on the skills required to diagnose a critically ill pediatric patient. My presentation stemmed from talks I had previously assembled that targeted "decoding vital signs." A physician had to use his existing skills to diagnose whether a child's condition was worsening. I knew the kind of equipment that these Nigerian physicians had available in their local clinics and hospitals so I acted as though I was working in those less than high-tech medical venues.

I took a chance to give this improvised lecture and was rewarded by its reception. I demonstrated simple skills to identify a pediatric patient having medical issues, as well as how to treat a child by employing the resources at hand. I worked with the audience and demonstrated the procedures. They were laughing and trying some of these techniques on each other. When my session was over, I was given a standing ovation!

After I took some challenging questions and repeated a few methods, we all moved outside. Two elderly physicians, who had been standing in the rear of the class, came forward to speak with me. We walked to an isolated two-story building with a ramp that led from the ground to a door on the second floor. When they opened the locked door, I was utterly astounded. Before me was a wall-to-wall critical care unit equipped with the latest monitors and resuscitation apparatus. Transparent plastic sheeting covered everything. An unidentified European nation had donated the equipment two years earlier.

This room had never been used. I was shocked and wondered why these physicians were showing it to me. In silence, I sensed their astute message. I could not imagine any of the physicians from my lecture audience knowing how to use this advanced technical equipment. I doubted that any of those doctors in the nearby hall even knew about the existence of this highly computerized room.[3] This level of medicine was beyond the training and capability of most Nigerian physicians, nurses, and technicians.

The long, embarrassing silence was finally broken when one man offered a subtle hint. The Nigerian military president, Ibrahim Babangida, who had visited the site, had suggested that moving the gurneys up the ramp would be too difficult. After a few moments, I noted relief in their faces when I agreed that it would be much too

---

3. Dr. George Little, Emeritus Professor of Neonatology at Dartmouth Medical School and a med school classmate, shared with me a similar experience. He had spent many months in developing countries as a global health expert. He trained neonatologists and pediatricians to improve health care delivery in newborn infants, as well as instructing physicians about new and useful skills. While teaching at an Egyptian hospital, he was shown a carefully covered laboratory device sent by U.S. donors. The equipment analyzed blood specimens for the study of infant metabolic disorders, a common problem in Africa. As with my Nigerian experience, Dr. Little could not find a local pediatrician with interest or training in the use of this expensive apparatus. In addition, the device was nonfunctional due to needed testing reagents and not having available maintenance.

Another Ministry of Health hospital in Egypt had received donated resuscitation equipment to stabilize newborn infants in respiratory distress. When Dr. Little attempted to use the free equipment to stabilize such an infant, the laryngoscope was not operational because it had no light source. One of the obstetric nursing staff walked to a window and pointed to the shop below where batteries could be purchased, but obtaining them in time to help this infant would have been impossible.

Providing continuous airway pressure is an established technology for treating infants in respiratory distress. But I found that implementing such training in Nigerian hospitals was unfeasible due to a lack of basic electricity and oxygen supply infrastructure. Also, the health care workers would not have had the training to know how to use this technology.

dangerous for gurneys to be pushed up this incline and far too hazardous to treat patients with this advanced equipment. Those words were all these men needed to hear. They thrust out their hands to vigorously shake mine. After replacing the plastic sheeting over the equipment, we rejoined the group of young physicians outside.

I looked for Alvin Crawford and briefly told him what had happened, restating that Nigeria was struggling just to provide primary care to its people. The well-intentioned donor nation of this state-of-the-art technology simply didn't understand the culture or Nigeria's basic health care needs. However, the recipients of this largesse didn't want to insult the donor. Now they could use me as an "expert consultant" to get their president off the hook as to why they were not making use of the contributed equipment.

The Forgotten

Later that day, I asked our driver to take me back to the hotel and show me downtown Lagos on the way. We moved at a snail's pace through the heavy traffic, encountering multiple blind children in body harnesses with leash-like tethers. They were being herded by their male handlers. The children pounded on the windows begging for money. The driver advised me to sit in the center of the back seat. One child climbed from the top of the car's trunk to pound on the sunroof.

While this incident was a jarring experience, it was a reminder of all the forgotten children worldwide left to fall through the cracks by systems and conflicts that weren't designed to prioritize them. A 2000 study of street children in Lagos found that poverty emerged as an important factor in how they ended up in these circumstances. Additional predisposing factors included large families, polygamy, child labor, and family disruption.[4] These factors, paired with a lack of eye care in the country, also contributed to the high level of blindness in street children, though the major causes of blindness in developing countries are largely avoidable.

Even in 2015, the cause of child blindness in Nigeria had not been well-defined, but very little fact-based information was known in the 1980s. However, diseases, such as rubella, have been linked to pediatric cataracts. Through the car's windows, I observed the child's thick, white, opaque cataracts that looked like two headlights, and I thought of the impact immunization campaigns could have here.

The main roadway we were traveling was divided by a 20-foot-wide grassy median totally occupied by homeless citizens. The driver said that every few weeks more than 2,000 newborns would come from this displaced population trying to survive in the middle of this main highway. These babies would add to the population of Lagos of 4 million, the capital at that time, and most likely also be forgotten.

---

4. A.A. Aderinto, "Social Correlates and Coping Measures of Street-children: A Comparative Study of Street and Non-street Children in South-western Nigeria," *Child Abuse & Neglect*, 2000 September 24(9):1199–1213. Available at https://pubmed.ncbi.nlm.nih.gov/11057706/.

When we later arrived at the U.S. Embassy, I picked up a copy of the local newspaper. The blaring headlines declared: "Dog shit can make you blind." The accompanying article spoke of the millions of children in Nigeria who had their lives ruined by contracting irreversible blindness through the feces of dogs and cats. This pet waste, the article affirmed, contained the common roundworm that caused the condition called "toxocariasis."

The editorial strongly suggested that more foreign aid and resources be directed to stem this scourge in African children. In November 1989, the United Nations General Assembly adopted the Convention on the Rights of the Child. Its purpose was to establish the civil, political, economic, social, and cultural rights of every child, no matter his race, religion, or abilities.[5] While this human rights treaty was a global acknowledgment of a glaring problem, Nigeria, as well as other countries, still has a long way to go to ensure the rights of every child.

On the evening of the conference, Ambassador Lyman and his wife held a reception in our honor. With a nod of recognition from the podium, the Director of the National Orthopaedic Hospital personally expressed his deep gratitude. The Ambassador then pulled me aside to convey his sincere appreciation for coming to the meeting with little advanced notice. He also thanked me for solving the embarrassing dilemma of the critical care unit. He went on to state, "We had hoped you would see the problem and help us save face." Lyman then stated in a follow-up letter that I had "quickly adapted to the 'situation,'" adding, "I was unquestionably the most popular speaker."

On the last day of our visit, Alvin Crawford met with the hospital staff to propose recommendations to the Minister of Health, using notes taken from my talk. Alvin then wrote me several weeks later that he agreed with me about what Nigeria's medical priorities should be. He had learned that while the advanced techniques and technology of the surgical management of orthopedics were of some "import to them, their major problem at this time is the lack of expertise in primary care of the critically injured child."

Before leaving Nigeria for home the next day, I once again experienced harassment at the airport. Several security guards stopped me just before I headed to the plane. Some prescription bottles in my carry-on luggage had fallen to the floor at the departure gate. Several men rushed to grab the bottles. Then one guard uncovered my Navy cap in the opened suitcase and immediately snapped to attention. I calmly told them they could take the medicine but it might kill them. The guards quickly put the bottles back into the suitcase and personally escorted me to the airplane door, giving me another salute.

I had gotten into Lagos based on being an expert on critical care, but it was my Navy captain's hat that gave me more importance and enabled me to get out of Nigeria. And strangely, I never learned why the speaker I replaced had been assassinated.

---

5. UN Convention of the Rights of the Child. Available at https://www.ohchr.org/Documents/ProfessionalInterest/crc.pdf.

A Love Affair with China

Although I had been to China in the late 1970s, my affiliation with the Chinese accelerated in the mid–1980s. China was struggling as an emerging nation, and the available epidemiological data indicated that the country was ripe for humanitarian intervention. But the level of outside needed assistance was unclear. At that time, an unprecedented 83 percent of the population suffered from poverty and malnutrition.

In the early 1980s, with its population at a billion, China had the highest infant and maternal mortality rates in the world. With the push for privatization of health care, government funding for health programs stopped, and the rural cooperative medical system essentially disappeared. Malnourishment among children outside the cities was one of the most pressing problems. Training programs needed to be quickly established to learn how to care for them. During my visits, I taught Chinese physicians techniques used to rehydrate and properly feed the younger generation.

I met Professor Zonghao Li, Director of the Beijing Emergency Medical Center, at a World Association for Disaster and Emergency Medicine conference. We began a lasting friendship. A learned and charming gentleman, Dr. Li became a committed colleague and an adopted member of our family. Through our partnership, I helped promote urgent care and then emergency care as a specialty.[6]

I distrusted the communist government but after many trips to China, I was increasingly drawn to this captivating, enigmatic country and its people. I was continually invited back to China to assist in the management of malnutrition in children and also in the development of emergency services at hospitals. Many of these hospitals are still thriving today in and around Beijing.

Dr. Li was proud of participating in the creation of the first Western-modeled emergency medicine department, located close to Tiananmen ("Gate of Heavenly Peace") Square in the center of Beijing. We co-lectured and co-authored articles on skills for this field, which was still in its infancy in China in the early 1980s. He was a prolific writer, publishing the first Chinese books on emergency medical care. We consulted on many new hospital emergency department services, both within and outside major Chinese cities. Dr. Li and I became "brothers" in these efforts by sharing plans and experiencing the apparent progress of emergency medical practices.

Knowing about my great interest in and love for Chinese culture, every visit was highlighted with some surprise. The Forbidden City, located to the north of Tiananmen Square, is a palace complex that served as the home of Chinese emperors, as well as the center of the Chinese government for 500 years. Until the 1980s, it had been closed for decades to all Chinese residents and outside visitors.

One day I was escorted by car to a back street and entered the former Chinese Imperial Palace. This excursion had been arranged by Dr. Li as a gesture of friendship. I was left alone to explore the royal premises, spending more than two hours

---

6. Emergency care is indicated for life-threatening situations. Urgent care is more suitable for patients requiring less immediate, less serious care.

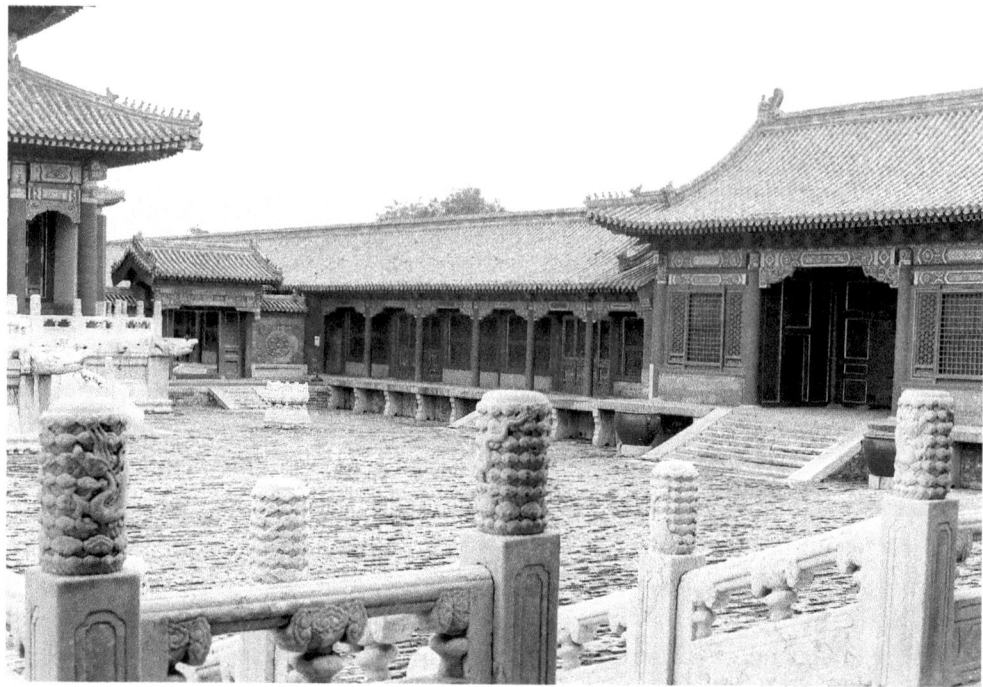

A rare visit to the Forbidden City, which had been closed for decades to all Chinese residents and outside visitors (author's photo).

strolling through magnificent courtyards and multiple smaller palaces. I tried to imagine the history that took place on this site centuries before I could leave my footprints. Even at that time, I recognized the honor and privilege of being able to walk these grounds. I also appreciated the high level of intervention required to organize this visit. Those few hours of wandering through time have been one of my lingering, incredible lifetime experiences.

Despite the frenetic traffic outside its tall thick walls, the Imperial Palace remained a quiet, immaculate, untouched beauty. Years later, Dr. Li, now acting as my translator, accompanied me on another visit to the Forbidden City. This time, however, work was under way to open the palace to the public. As he and I walked through the halls, laborers were carefully replacing worn or weakened paving stones near the entrance that covered its vast floor space.

In silent awe, we stopped to observe the workers' skills. One of them suddenly motioned me to take his tools and replace several worn pavers. Nodding with a cautious smile, I set to work to hopefully leave a mark of my amateur craftsmanship at this historic entrance. Without a single word between us, his fellow workers, sporting wide grins, joined in the laughter and appreciative nods at my clumsy lack of expertise. Since it was difficult to find opportunities to meet ordinary people on these trips, this shared engagement behind the massive doors of the Forbidden City proved to be the highlight of this palace visit.

Soon the Imperial Palace would be opened to all and mobbed by millions of

7. Becoming a Global Health Professional

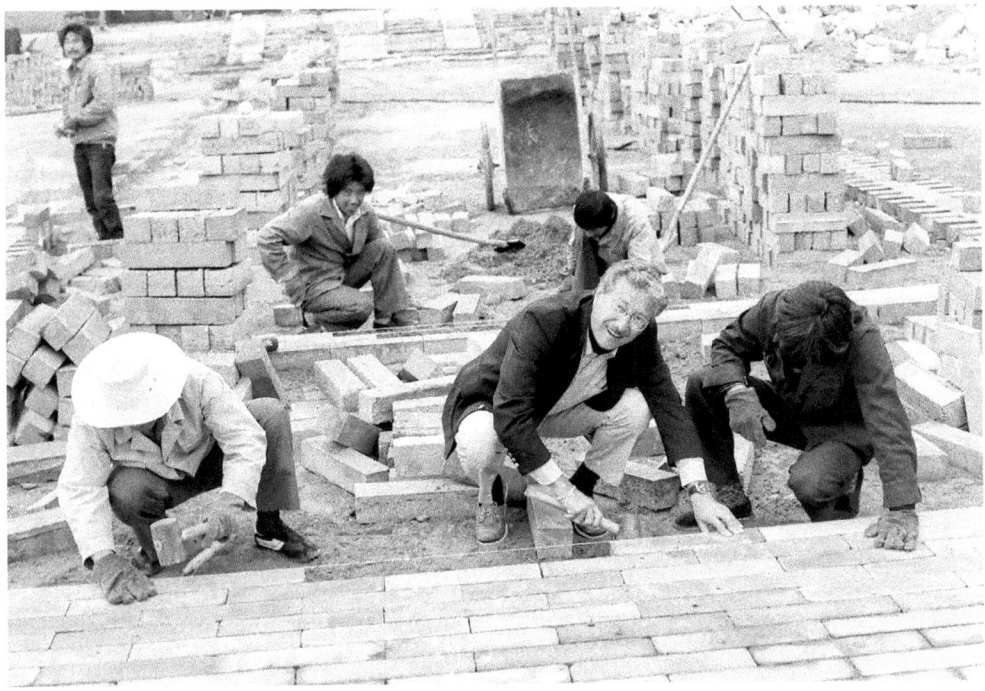

Skip lays a tile in the Imperial Palace (author's collection).

Chinese and foreign visitors who had never been permitted to enter what is now designated a "World Heritage Site" as of 1987. When I returned years later, the building showed much wear and tear from the flood of tourists. The paving stones, now supporting multiple shops and eateries, had not held up well.

To record my very personal contribution to the renovated palace, I had taken photos and painstakingly memorized the location of the pavers I had laid down so long ago. Thanks to my on-the-spot documentation, I was now able to find them again. Remarkably, the "Burkle floor pavers" were still intact despite the heavy foot traffic during all those years. Nowadays, the palace must be periodically closed to repair the damage caused by endless human and bicycle use. Preferring to remember the palace as it once was, serene and quiet, I chose never to return.

Tiananmen Square

Worldwide attention was focused on a million Chinese students protesting in Tiananmen Square from mid–April to early June 1989. During the rapid economic development in post–Mao China, the demonstrations reflected the students' anxieties about the country's future and their fundamental grievances against government inflation and corruption. The young activists wanted democratic reform, an immediate end to government corruption, and an improved economy.

By mid–May, Deng Xiaoping's government, deciding the protests were getting out of control, declared martial law, and brought in 300,000 troops. On June 4, 1989, soldiers, supported by tanks, entered the square and fired indiscriminately into the crowd. Tiananmen Square, which was anything but the "Gate of Heavenly Peace," ran red with the death and wounding of several thousand students and bystanders. The Beijing emergency department and more than 40 other hospitals had to deal with the aftermath beyond each of their capacities.

A second World Association for Disaster and Emergency Medicine meeting had been scheduled to take place in Hong Kong a few weeks later, but a regional meeting was due to convene in Beijing in mid–June 1989. International outrage over the very recent massacre resulted in a large majority of physicians and scientists canceling their attendance at the Beijing conference. However, Dr. Matthew Rice, an emergency medicine physician, and I decided we needed to carry out our teaching commitment at the Beijing meeting. We had to assess the emergency medical response kept secret from the outside world. Our conference hosts were nervous, cautioning us to stay away from Tiananmen Square.

Matthew had never seen Tiananmen Square or the adjacent Forbidden City that I had talked about so much. We hired a taxi parked outside the hotel, and, in broken Chinese, I asked a very old and weather-beaten driver to take us to Tiananmen Square. I assumed we could get reasonably close, and then we would be able to walk to the nearby square. Without any verbal exchange, except to say "Tiananmen Square," the white-haired driver with a jolly smile confidently drove off.

We traveled down the main boulevard with separate lanes for vehicles, bicycles, and human traffic, but all driving lanes were empty except for

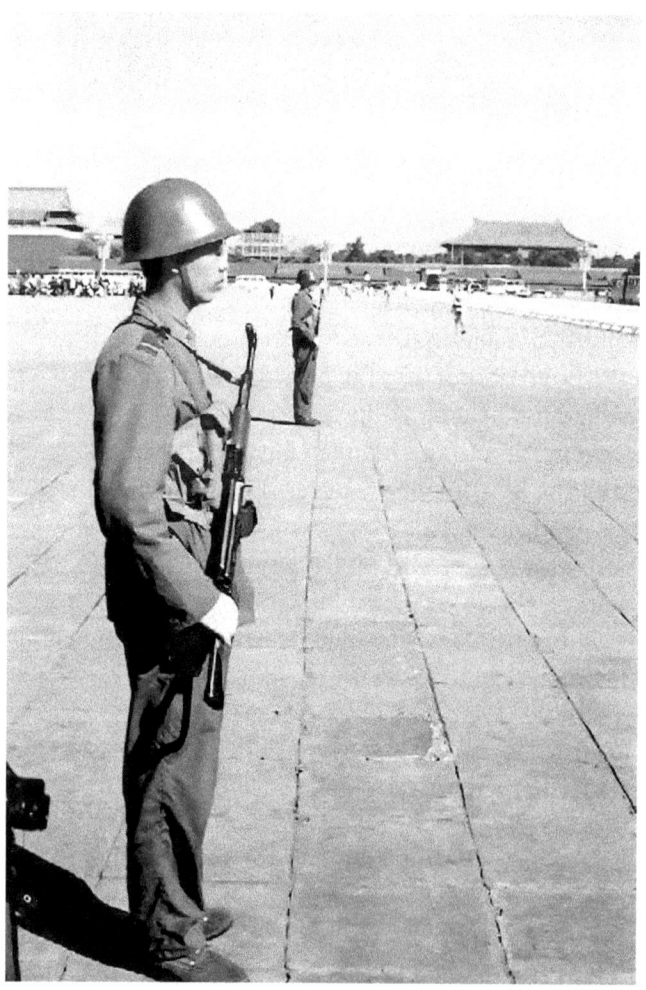

Tiananmen Square was deserted but for an uncomfortably empty silence. Armed soldiers guarded Skip and Matthew Rice's singular presence (author's collection).

our taxi. We were rapidly closing in on Tiananmen Square without any visible barriers. The taxi driver sharply turned into a narrow, tree-lined street bordering the square, and then he slowed down to where a small number of Chinese officials and soldiers were casually milling about.

The troops came to strict attention as we exited the taxi. Smiling city officials offered their outstretched welcoming arms and guided us into the vast and empty square. Without saying anything, we continued to walk silently toward the center of Tiananmen Square so as not to draw attention by word or gesture. We both realized that the exuberant welcome we had received might have been a major misunderstanding.

The entire 100-acre paved square was deserted—from the Forbidden City on the north side of the square to the People's Heroes obelisk on the south side. In Tiananmen Square, one of the largest public squares in the world, all we had before us was an uncomfortably empty silence and hundreds of armed Chinese soldiers guarding our singular presence.

We spent an hour walking around the square. Strangely, Matthew and I did not feel any sense of threat from all those nearby armed guards whose backs we faced. The tank treads had made their indelible imprint on the concrete surface and up the steps to the 10-story Monument to the People's Heroes. We took the customary photos of each other smiling. We abruptly stopped snapping photos, however, after realizing we were standing on recently bloodied sacred ground. Workers, by order of the government suppressors, had scrubbed the pavement and removed the bloodstains immediately after the massacre. But awareness of recent death and injury surrounded us. No evidence existed outside the square that a bloodbath on a massive scale had recently occurred in Beijing.

The silence was overwhelming. While retracing our steps across the wrecked pavement, we were distracted by a large bus slowly entering the same narrow lane our taxi had entered. The bus discharged a large contingent of Caucasian foreigners looking very official. Within minutes, all attention focused on us with some bureaucrats pointing in our direction. A group of soldiers hurried out and impatiently motioned us to follow them. Someone called for a car to take us back to our hotel. A rather sullen foreigner from the bus, having mistaken our nationality, muttered that only Yugoslavian visitors were being allowed into Tiananmen Square. The face of China in June 1989 was the carnage in Tiananmen Square. Being there in person was surreal as the world remained in shock over this military crackdown.

* * * *

The following year, 1990, marked 25 years since I had graduated from medical school. At age 50, I was now certified in emergency medicine, pediatrics, adolescent medicine, public health, and a fifth specialty, psychiatry. I thought at the time that all these specialized areas would be essential for my vision of what a career in global health would require. Between these skills and my time in Vietnam and China, my dream of working internationally in this field was beginning to take shape.

As I was poised to practice global health and disaster medicine on a grand scale, however, an unexpected event interrupted my plans. In early August 1990, Saddam Hussein's army invaded Kuwait, triggering the Persian Gulf War. As a captain in the Navy Reserve, I knew it was just a matter of time before I would be called back to duty and head into my second war.

8

Back to War—Iraq
December 1990–March 1991

> *"I stood above the assembled personnel on a Conex box with the wind whipping up the corners of the large and crowded tent. In a loud, purposeful, confident voice, I declared that I expected all medical personnel to perform their duty and work to their full potential to accomplish our mission."*

News of another world crisis crackled across the airwaves on August 2, 1990. On that searing hot morning, columns of Iraqi tanks rolled south into Kuwait, initiating a violent takeover of this oil-rich nation. Saddam Hussein was up to his old tricks. The Iraqi dictator had demonstrated his penchant for invading neighbors the previous decade when Iran had become his victim in 1980. Before that conflict ended in a draw eight years later, hundreds of thousands of Iranians and Iraqis had been killed.

From the South Lawn of the White House on August 5, President George H.W. Bush angrily asserted, "This will not stand, this aggression against Kuwait."[1] Under the code name "Operation Desert Shield,"[2] U.S. troops were dispatched to Saudi Arabia on August 7 in response to a request from King Fahd, that nation's monarch. Three weeks later, Saddam proclaimed Kuwait as Iraq's 19th province. The Persian Gulf War was about to begin.

Phyllis and I had been in Micronesia, where I was teaching an advanced trauma life support course when Iraq invaded its sovereign neighbor to the south. Kuwait was definitely in the news and on our minds. When we returned to Oahu, and still being in the Navy Reserves, I knew I would be called up—and I was. My heading halfway around the world didn't come as a shock to Phyllis, as she told me, and her life wouldn't go all "topsy-turvy." She understood I had this military obligation to go.

And then I was off in December, headed to yet another war. I started the trip, however, with a painful instep. The night before I left, Phyllis gave me some Tylenol to ease the agony. Our son Chris took me to the airport, but on the way, I started having severe breathing problems. I had inadvertently taken Motrin, which contains

---

1. President George H.W. Bush's remarks to reporters, August 5, 1990, in front of the White House. Full text available at https//www.margaretthatcher.org/document/110704.
2. "Operation Desert Shield" was the designation for operations leading to the buildup of troops and defense of Saudi Arabia. "Operation Desert Storm" was the Persian Gulf War's combat phase.

aspirin, several hours before I left. I am highly allergic to aspirin. I went immediately to the airport's medical facility and was given an adrenaline shot and then rushed to the gate. I was the last one on the plane. During the flight, the breathing issues continued. I had to convince the flight attendant I was all right. Certainly not a good way to feel going into a war zone. My seat companion was a local Hawaii judge who later phoned Phyllis about my health difficulties on that leg of the flight but that I eventually recovered.

The Winter of Our Discontent

Because the United States had not been involved in a true ground war since American troops left Vietnam in March 1973, many members of the military had never seen combat. As a Navy reservist, I was called up to join a Navy-Marine Medical Company in Saudi Arabia, attached to the 2nd Medical Battalion and the 1st Marine Expeditionary Force (MEF). When I arrived in late December 1990, I joined a medical group occupying an abandoned boys' school not far from the Kuwaiti border. Some of the unit's medical personnel had arrived weeks before. Many medical professionals in this company had been in Saudi Arabia for months, ostensibly preparing for a war that had as yet not reached the shooting stage. This state of affairs during these winter months smacked of the timeless military dictum, "Hurry up and wait."

I immediately noticed pervasive discontent among the staff. Supplies were generally lacking, but after recalling the paltry resources we had in Vietnam, I didn't think the situation was that limiting. The real problem was the long-winded preparatory stage. Physicians and other medical personnel were becoming progressively frustrated with the lack of leadership and no visible plan. Often idle, the officers began backbiting among themselves.

One surgeon explained to me why everyone was grumbling and why the morale was so low. After giving him my full attention, I inquired, "And how about you?" I didn't expect his very unorthodox and noticeable answer. He had become so disgusted that he removed his captain's silver eagle devices and replaced them with an enlisted chief's devices. He added that he wasn't crazy, but was tired of listening to so many disputes among the physicians, Medical Service Corps (MSC) officers,[3] and nurses as to who was and was not in command.

Complaints were not without reason. A few doctors feared losing their sharply honed medical skills. Other physicians, who had left their medical practices to go to war, wondered if they would have livelihoods when they returned home. All the medical personnel worried about how their families were faring without them. Low confidence and restlessness had become infectious and the tension was palpable.

---

3. The Navy Medical Service Corps consists of officers who serve in health care administration, patient care, and the allied health sciences.

I didn't realize the circumstances at the time, but, in some ways, this deployment would prove to be more challenging than my year at Delta Med back in 1968. And now, once again, I found myself close to the edge of battle amid professional bickering.

Endless Sand

After two weeks in the northeastern corridor near Kuwait, our unit began heading northwest. We left in phases to regroup at a larger trauma hospital secretly being built in a remote Saudi desert location. Our commercial buses kicked up so much dust that visibility was near zero, especially when following the first bus. We made stops only to relieve ourselves in the sand.

Eventually, after losing count of the hours and finding grit in every known orifice, we reached an apparent construction site about 300 miles from first setting out on this desolate journey, overwhelmed by sand and more sand. Most of what we observed was underground with raised sandbanks known as "berms." Tents within the berms flapped in the stiff wind. I had seen a picture of the plans for a circular facility with a surrounding berm. The future hospital post looked functional and secure, but everyone else seemed to think otherwise. With sunset, the temperature kept dropping. On winter nights, the Saudi desert gets bitter cold.

At this point, we joined up with three other companies, including Delta and Kilo, to officially become the 2nd Medical Battalion, Al Khanjar Navy-Marine Corps Trauma Center. The addition of these new medical companies should go well, I thought somewhat sarcastically, as if my team hadn't displayed enough squabbling and friction. Now we can add even more disgruntled individuals to this mix of short-tempered professionals.

The U.S. Marine Corps would now have the largest field medical treatment facility since the Second World War. At this point, however, the emerging setup certainly didn't look like much, but the site would in time have an interesting but very brief history.

On February 6, 1991, Brigadier General Charles Krulak, commander of the 2nd Force Service Support Group, had received orders to begin construction of a huge desert base just 22 miles southwest of the "elbow" of southern Kuwait. In the next two weeks, the Marines performed a seemingly impossible feat. They constructed 26 miles of a blast wall berm containing the Marine Corps' largest ammunition supply dump that the service had ever built. The site covered 768 acres with a 5-million-gallon fuel farm. When the Trauma Center was completed as part of this vast compound, it would have 12 operating rooms and 270 beds, including a 36-bed intensive care unit. Two mile-long packed sand airstrips, capable of handling C-130 transports for resupply and medevac, were also part of the complex.

The area was so remote from any settlement or feature that it had no name or

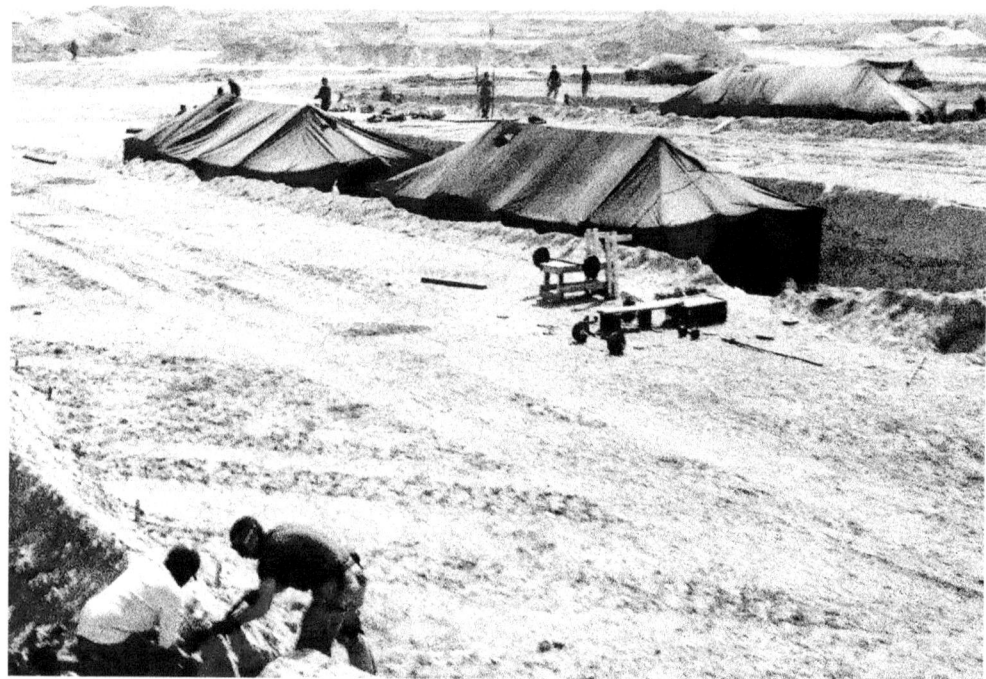

Sinking tents within a sand berm was the only protection from incoming fire (author's photo).

designation on maps except "gravel plain." Even though Al Khanjar was considered desert terrain, the gravel, ranging from sand grains to pea-sized pebbles, was too heavy and dense for the wind to blow the gritty desert mixture into dunes. General Krulak's staff named the place "Al Khanjar," Arabic for a "curved dagger." By February 12, this Trauma Center was providing combat service support for the Marines in the theater.[4]

Al Khanjar was remote and farther from supply lines than any other existing Navy-Marine facility. Numerous evacuation schemes were prepared, given the potentially insecure, hostile, and contaminated environment. Navy records reflect the unspeakable prospect of mass casualties—from both conventional and chemical

---

4. *U.S. Marines in the Persian Gulf, 1990–1991: With the I Marine Expeditionary Force in Desert Shield and Desert Storm*, Col. Charles J. Quilter II, History and Museums Division, Headquarters, U.S. Marine Corps, Washington, D.C., 1993, p. 56. Available at https://www.gulflink.osd.mil/histories/db/marines/usmcpersiangulfdoc5_005.html.

weapons—to be the major concern of Navy Captain Jerry R. Crim, 1st MEF Surgeon. To counter a threat of biological warfare, specifically anthrax, Crim initiated preventive measures throughout the force. To mitigate the effects of nerve agents, all members of the medical staff began taking pyridostigmine bromide tablets three times daily in mid–February 1991 shortly before the ground war began.

Regardless of continuing impatience and anxiety among the medical staff, the Marines made progress to make the facility serviceable. Work suddenly stopped one day when it became obvious, despite the protective circular berm, that the tents were too exposed to possible incoming fire. We then dug deeper and ended up with just the tent tops peeking out of a large dugout depression in the sand. For the war's duration, those tents would house us officers with just barely enough space between each cot—shades of my cramped sleeping arrangements at Delta Med in Vietnam. It would certainly be beneficial to have a good relationship with your neighbor.

Regardless of the restlessness and friction among the officers and enlisted personnel, the medical staff members eventually got to know each other well. I had a small circle of friends. We had about 60 physicians among a total of approximately 500 medical personnel. Two women, one being a Marine and the other a Navy psychologist, were also part of our group. I was one of the few physicians who had previously served in a war zone, and therefore I knew what to expect in terms of triage and living conditions. My experiences in Vietnam came through for me again.

This new landscape was totally unfamiliar. Serving in Southeast Asia, our main concerns were heat, humidity, and other threats that came with the jungle territory, such as malaria, snakes, and insects. In Saudi Arabia, the surroundings were completely different. We were in a cold, dry, bleak environment. Water was a hot commodity, and, thankfully, the Marines would occasionally truck water to us so we could wash our hands and faces. We had no showers, not that the medical personnel wanted to bathe anyway because of the freezing temperatures.

Roughing it was a daily routine. Going to the latrine in the middle of the night was an adventure, made more so by the presence of vipers and other menacing desert creatures. Latrines were not much more than holes in the desert floor just inside the perimeter. If nature called in the middle of the night, we had to rely on starlight or moonlight to find the way to these so-called "latrines." We were never issued flashlights.

For the most part, irritation and idle time lingered, the only difference being that we were at a new location with more people. One of my comrades, Commander Gary Breeden, pointed out a recipe for disaster among medical professionals. He said that when general and orthopedic surgeons are in one place with no pecking order, no schedule, 15-year-old supplies, and just waiting for the war to start, tensions are bound to arise.

I tried to keep my distance, but we didn't have much to do except watch this forward Trauma Center being built. Small talk indicated that many of the doctors had limited experience in trauma care since military hospitals largely serve healthy military populations and their dependents. Falling back on my experiences in Vietnam, I gave several impromptu talks on wartime triage and other subjects. But otherwise, I stayed in the background and remained fairly unknown to the group. And the waiting continued for the ground war to begin.

The Middle-of-the-Night Order

One night around 2 a.m., asleep with 17 of my physician colleagues massed together in our tent, I was awakened by Commander William Brown, the hospital's commanding officer. "Come with me," he grunted. "We're going to see General Krulak."

I didn't know the general personally, but I groggily climbed into a Humvee with a Marine driver. The vehicle had slits for headlights. Not showing any light was vital for security. After a fair distance, we reached another site within the base where Marines were working with great speed both above and below ground to finish the construction.

A Marine led the Commander and me into an underground bunker complex dimly bathed in red light. Brigadier General Krulak sat imposingly behind a makeshift desk. At this early morning hour, he got right down to business, and, with some urgency, affirmed that the Marines were ready for the ground war to start—except for the medical component. Krulak contended that once the war began, the Iraqis might deploy biological and chemical weapons. He pointed out that if we weren't ready medically, we could lose this war.

And to underscore what Commander Brown and I already knew, Krulak revealed his knowledge of what was going on at the hospital. Stories had come to his attention that the Trauma Center was rife with dissension and infighting. Leaning forward over his desk for emphasis, he snapped that medical leadership at Al Khanjar was a mess, adding that no one at the Trauma Center seemed to know what to do.

Brown and I shot embarrassing glances at one another, both wondering how Krulak was so aware of the shocking state of affairs at Al Khanjar. After a momentary pause, he suddenly dropped the name of a Navy surgeon from Vietnam days. I remembered Bob Glass but I didn't know him well. Glass had been a physician at Alpha Med when I was at Delta Med. According to General Krulak, Glass had reviewed the roster of available physicians at Al Khanjar, and, without hesitation, told Krulak to put Skip Burkle into this top position because he would get the job done. With this strong recommendation, Krulak cleared his throat and then declared that I was to be the Senior Medical Officer of Al Khanjar. Caught completely off guard, a cold chill went down my spine, and I didn't respond right away.

I hadn't initially made the connection with the "Krulak" name. But I suddenly realized that this strapping Marine before me was the son of the famous World War II general, Victor "Brute" Krulak. It also dawned on me that I had triaged this younger Krulak when I was in Vietnam. As a lieutenant, he had come to Delta Med with shrapnel wounds to his hand that required delicate orthopedic surgery, a procedure that we could not perform at Delta Med. Therefore, we sent him on for treatment to one of the two hospital ships or to the naval hospital in Da Nang.

My attention then quickly returned to the mind-boggling scenario before me, wondering if I was even capable of this wartime assignment. Could I bring this increasingly quarreling group of medical professionals together as a team? It would be an enormous task, and I realized I didn't have the luxury of time. The ground war could begin any day, yet saying no to General Charles C. Krulak wasn't an option.

The General never took his eyes off me. After an uncomfortable silence, he proclaimed in the strictest confidence that the ground war would kick off in six days. My only thought at that instant was that "six days" translated into one glaring fact: I wouldn't have much time to turn Al Khanjar around to become a smooth-running trauma center.

In the middle of that blurred night, I heard myself responding, "Aye, aye, sir! I'll take the job and do the best I can." At least I had the rank and background to do the job, but this new duty was on an epic scale. Krulak nodded approvingly. We saluted and our meeting ended as abruptly as it had begun. Arriving back at our camp, Bill Brown left me at my tent with the same brusqueness he had displayed at 2 a.m., bluntly saying, "We'll meet in the morning. We have a lot of plans to go over."

In Charge

Later that same day, everyone involved in the emerging Trauma Center showed up for our first "all hands" meeting. After many weeks of disagreement and unrest, the crowd was eager to learn what to expect from their new Senior Medical Officer. They wanted to know, understandably, what kind of environment they'd be thrust into for the foreseeable future. The main contention among the physicians was that they had hoped to have complete control of the Trauma Center, including being able to oversee all administrative duties. Many even thought the hospital's commanding officer, Commander William Brown, a Medical Service Corps officer, should be replaced by a physician.

I stood above the assembled personnel on a Conex box with the wind whipping up the corners of the large and crowded tent. In a loud, purposeful, confident voice, I declared that I expected all medical personnel to perform their duty and work to their full potential to complete our mission. In the end, we would all be judged by our accomplishments. Every person knew the shared goal was to save as many lives as possible. Personalities were to be checked at the door.

I stated straight out, "We have enough to do as physicians. I have no problems with the current structure so that's how this hospital will be run."

Changing the subject, I began to share what I knew about combat medicine,

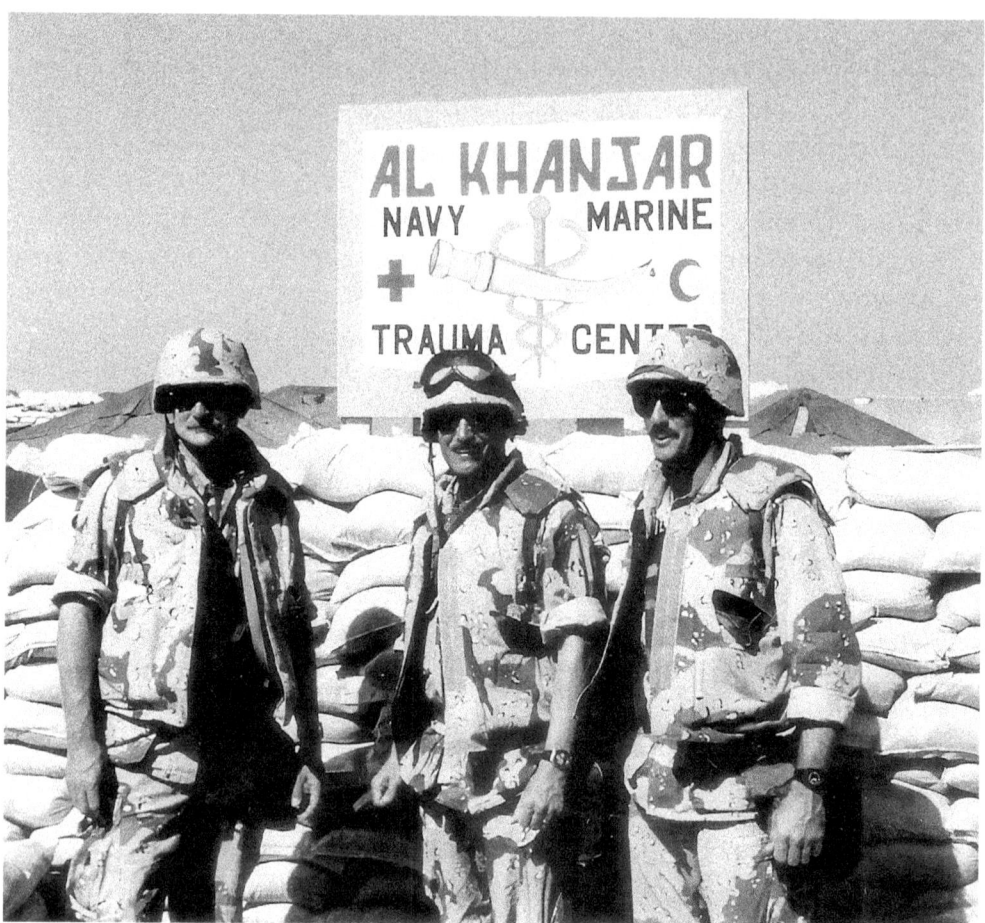

Captain Skip Burkle, Senior Medical Officer, flanked by two medical colleagues (author's collection).

focusing on how we should conduct triage and the challenges we might face. I pointed out that most of the casualties would probably be Iraqi troops—not U.S. Marines, not U.S. Army soldiers, and not other Coalition troops.[5] The staff had not considered this scenario. I emphasized that Iraqi prisoners of war, who were to be designated as "enemy prisoners of war" or "EPWs," would not have dog tags or identified blood types. A simple surgical counter, to be set up in the triage area containing "anti–A" and "anti–B" serum, would suffice for immediate transfusion decisions. This stand would allow the laboratory technicians to better cope with doing the anticipated cross-matches.

I ended my soapbox briefing and dismissed the staff. Then the chief of nursing, company commanders, several corpsmen, and I began evaluating the center's layout. We identified the optimum location for triage, chose a decontamination area in case of chemical or biological exposure, and determined the site where casualties

---

5. Nearly 40 nations contributed troops to what became known as the "Coalition" forces.

would be directed. I also wanted to become more familiar with the medical staff. They likely would be invaluable in upcoming crises. I took down each of their names and inquired about their prior involvement in advanced trauma life support.

None of the corpsmen, unfortunately, had ever had any experience in this field of combat medicine. Even more alarming, only a handful of physicians had attended a training program in acute trauma life support. Naval hospitals were not trauma centers. I made a mental list of the fundamental tasks that needed to be done to get this group up to speed.

We had five days left, and I realized I still hadn't conferred with most of the physicians. Estimates indicated that at least a thousand casualties were expected on the first day of the ground war. At the time, the media and official sources put great credence in Saddam Hussein's threat that the war for Kuwait would be "the mother of all battles." Based on what weapons he had unleashed on Iran several years earlier during the Iran-Iraq War—and even let loose on his own people, the Kurds—the use of biological or chemical warfare was a high probability.[6]

My next order of business was to evaluate our current blood supply. Al Khanjar possessed about 80 percent of all blood in the theater—about 2,100 units[7]—but I knew that a few of those units were already out of date. I decided to adopt a modified Israeli team approach in terms of triage and blood allocation by dividing the staff into blue and gold teams. The Israel Defense Forces had perfected this efficient system in combat, and it proved very effective in several of their conflicts.

The average number of blood units a wounded patient required was 2.4 units. I told my staff they could order only two units at a time. If a casualty had to have more than that amount, he would have to be reprioritized. The triage personnel would then need to decide if a patient's condition was futile, otherwise we would quickly run out of blood. As dark and harsh as this imposed restriction seemed, without a limitation I knew our blood supply would rapidly disappear. I also wasn't sure how soon we would be able to obtain more units.

After the initial classification of wounds, which included confiscating personal weapons outside the larger triage tent, the injured would be moved to resuscitation. If a wounded soldier needed surgery, he would be handed over to a new blue or gold triage team, each consisting of a surgeon, an anesthesiologist, and an orthopedist. The 12 narrow operating rooms were icebox-like containers set up right next to each other, so an organized process had to be in place to use these ORs as proficiently as possible.

Monitoring surgery would be my next most important job. I met separately with my two blue and gold teams, walking them through each procedure. I emphasized

---

6. Saddam had launched chemical attacks against 40 Kurdish villages and thousands of innocent civilians from 1987 to 1988. The worst use of Saddam's many poison gas attacks was on the Kurdish city of Halabja on March 16, 1988. Almost 5,000 civilians died from a nerve agent. Available at https://2001-2009.state.gov/r/pa/ei/rls/18714.htm.

7. One unit of blood is roughly equal to one pint. The average adult has between 8 and 12 pints of blood.

that they needed to be aware of the patient's status at all times, as well as how much blood was being used. I stressed that they discuss those questions before they came to see me. They needed to make a decision among themselves about removing a patient from surgery and putting another wounded patient in his place.

Having to take a patient out of surgery had occurred in Vietnam, but, hopefully, that situation would not occur at Al Khanjar because we had enough operating rooms. The possibility of an inadequate number of surgeons and ORs existed since it was predicted that 1,500 to 3,000 casualties would swamp our facility in the first 12 to 24 hours. Those large numbers of casualties would greatly exceed what we could handle.

As I was putting a workable system in place, the morale issue again caused problems when a small group of corpsmen asked if they could speak to me about an issue that concerned the triage team. Even though they were now feeling more confident in their roles and were working well with the physicians, one orthopedist had constantly been berating the corpsmen and criticizing the agreed-upon casualty management system. They were discouraged and felt they hadn't deserved his abuse. Listening intently to their concerns, I then asked questions to clarify their grievance. I had to assure myself that this complaint had some substance that needed an immediate response. I promised to look into this problem.

That afternoon the blue and gold team physicians and corpsmen met me in the triage area. As they gathered around, I emphasized that everyone would have to work with the triage corpsmen to fully understand the status of every casualty. Once the patient's condition was specifically identified, then he would be assigned to one of the 12 operating rooms.

As I spoke, I noticed a few corpsmen attentively taking notes. I also sensed the doctor in question was not paying much attention. When I finished, I turned to the orthopedist and warned, "For the duration of the war, you are to grow up, keep your mouth shut, and stop complaining or you will be sent out of the theater. After the war, you can start being a child again. That's an order!" I broke the silence and ended the impromptu gathering. "That's all. I expect nothing but the best and I chose you all because you *are* the best."

Despite the driving winds and flapping of the triage tents, the silence was deafening. I witnessed a confirmatory wink from the surgeon on the team, but said nothing more as I walked away. I was sure this confrontation would spread like wildfire among the medical personnel.

I considered that the behavior of this officer in question may have been a cover for anxiety felt by many others. After all, a war was about to commence and we would be dealing with the consequences so I had no choice. That doctor never caused a single problem after my talk. Six months after I returned home, he sent me a letter of apology, thanking me for reprimanding him, adding that serving at Al Khanjar had been a life-changing experience for him.

Even after I had taken the bull by the horns, that is, the orthopedist, I felt even more isolated as I returned to my bunk that night after my team talk. I knew, though, that I had to let my tough words percolate and settle in. In the days that followed, I was proud of the coordinated performance and the feedback many were giving me. They now felt prepared. My main concern was just how long I could hold out with the supplies at hand.

The orchestration of stocking provisions in war may often seem like an afterthought, but the success of both fighting and health care delivery depends on an effective supply chain of required provisions and medications. The inflow of medical necessities competes with the requisite bullets and tanks. The other challenging logistical picture is the outflow of patients waiting for cargo planes. These planes had to be reconfigured as litter planes to get critical patients out of Saudi Arabia, then to medical facilities in Germany, and eventually to the United States.

During the height of the buildup and war, planes were landing so frequently that five planes might be on the runway at one time. Organizational prowess was much needed to manage this massive effort. But being in the most isolated area of Saudi Arabia, we were not privy to these events occurring many miles farther south. Our physicians, who had never practiced medicine in time of war, were waiting near the front lines with out-of-date supplies, as well as an outmoded network for getting those necessities. Not surprisingly, some chaos existed at this northernmost field hospital, but we were determined to improvise with what supplies we had.

Fortunately, we were not alone in delivering health care in this desert remoteness. A land-based Navy Fleet Hospital was located near the Persian Gulf coast, about 120 miles south of the Kuwaiti border, and two Navy hospital ships, *Mercy* and *Comfort,* cruised just off the coast of Kuwait. Additional corpsmen were assigned to field units in support of their combat mission. As we developed routines, the beginning of the ground offensive approached.

"The Mother of All Battles"?

I had dutifully maintained the secret General Krulak had entrusted to me, not sharing it with anyone else until two hours before the beginning of the ground attack at 6 p.m. on February 24, 1991. The prevailing wind, which was blowing toward our troops, delayed the start a few hours due to concern about Saddam's threat to use chemical weapons. But once the wind shifted, the troops moved forward. We observed the exhausts from the Iraqi Scud[8] missiles streaking across the sky at high altitudes. They were headed for targets farther south. Meanwhile, artillery barrages and bombing became more intense.

The first casualties arrived at night: several Marines who had been sent north

---

8. Scud tactical ballistic missiles, originally developed by the Soviet Union, were purchased by several Communist Bloc and Third World nations. During the Persian Gulf War, Iraq fired dozens of Scuds at targets in Saudi Arabia and Israel.

in advance of the assault. However, the tempo quickly picked up. Two days later, incoming casualties demanded all hands on deck when Al Khanjar Navy-Marine Corps Trauma Center received its first enemy prisoner as a patient. As U.S. military forces breached Iraqi defenses within hours and made their assault into Kuwait, the Trauma Center received 21 Coalition casualties.

Most victims were brought in by air and some by ground transportation, many receiving treatment for extremity trauma, penetrating shrapnel fragments, and high-velocity bullet wounds. Lieutenant Commander Jamie Whiteman, Executive Officer of Company A, later reminded me that Dr. John Atkinson had also performed a few brain surgeries. Less than six months before, Dr. Atkinson had completed his neurosurgery residency at the Mayo Clinic. We treated more than 95 percent of the Marines who received major injuries during the breach. They remained with us for about 24 hours, but no more than two days.

"But sadly, we lost a few patients," Whiteman recalled. "We received two Marines who were dead on arrival, and another Marine died after an operation. We also had a small number of Iraqi soldiers who didn't make it."[9]

Once trauma patients were treated and stabilized, they were sent to fleet hospitals in the rear. From that point, the cases requiring more definitive care went back through the evacuation system. That process began at the airstrip built about a mile from the Trauma Center. The landing strip served to evacuate casualties either by helicopter or by C-130s.

All the first casualties transferred to the landing strip were all returned to us, unfortunately, by Air Force personnel because no straps were available to fasten the wounded to the stretchers. We didn't have any kind of constraints so I ordered every male staff member to donate his belt to secure the casualties as best as possible. These belts were then immediately sent back to the airstrip. One belt could hold the legs down, but we had to double up for the chest or abdomen. This time our patients did not return, and we could hear the plane roaring down the sand-packed runway.

I tried to imagine the expressions on the faces of those Air Force personnel when they realized that those makeshift straps were simple belts that once had held up the trousers of corpsmen and other medical personnel. I never heard any more talk about our contrived belt technique, but I know the incident was included in an after-action investigation.

Cannon Fodder

In addition to combat troops, including both Coalition soldiers and Iraqi prisoners, the Trauma Center also assisted Iraqi and Kuwaiti refugees fleeing war-torn areas. Iraqi civilians suffered gunshot or shrapnel wounds, some from mortar fire

---

9. *Hawaii Marine*, Vol. 20, No. 19. May 9, 1991, A-4. Available at https://www.dvidshub.net/publication/issues/20975.

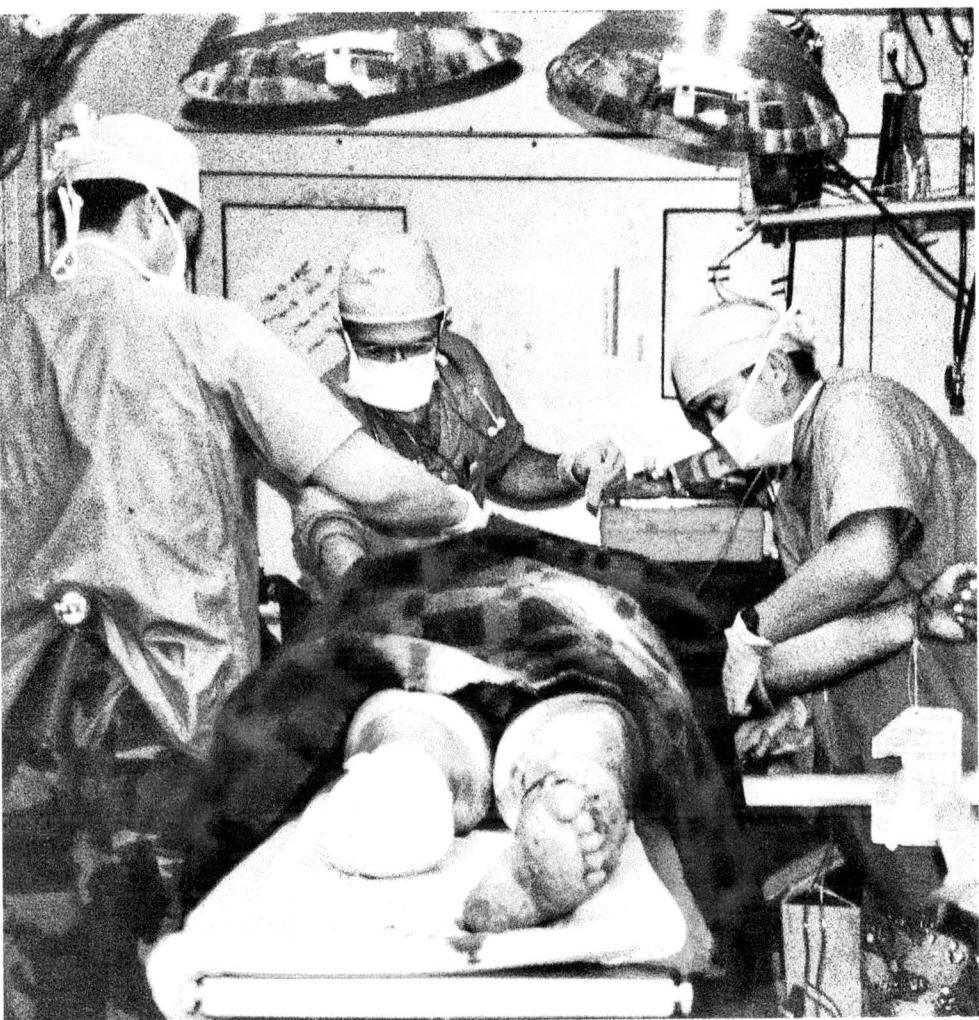

An Iraqi POW receives life-saving surgery (author's collection).

or other artillery. Regrettably, as more Iraqi EPW casualties arrived, we found that most were young and of Islam's Shia sect. With Saddam being Sunni, most of his frontline troops were Shia Muslims. Saddam considered this other branch of Islam expendable cannon fodder.

Some Shia soldiers, who had suffered months of bombardment from the air and were starving, now threw in the towel and began running in our direction to surrender. Their Sunni commanders ordered these escaping troops to be shot in the back. Several Iraqi casualties had taken shelter in underground bunkers built by the Iraqis in occupied Kuwait. They sat in a wedged sitting position for weeks as the air war pounded their positions. These prisoners of war arrived frozen in these positions, wearing foul-smelling, vermin-infested uniforms. They lacked any water and food. Several died from malnutrition and apparent kidney failure.

Lieutenant Commander Whiteman told me about a 40-year-old Iraqi army private whose commander claimed that if he and his comrades were captured, the bloodthirsty Americans would summarily execute them. As with all the other prisoners, he was lice-infested, without shoes, and had not eaten for days. When offered food, he refused, thinking it was poisoned. But once this prisoner saw Whiteman eating, he took a few bites and began to talk. Then the EPWs began to show their gratitude with smiles and gulping down American food.

As Whiteman recollected, "It became more of a humanitarian affair and thoroughly heartwarming as both Marines and sailors gave away their food and clothing to make life for these defeated Iraqi soldiers just a little more comfortable. This personal generosity and sharing took away some of the pains that come with war."[10]

The war's prognosis became obvious in almost a matter of hours. Once it was clear to Saddam that he would lose the "mother of all battles," his retreating troops torched more than 600 oil wells on their withdrawal back into Iraq. These towering infernos, which dotted the Kuwaiti desert landscape, covered the horizon and shrouded our Trauma Center in thick, acrid, black smoke, making it difficult to see or to breathe.[11] High noon appeared as midnight. I took a photo of our Humvee but only its outline was visible. This smoke-filled darkness went on for almost three weeks. I frequently had to use an inhaler for my asthma.

In the days following the Iraqi retreat, the desert from Al Khanjar up into Kuwait was strewn with unexploded mines and respiratory inhalers normally used by asthmatics. The damage done to the Kuwaiti people, not to mention the devastation of the landscape from the burning wells, was devastating. In 2010, *Time* magazine included these burning oil wells as one of the world's top 10 environmental disasters.[12]

False Alarm

During the so-called "100-hour" ground war, we saw several frontline troops with respiratory distress who declared they had been gassed. This claim was terrifying. All staff members were justifiably anxious and frightened. But no gas was detected. Without my knowledge, an Army chemical detection sergeant showed up at Al Khanjar. Covered with a face mask, he began to probe the triage wards and surgical spaces. He then entered an OR where a patient, already anesthetized, was being readied for surgery with the staff gowned and gloved. He shouted through his heavy-duty mask that the casualty was contaminated and ordered all persons out of the OR.

---

10. *Ibid.*
11. This condition, known as "Gulf War Syndrome," affected many war veterans with fatigue, persistent headaches, muscle pain, and neurological symptoms, such as tingling and numbness in arms and legs. Some sufferers also experienced short-term memory loss and an inability to retain information. Smoke from oil well fires, pesticides, depleted uranium used in tank ammunition, or exposure to solvents and corrosive liquids may all have played a role in troops' post-war symptoms.
12. Gilbert Cruz, "And the Earth Cried: Kuwaiti Oil Fires," *Time*, May 3, 2010. Available at http://content.time.com/time/specials/packages/article/0,28804,1986457_1986501_1986442,00.html.

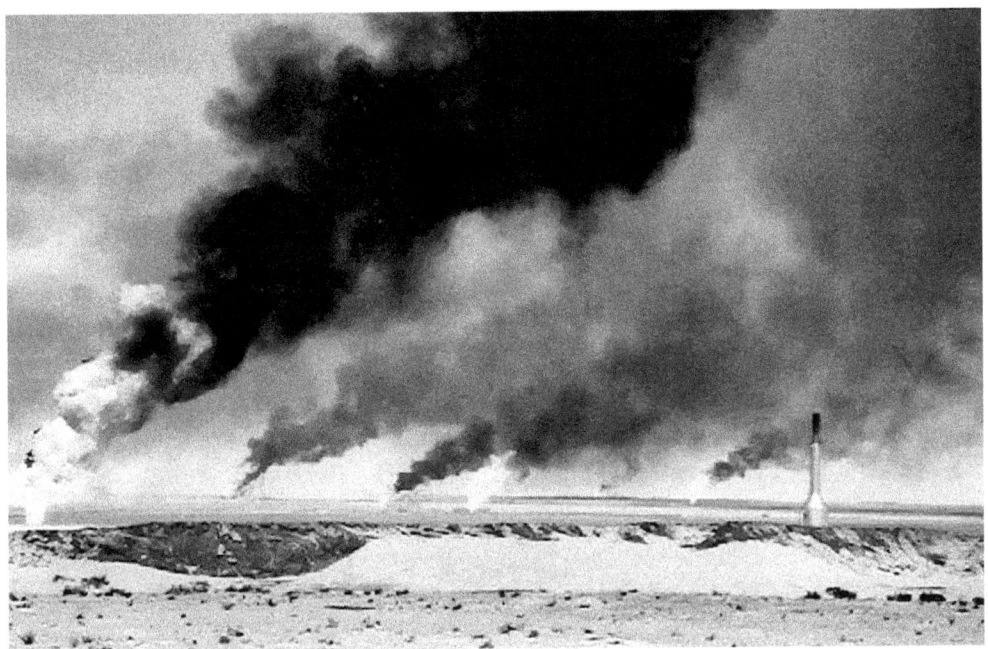

Oil fires, which were set by fleeing Iraqis, became a serious, long-standing breathing hazard (author's collection).

The surgeon rushed to triage to tell me that this sergeant was closing down the hospital. I ran to the surgery area, now abandoned except for the one operating room he had tested. In that OR I found an anesthesiologist, who, refusing to leave, was artificially breathing for the unconscious and intubated casualty. The anesthesiologist saw no symptoms of any chemical infiltration and no indication of a nerve agent. Trying to quickly calm him down, I said anesthesia gases could set off detection devices.

I hurried back to triage to find the sergeant, now surrounded by multiple officers. He ordered the hospital to be closed and evacuated immediately due to contamination in the air. I forced myself into the small crowd and declared, "Over my dead body you will! Anybody worth his salt knows that anesthesia gases set off detection-level machines at very high levels. And nowhere else have you encountered this but in one OR where a surgical patient was being treated. Did you know that?"

"No," the sergeant said, showing some embarrassment.

"The hospital stays open until we can confirm that this chemical contamination is real," I firmly stated.

Luckily, it was the anesthesia gas that had triggered the detection levels, not poison gas. I purposely thanked the sergeant for doing his job, but emphatically stated that the next time he came by, he first had to contact me to make the rounds together. I never heard another word about exposure. It took a while for our compound to settle back down as everyone was naturally on edge. All medical personnel eventually felt reassured that the scare was a false alarm.

After all the massive buildup and planning, and given my year of constant fighting and triage in Vietnam 23 years earlier, I hadn't expected this war to be over in such short order. Following weeks of bombing, the ground offensive lasted only 100 hours. During that mercifully brief conflict, Al Khanjar Navy-Marine Corps Trauma Center admitted 466 patients and conducted 88 major surgeries. Those figures included Iraqi soldiers, Coalition forces, 1st and 2nd Marine Division personnel, and members of the U.S. Army's Tiger Brigade.

A week after the war ended, we began shutting down the hospital's operations and vacated the area on March 11. By then, the morale of this large group of medical personnel had soared. Moreover, I was impressed with the great work they had all done. Everyone was proud of his or her accomplishments. I was quite moved they felt this way about themselves and the Trauma Center's teamwork. We never discussed the unsettling lack of direction that existed before the war began. At every opportunity, I conveyed to them that they did a damn good job. I had brought these people together, who had never been in a war zone, to do their respective assignments and they excelled at doing it.

* * * *

Before decommissioning the Trauma Center, we held a "rating meeting" under a tent attended by medical officers composing all Marine Medical Units in the theater. To my surprise, I was rated "Number 1." I reminded those present that I was a reservist and would soon be retiring. Instead, I recommended that the honor be given to an active-duty physician whose career would be greatly enhanced by this accolade. But they were adamant, maintaining that I had earned the rating they had conferred on me.

Several days later, we left for Kuwait City. From there, I flew to Spain on a C-141 transport, and then on to Otis Air Force Base on Cape Cod where we landed in the middle of the night. The temperature was frigid when we deplaned, but I could see the outline of a hangar with just one light over the door. We all rushed to the darkened building to get warm. Suddenly the lights went on and a massive number of people, all local citizens and families of military personnel, cheered us as we entered. It was past midnight yet all those folks were eager to greet us in a very cold airport hangar. Hugging, taking photos, and devouring great food went on for hours. This welcome home in March 1991 was an entirely different experience from my silent return from Vietnam in 1969.

I then made my way to California and finally back to Hawaii and into Phyllis's waiting arms. As it turned out, any downtime or return to a "normal life" as a professor of medicine would have to wait. A new crisis soon awaited me, and once again, it was in Iraq. Just a few weeks later, I found myself actually in the so-called "Cradle of Civilization," but at that time Iraq was anything but "civilized."

9

Operation Provide Comfort

Spring 1991

"Cultural lessons are always learned the hard way, a fact I already understood."

The nation cheered about the victory over Saddam Hussein in late February 1991, and I greatly appreciated the warm welcome home from the short-lived Operation Desert Storm. But the many Iraqis left behind in the wake of destruction were just beginning a new chapter of struggle and deprivation that still endures today.

In the spring of 1991, immediately after the Persian Gulf War, Shia in southern Iraq and Kurds in northern Iraq rebelled against the Iraqi leadership, with the encouragement of President George H.W. Bush.[1] Saddam's response was quick and brutal. Despite being weakened militarily, he sent his remaining tanks and aircraft to put down the rebellions.

An estimated 200,000 Kurds fled even farther north to take refuge just south of the Turkish border, but their survival in wretched mountain camps was tenuous. Within days, 1,500 Kurds had died of exposure. Despite a strong determination not to be involved militarily in any post-war internal struggles, the U.S. established a northern "no-fly zone" and offered humanitarian assistance to deal with the crisis.

Understanding the complexity of the Kurdish situation is essential. The Kurds are not a homogenous people, and the many factions are not necessarily connected culturally or politically. Kurdistan is not a nation state.[2] The Kurdish ethnic groups, consisting of 25 to 35 million Kurds, are spread across several nations—Turkey, Iraq, Iran, Syria, Jordan, and portions of other nations. The Kurds are not of one religion. They included many religious factions from Sunni Muslim to Shia Muslim to

---

1. On February 15, 1991, President George H.W. Bush spoke at the Raytheon Corporation plant in Andover, Massachusetts, which, at that time, produced parts for the Patriot surface-to-air missile system. He urged the Iraqi military and civilians to "take matters into their own hands" to expel Saddam Hussein. Available at https://www.c-span.org/video/?16518-1/persian-gulf-war.

2. The "Kurdistan Region" is considered independent and consists today of four Kurdish-majority governorates of Erbil, Sulaymaniyah, Duhok, and Halabja. But Halabja wasn't created until 2014. An Arab governorate is a separate administrative division of an Arab sovereign nation. The four governorates, which exist in Iraq, border Iran, Syria, and Turkey.

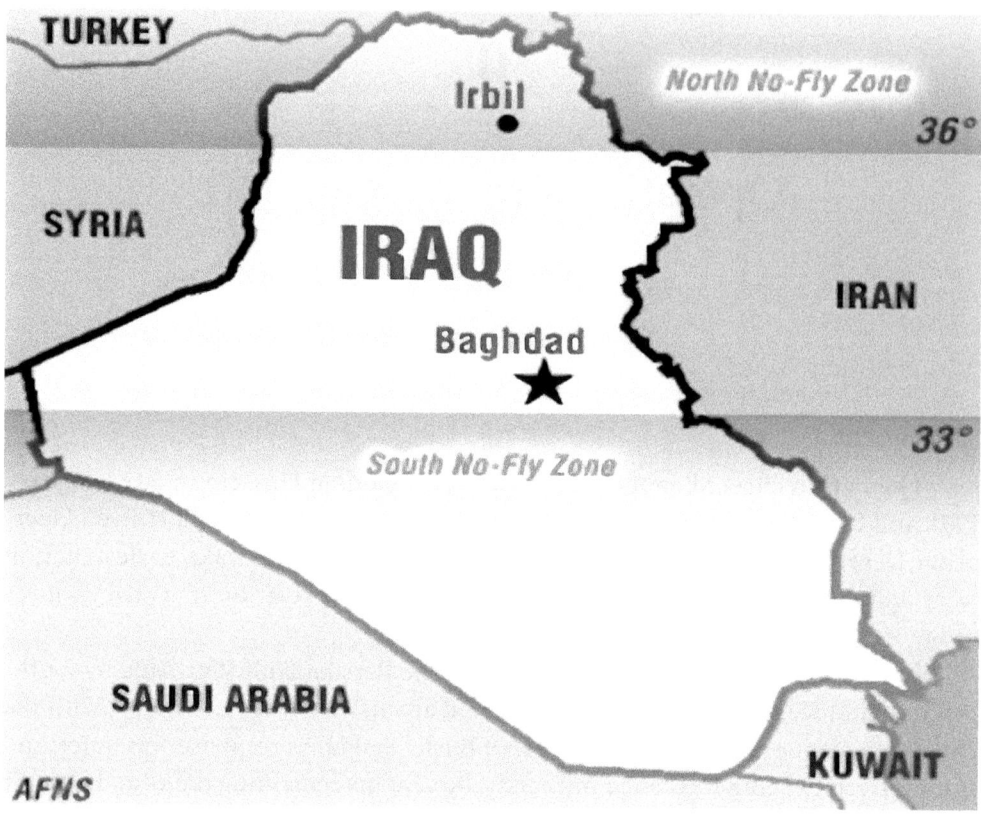

The April 11, 1991, armistice, signed by the Iraqi Army and the Coalition forces, ended the Persian Gulf War. No-fly zones were imposed in northern and southern Iraq, designed to protect Iraqi minorities from Saddam's retaliatory air force (author's collection).

Christian, among other sects. Within each of those countries, this ethnic group lives in what is called the "Kurdistan Region."

Iranian Kurds have been easily assimilated and have caused no problems to the Iranian government. The Kurds in Turkey, the largest ethnic group in that country, comprise almost 20 percent of the population. They have demanded separation from Turkey for decades, aspiring to create either an independent Kurdistan or to have autonomy and greater political and cultural rights in that country. These 10 to 15 million Kurds have been represented by the Kurdistan Workers' Party (PKK), designated by the Turkish government as a "terrorist group" since 1978.

Syrian Kurds have inhabited land across a narrow corridor in northern Syria close to Turkey and Iraq. These Kurds have intermingled with many non–Kurdish minorities. The Syrian Civil War that began in 2011 gave some Kurds a slim hope of improved self-rule.

In Iraq, the Kurds are the largest ethnic minority. In 1991, Masoud Barzani, leader of the Kurdish Democratic Party (KDP), and Jalal Talabani, head of the burgeoning Patriotic Union of Kurdistan (PUK), vied for control of the Kurdistan Region in Iraq. The two men, having differing goals, had clashed for many years despite having been allies during the Iran-Iraq war in the 1980s. With Iranian encouragement, the KDP and PUK militias then joined forces to oppose Saddam, who brutally put down the rebellion with large-scale bombing and the use of chemical weapons. Saddam waging war on his people, the Kurds, was just a precursor to what would occur in 1991 following the Persian Gulf War. Competing claims between Talabani and Barzani arose as to who would lead the Iraqi Kurds in the Gulf War's aftermath.

New Job Titles for New Challenges

In late March 1991, just three weeks after I returned home to Hawaii from the Persian Gulf War, I received a call from the American Red Cross asking me to join a small executive-level group headed for northern Iraq. Our team's goals were to evaluate the Kurdish refugee calamity, and then try to negotiate with Saddam for better conditions for the Kurds. At that time, I held the title of Medical Advisor to the World Health Organization, but I was also named the first Senior Medical Liaison for European Command for the Red Cross. That elongated title put me in the position of a civilian-military liaison.

So just weeks after arriving home from my deployment at Al Khanjar, I found myself traveling with the American Red Cross party to the Persian Gulf—first to Ankara, Turkey, and then on to the refugee camps in northern Iraq. At that point, Saddam had not surfaced in the press for a while, and rumors were widespread of him being dead or injured.

Besides myself, the team consisted of two American Red Cross leaders plus a minister from the Libyan government. My focus was to assess the influence of the large UN military presence that was protecting the fleeing Kurds, as well as the potential of the humanitarian community beyond that of the American Red Cross.

"Operation Provide Comfort" was organized by the United Nations with a military component to give direct assistance to the Kurdish population until the region was secure for the humanitarian coordinators to take charge. American troops would then provide security for the humanitarian organizations to operate, including such support agencies as logistics, transport, and communications. At that time, the humanitarian community considered the UN military as an ally in the struggle to provide security and assistance.

Chapter VII of the United Nations Charter requires military intervention to stop the violence. But the military must also participate in decreasing civilian mortality and morbidity[3] until it is safe for non-government agencies (NGOs) to operate. Consequently, strict monitoring of human rights and observance of international humanitarian law (IHL) must also take place. Once a peace agreement or accord is

---

3. Morbidity refers to the condition of having a disease or a symptom of disease, or to the amount of disease within a population.

signed, a transition to UN peacekeeping forces takes place under Chapter VI of the United Nations Charter.

Suffering on a Mountainside

When we arrived at the refugee camps, the Kurds had just endured a terrible situation, precariously perched on the side of a mountain in the northeast corner of Iraq. Although it was already spring, winter-like conditions on these slopes subjected the refugees to freezing nighttime temperatures. By the first week of April 1991, 800 to 1,000 deaths per day were being reported, primarily among children and the elderly. What immediately struck me visually was the total absence of young men. They were either off fighting or had already been killed. The population breakdown in these camps was about 50 percent children, 30 percent women, and 20 percent elderly men and women.

Several NGOs were already functioning in the region and were doing an extraordinary job under extremely challenging circumstances. I was quite impressed with the level of teamwork. Working together with European NGOs operating field hospitals, the U.S. military was sending in food and medical supplies and taking

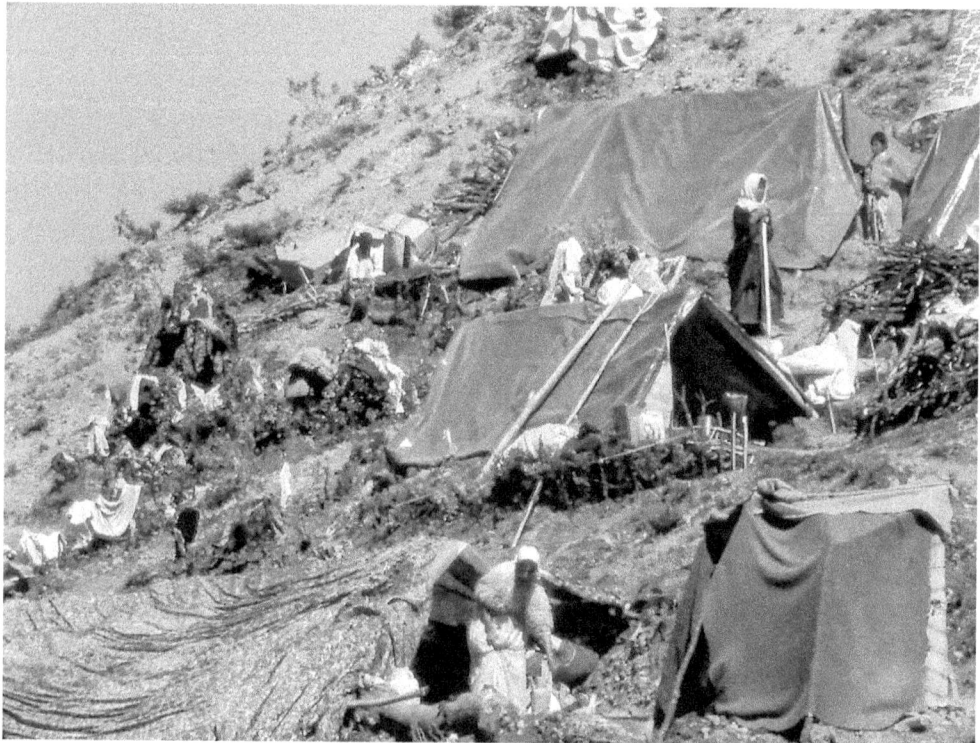

Thousands of Kurds were forced to live in the bleakest conditions on the precarious slope of a mountain in northern Iraq. Sanitation was non-existent (author's collection).

out garbage by helicopters. Although this humanitarian cooperation was gratifying, it was clear that this way of life among the Kurds was not tenable. We had to get the refugees off that mountainside.

Our group then began supervising the construction process of the first of many planned camps. I insisted that the military personnel, who had been assigned to dig latrine holes, reconfigure those communal toilets to face away from Mecca. But an inexperienced officer waved me off, contending, "They're fine. We'll just keep them as is." As predicted, the Kurdish refugees arrived and they intensely objected to the latrines' direction that looked toward their holiest of cities, so new latrines had to be built. Cultural lessons are always learned the hard way, a fact I already understood.

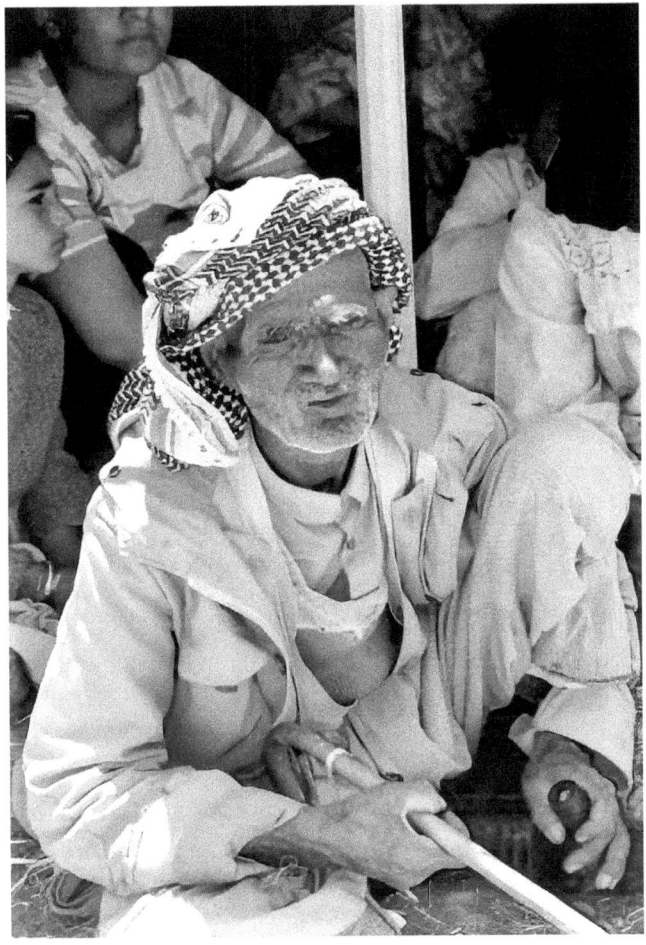

The majority of the Kurdish camps' refugee inhabitants were women, children, and the elderly (author's collection).

Then a bizarre series of inscrutable political and diplomatic maneuvers occurred. Since negotiations to get the Kurds back to their homes had already begun, our American Red Cross team boarded a helicopter to Istanbul. Arriving at the airport, we immediately got into cars awaiting us on the runway. The cars' windows had been blackened for security. Our caravan then proceeded to drive around the inside of the airport boundary for 30 minutes, skirting parked planes along the way. We had no idea of our whereabouts, but this maneuvering, apparently, was to ensure that no one knew our team was back in Turkey. This secrecy was also a cover for Turkey's cooperation.

Following that little perimeter detour, we boarded a plane to fly south to Amman, Jordan, to meet with the Jordan Red Crescent Society[4] and the Jordanian

---

4. The International Federation of Red Cross and Red Crescent Societies (IFRC) is a humanitarian aid body with 192 members, including the Red Crescent societies of Jordan, Iraq, Iran, and Turkey.

Crown Prince to discuss the refugee crisis. We then went first to the eastern part of Jordan, which had massive refugee camps being run extremely well by the Jordan Red Crescent Society. These sites were some of the most well-managed camps I had ever observed.

Next, we drove east for a 13-hour drive across the desert to Baghdad, and, of course, our caravan was halted at the border. While waiting for soldiers to inspect our truck, another vehicle heading back into Jordan was stopped. A soldier opened the trunk to reveal a supply of AK-47s and rocket launchers. The border guards barely blinked. Gunrunning was openly taking place in both directions.

Continuing our trip east, we passed through Ramadi and then to Fallujah to inspect a camp. Both cities would play a major role in the next Iraq war, but these hostilities would be 12 years in the future. Fallujah, about 35 miles west of Baghdad, had a long-term refugee camp inhabited by Kurds, and this site was quite a contrast from what we had just witnessed in Jordan. This camp, by far, was the worst refugee center I had ever seen. Its occupants were starving, their water was laden with oil and feces, and they were living in hovels—if the word "living" can be applied.

Our American team finally made it to Baghdad. We checked into the Rasheed Hotel, which was located adjacent to a blasted-out Iraqi armed forces headquarters building, the bombing courtesy of American forces in the months prior. A short line led to the hotel's check-in desk. Not out of the ordinary, an Arab, nonchalantly carrying an AK-47 slung across his back, stood in front of me in that line.

As was to be expected, the elevators didn't work. Already exhausted from that 13-hour bleak, dismal drive, we had to climb the stairs to our rooms, mine being on the seventh floor. Curiously, each of us had rooms on different floors. The toilets flushed but they were the only fixtures that worked. The room itself was adequate but an air-water mixture churned out of the tap and spit at me. When the "water" finally came out, it was as thick as dirty chalk.

The "Meeting"

Our first meeting took place the next morning. The infinitely long conference consisted mainly of Iraqi officials ripping into us Americans because of the devastation we had caused to their country. They also accused us of being in bed with the Iranians, asserting that one-half hour after the ceasefire had been signed on February 28, 1991, the Shiites (Shia) orchestrated fighting throughout all the cities in Iraq.

These authorities, literally and symbolically on the other side of the table, added that the U.S. had planned this entire scenario of uprisings. The Iraqis insisted they were peace-loving people and made known that the U.S. was pushing them down on their knees. We all tried to stay calm and focus on our mission at hand to convince Saddam to let us bring the Iraqi Red Crescent Society (IRCS) through American lines and begin negotiations with the UN.

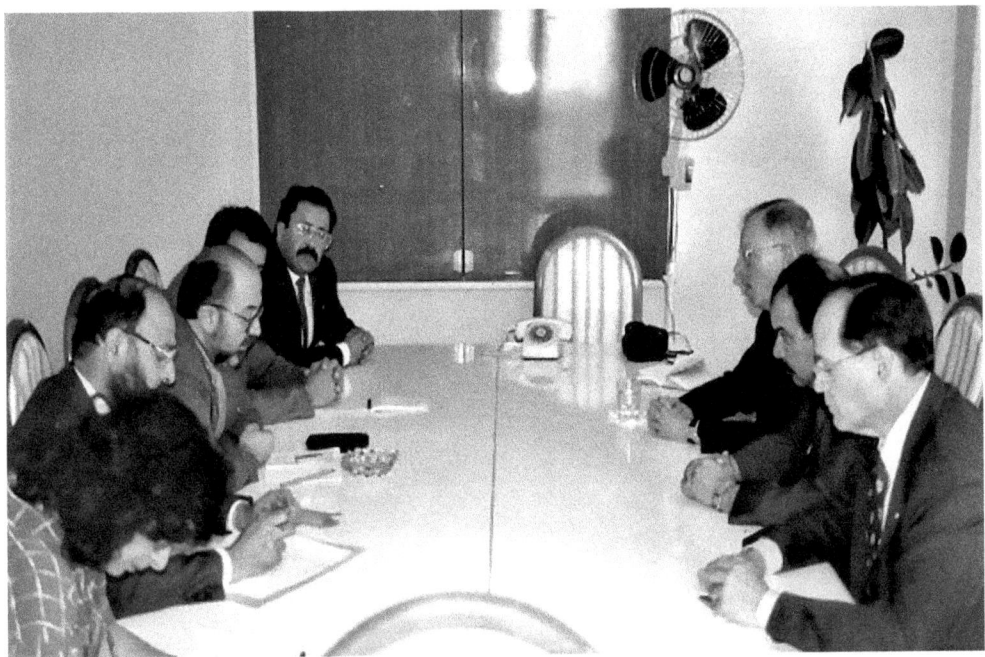

Negotiations with the Iraqis were often tense and unproductive. The line where the two tables joined symbolized the great divide between Saddam's underlings and Coalition representatives (author's collection).

After lunch, the Libyan minister in the room asked for Saddam, expressing everyone's frustration about him not being present. We were told he was in the building, but I noticed a woman at the table periodically leave the room. When she returned, she would whisper something into the ear of a top Iraqi official. This arrangement, however, was not acceptable to the delegation, and the Libyan member eventually blurted out, "No one makes any decisions in this country except Saddam. We need to talk to him."

Nevertheless, negotiations continued in circles. By 4 p.m., we had made absolutely no progress, and I had yet to say anything. After standing up and moving around for a few minutes, I finally felt it was time to speak up. Only four of us sat on one side of the large table. The other side was crowded with unnamed Ba'athists, both men and women, from Saddam's Iraqi Ba'ath Party who stood for promoting Arab nationalism.

I began talking slowly, carefully choosing my words. "It seems to me that after all that has happened," and then I paused for effect, looking directly at my adversaries across the table. I purposely did not mention the loaded word "war," which might be an offensive reminder of what Saddam had lost. I was also aware that Saddam, a narcissist, would always be looking for something to satisfy his egotistical needs. Furthermore, he had to be perceived as a benevolent leader once again. So I continued, "Saddam would want to be seen by the world as a humanitarian." I then added, "These are his people," referring to the displaced Kurds.

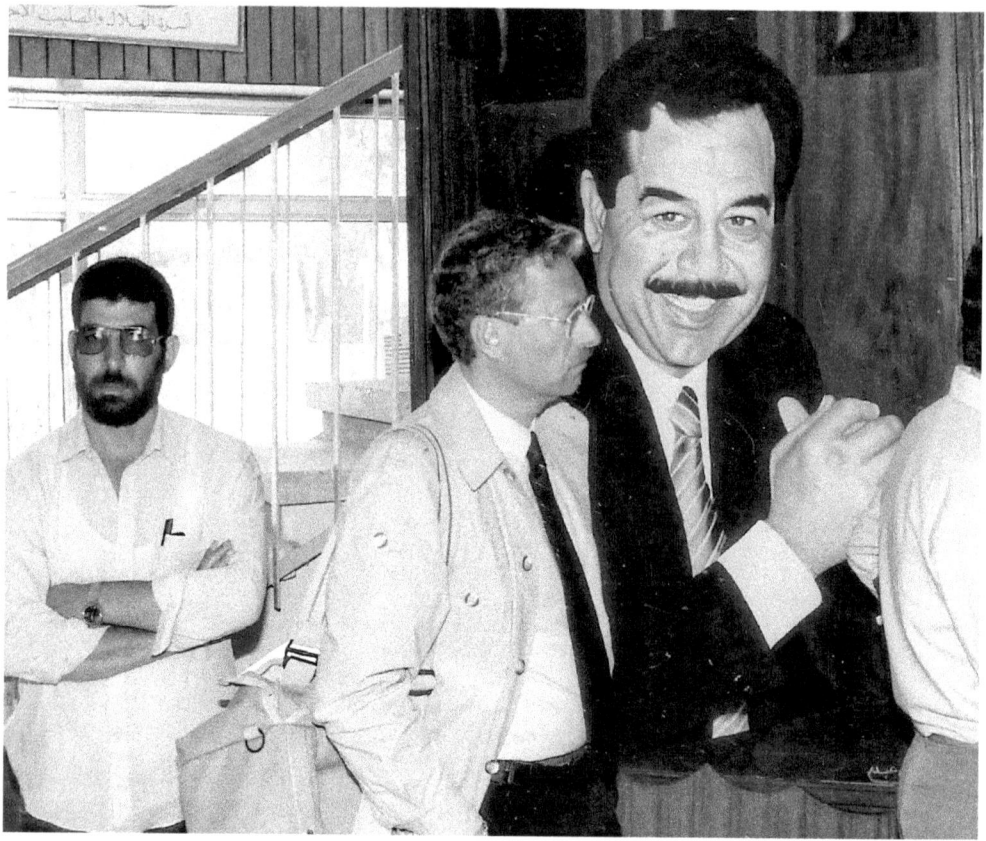

Skip's assigned and staunchly determined bodyguard (left) never let Skip out of his sight. Saddam Hussein always knew Skip Burkle's whereabouts (author's collection).

After I spoke, the Iraqi side of the room buzzed with frenzied debate. The same messenger woman stood up and left, returning 20 minutes later. She announced that Saddam had invited us to stay for the next week, and he would also consider our proposal. The Iraqi officials knew I was a doctor and carried a camera, but that was the extent of their knowledge about me. After hours of silence and then making my definitive statement, I think I piqued their curiosity.

They had no idea I represented the military but never asked me any questions. I carried my military ID in my shoe. Nevertheless, after my few short observant words, for whatever reason, they decided to provide me with my own personal guard, a large thug who never left my side. The next day we headed to the Iraqi Red Crescent Society to confer with their officials.

Ghost Cities and Wooden Jets

The following week, Saddam invited us to witness firsthand, by helicopter, the war's tangible destruction. On our first chopper excursion, we flew low over the countryside to satisfy Coalition demands that no Iraqi aircraft could fly higher than 1,000 feet. We observed what the Iraqis claimed were crashed U.S. jets and a large assemblage of Iraqi tanks on the border with their arch enemy—Iran.

One day, flying low, we spotted a monstrous tank, which stood out from all the other armored vehicles parked on the border. In place of the turret was a massive metal Pegasus horse head. As I reached for my camera, I asked one of the Iraqis on board what the head signified, but he quickly pushed the camera aside. "No picture!" he barked, explaining that the tank belonged to Uday, Saddam's eldest son. The tank had huge speakers on each side from which Uday had blasted heroic music while leading the tank charge into battle against the Iranians.

Our next stop was Karbala, considered a holy city to the predominantly Shia inhabitants. The aftermath of the recent Shia revolt in this city was evident with burned-out buildings and rubble filling the streets. Our Red Cross team met with several of Saddam's generals in one of the buildings still intact. The scene in the hot conference room was quite peculiar. At the outset, no one from the other side spoke. The awkward silence went on for more than 20 minutes until an Iraqi guard entered the room carrying a large photograph of Saddam and placed it on an empty chair. With Saddam now present, so to speak, the negotiations could begin.

We then flew several hundred miles down to Basra, the port outlet to the northern end of the Persian Gulf. Multiple large ships had been sunk or were lying on their sides, blocking the entrances to the harbor. The hospital in Basra was in a deplorable condition. The neonatal critical care unit was bombed out, and the staff told us this barrage was not from Iraqi forces but shelling from Coalition forces.

Before leaving Basra, we met with more Iraqi officials in a former government building. Many of the rooms had been destroyed by fire, and the acrid smell of smoke still lingered. In this port city, we also witnessed the same "Saddam ritual" we had experienced in Karbala. After waiting some time in virtual silence, someone finally located a child's painting of Saddam and placed it on an easel. The talks then proceeded.

The whirlwind schedule continued after we returned to Baghdad for a short stay. We next flew north to Mosul and then on to the Turkish border. As we were boarding the helicopter, I was finally able to temporarily slip away from my ever-present guard. At the last moment, I grabbed the one remaining seat along the side of the helicopter, which gave me an unobstructed view of the countryside. The guard was visibly angry and had to maneuver over to the opposite side to get the last seat available. This opportunity allowed me to take some photos. Approaching the airport in Mosul, we saw full-size bogus, wooden fighter jets built to straddle the runways of the Mosul military base. They looked real but on closer inspection, we could detect that they were a good imitation of modern-day jets on stilts.

Throughout our time in the Iraqi countryside, we never actually saw Saddam, and wild rumors flew that he had either been killed or severely wounded. But on the day we flew to Mosul, he emerged brazenly on the balcony of his presidential palace, brandishing a rifle and firing into the air. Saddam reveled in photo ops of himself wielding guns. He appeared thin and ill, but this display of defiant bravado was his way of showing the world he was still alive and in charge.

From Mosul, we were all placed into one vehicle and driven up to Dohuk, a beautiful mountain city in the northern Iraqi Kurdistan Region near Syria's northeast corner. Now eerily empty, Dohuk, the provincial capital, was one of three Iraqi autonomous Kurdish Regions in 1991 that had its own language and customs. The two other Kurdish provinces, Erbil and Sulaymaniyah, were experiencing intense fighting with Saddam's troops. It was normally home to 350,000 people, mostly Kurds and Assyrians. After the Persian Gulf War, the Iraqi army drove Kurdish insurgents from Dohuk. The region was almost totally depopulated in a month with more than 1.5 million of the 3.5 million Kurds in Iraq fleeing even farther north as Saddam's army moved in. The urban structures remained intact but not a soul was living in Dohuk at this point.

In this abandoned city, our Iraqi "hosts" ushered us individually into separate unmarked vehicles, each with Iraqi guards wearing civilian clothes. I sat alone in the back seat. No one in my group spoke English, but these guards were members of Saddam's trusted security force.

From Dohuk, we drove northwest toward Zakho, located a few miles from the Iraqi-Turkish border and very close to the Syrian border. Zakho was a major economic center serving the Kurds in this area of northern Iraq. Before the American military arrived, most of the local inhabitants had fled to the mountains. Zakho soon became a "ghost city."

As we approached the Turkish border, we began to make out a U.S. Marine checkpoint in the distance, just south of the border. One of the vehicles in our group suddenly signaled and stopped. Several guards got out, began talking among themselves, and gestured back toward my car. Then, inexplicably, we all turned around and drove 30 minutes back to Dohuk. When we reached the city, I realized what had happened after watching the guards open the rear of my car and take out several loaded rocket launchers. Once that contraband was removed from the trunk, we turned around and headed back to the border. Without a doubt, Saddam's security guards didn't want those checkpoint Marines to see their stash of rockets when stopped for inspection.

Nearing that Marine checkpoint again, a very impressive sight awaited us. The Marines were flying the largest American flag they could find. General Anthony Zinni, USMC, who was Deputy Commanding General of Operation Provide Comfort in Turkey and Iraq at that time, later told me, "Air reconnaissance knew where you were all the time and we knew you were coming." Their intelligence system was extremely well executed. I never knew our caravan was being tracked.

Hope for Humanitarian Cooperation

The convoy then traveled north of Zakho to the wide and uncultivated fields that later would house the new refugee tents. But a negotiating tent had been hastily erected using ration boxes to support a UN flag. Discussions began almost immediately with the delegates we had brought from Mosul and the UN special envoy Staffan de Mistura from Italy, who had just arrived a few hours before.

The Kurds were in a terrible situation. Had they been allowed to cross the border into Turkey, they would have found fertile valleys with plenty of water. But Turkey had posted guards all along the base of the mountains preventing any refugees from crossing into their sovereign domain. Instead, the Kurds—women, children, and the elderly—were trapped in those inhospitable mountains. Because of the sloping topography, they had pitched small tents tilted at an angle. The ground beneath those tents consisted of volcanic, grayish-black sand.

These destitute people had no water and no options for sanitation or hygiene. The sickening, tangible effects of such appalling conditions were clearly visible. Eighty percent of the children had or would die from dehydration and diarrhea. These youths weren't suffering from any bizarre infectious disease. They were experiencing the same viruses and common bacteria that would hit any population—even our own—if sanitation was substandard.

But what gave me hope was the exceptional humanitarian response I observed. French and German national teams, World Health Organization teams, and NGOs cooperating with the military were all on the scene. They came together for the multi-tasked Operation Provide Comfort. Even Médecins Sans Frontières (Doctors without Borders), an organization that typically prefers to distance itself from any military operation, noted that the American forces were doing a superb job heading Operation Provide Comfort under the auspices of the UN. American military personnel provided security, transportation, logistics, and communications—skills in which they excel—and let the other NGOs carry out their respective humanitarian duties.

When the negotiations ceased in the late afternoon, we silently returned to the cars and retraced our route to Dohuk. Leaving that deserted city, our team came together once again in a single vehicle and quietly mused to ourselves whether any progress had been made.

After arriving in Baghdad close to midnight, the plan was to meet with our Iraqi Red Crescent Society handlers the next day. The intention was to have those supervisors of the Iraqi Red Crescent Society participate in camp functions, hoping the Kurds could eventually return to their homes. The causes of the Kurdish rebellions had not yet been resolved. Unknown to our team, Saddam had offered deals to both leaders of the KDP and PUK militias to share responsibilities in the government in exchange for their loyalty to him.

Any chance for a quick answer on resettlement for the Kurds in the mountains were smashed the next morning. In a meeting with the IRCS leadership, they announced that Saddam had just signed a pact with the Kurdish KDP's Masoud Barzani—but not with the PUK's Jalal Talabani. Saddam was not interested in the Iraqi Red Crescent Society participating in the relief efforts, ending any possible peace plan with the UN. The Kurds would remain in the Iraqi camps for many months.

In July 1991, the U.S. military Task Force moved out and the UN assumed responsibility for the refugee camp and Operation Provide Comfort. Five years later in August 1996, the Barzani-led KDP invited the Iraqi army to attack the PUK, which eventually turned the battle in favor of the KDP, actively ending Operation Provide Comfort.

Breakdown of Politics and Humanitarian Aid Cooperation

Only a year later in 1992, however, during the crisis in Somalia, everything learned and gained from the Kurdish Crisis had been forgotten. During that Somalia operation, the U.S. military relationship soured with humanitarian NGOs, and then that once remarkable cooperation fell apart. Politics had invaded humanitarian aid and care, making coordination nearly impossible. Operation Provide Comfort looked to be the first and last time such a multifaceted effort worked so smoothly and efficiently.

When our team's negotiations in Iraq ended, we left Iraq and began our return journey to Jordan. On arrival, as the others left to meet again with the Crown Prince, I was shuttled to the airport in anticipation of ending up in Germany to brief the military at the headquarters of EUCOM (European Command).

Inconveniently, I had come down with food poisoning that resulted in gastroenteritis. The commercial flight, which had been hurriedly arranged for me, was delayed in expectation of my arrival. I was conspicuously seated in the last row of first class. The Jordanian flight crew knew I was someone seemingly important, but they were unaware of the details. Jordanian security guards were also present and never took their eyes off me.

Before long, gastric urges took over. Being pale and sweaty, I was rushing to the lavatory every 10 to 20 minutes. As soon as I returned to my seat, the guards and flight attendants rushed to inspect the lavatory. They feared I had stashed a weapon or another kind of lethal device inside, drawing even more attention to my plight. I was tempted to yell out, "Dammit, I've got the runs!"

Dashing up and down the aisle went on for the duration of the flight. The crew members had no idea who I was or why they had to delay their departure. But I imagine they were very relieved when we landed, and they saw this strange ailing American leaving their plane.

A small Air Force military passenger jet awaited to take me to Stuttgart, Germany, to brief the commander of the European Command, Vice Admiral Leighton Smith, before I headed back to Washington. The officials at EUCOM were aghast by my gripping accounts of the Iraqi camps and seeing the hard evidence in my photos. But I'm also not sure I told them anything they didn't already know. Vice Admiral Smith and his aides took copious notes. He was especially interested in our combined insight and accrued knowledge that our unique operation had gathered. He said the information we had collected was "completely unfamiliar to him and was extremely valuable."

Our visit to Dohuk gave the admiral an eye-witness account of the conditions in Iraq and, more specifically, Dohuk's environs. This report started a critical debate among the military officials. They had to decide whether or not the area of security should be extended to provide a level of confidence sufficient to attract the Kurdish refugees back to that area. I had to balance my briefing between the needs of the humanitarian community and the security aspects that this conflict had caused. I also had to be sure the military officials understood the requirements of International Humanitarian Law and the role of the International Committee of the Red Cross. Following the meeting and after beginning a course of antibiotics for food poisoning, I slept for 12 hours straight.

It was only later that Admiral Smith learned that I was a Navy Reserve captain. In a letter[5] to the Navy Department, he flattered me by stating that he "was very impressed with this energetic, enthusiastic, and dedicated officer. Despite having food poisoning and being exhausted, this challenging assignment demanded a unique mix of stamina, intellect, decisiveness, and just good old fashion horse sense. Skip is representative of the very best of officers with whom I have served. I would actively seek his services again in any challenging assignment; he should be flagged for Command."

When I arrived in Washington, I reported my findings at the national headquarters of the American Red Cross. After my return to Hawaii, I kept busy working and writing to support the many efforts of the humanitarian community to bring stability to Iraq and to work toward a more independent Iraqi Kurdistan. With their adopted capital of Erbil, the Kurds have shown increasing promise as the only stable part of a still disrupted post–2003 war in Iraq.

"No Friend but the Mountains"

But what of the Kurds today? After World War I, the victorious Western Allies promised the creation of a Kurdish nation. But when the Treaty of Lausanne was signed in 1923, absent was a provision for a Kurdish state, leaving the Kurds spread across the new boundaries of Turkey, Syria, Iraq, Iran, and Armenia. The Kurdish quest for an independent state of their own has been one of the longest unfulfilled struggles in Middle East history. For decades, the Kurds have demanded separation from Turkey to create an independent Kurdistan, resulting in a continuing and bloody conflict between Turkey and several Kurdish insurgent groups, most notably the Kurdistan Workers' Party (PKK).

---

5. Letter dated May 23, 1991, from Admiral Leighton W. Smith, Jr., USN, Commander in Chief U.S. Navy Forces Europe and NATO Allied Forces Southern Europe, to Rear Admiral James E. Taylor, Director of Naval Reserves.

In Syria, the Kurds, along with Arabs and other ethnic factions, revolted in 2012 against Bashar al–Assad, the Syrian dictator. This uprising quickly became a complex international conflict represented by many local factions, including the Kurds and their strong People's Protection Units (YPG) plus Russia, Iran, and the Islamic State, now known as "ISIS."

The Kurdish militia forced ISIS from northern Syria, eventually occupying most of the border with Turkey. The YPG, the armed wing of the Kurdish leftist Democratic Union Party, has been seen by the Turkish government as allied with the Turkish-based PKK, and therefore labeled as "terrorists" and a "major security threat." Even more worrisome to the Turks was the YPG militia's control of Syria's northern border.

The U.S. entered this increasingly complicated state of affairs when the Obama Administration sought allies to help defeat ISIS. The most able and effective fighters were the Kurdish militia. Even with heavy losses, the Kurds drove ISIS to the brink of defeat, snatching most of the territory that ISIS had occupied during the height of its power in 2015. Despite that victory, the U.S. was caught between two allies—the Kurds and Turkey, a NATO ally determined to end the perceived Kurdish threat on its southern border.

Whatever level of stability existed ended abruptly in October 2019 when President Donald Trump gave Turkish President Recep Tayyip Erdoğan the green light to invade northern Syria by withdrawing U.S. troops. The Kurdish militia, no longer supported by the U.S. and overwhelmed by Turkish military might, withdrew from the border. Many Kurds crossed into Iraq, while others remained in Syria with their future very much in doubt.

Dissension among themselves, betrayed by their U.S. ally, and under attack by Turkish forces, the Kurds again have lost the opportunity to realize an age-old dream: the creation of a Kurdish nation-state. Still ruled by bleak circumstances, this hardy, determined, and long-suffering people must now take comfort from one of their most enduring proverbs: "No friend but the mountains."[6] It is tempting to speculate what this area of the Middle East would be today if the original map drawn by the British after World War I had included a country named Kurdistan.

* * * *

When I returned home following the Kurdish crisis, I kept asking myself the question: Was it possible to pursue my career in global public health while remaining in the Navy Reserve? Several years went by before I contemplated doing both. Although I had been away from home for too long and much too often in harm's way, I also had a dream I wanted to fulfill that would hopefully bring together the various actors in conflict and humanitarian assistance.

---

6. The proverb "no friend but the mountains" exemplifies the timeless feeling the Kurds have had of unending duplicity and rejection due to their history as a semi-stateless ethnic minority throughout the Middle East. Their military support has still left them with no friends to uphold their right to nationhood.

9. Operation Provide Comfort

In 1995, I contemplated the possibility of achieving flag rank—a Medical Corps rear admiral in the Navy Reserve. That rank would improve the odds that I could influence decisions that would help bring the civilian and military communities together in promoting more effective worldwide humanitarian cooperation. General Charles Krulak, who had overseen my performance at Al Khanjar during the Persian Gulf War when he served as the Marine Corps theater commander, wrote on my behalf. By then, he had been elevated to Commandant of the Marine Corps.

General Krulak penned this remarkably strong letter on my behalf: "A seasoned Medical Corps Officer, Captain Burkle's command presence garnered immediate respect from all medical staff. Captain Burkle was chosen, <u>above all others</u>, [his underline], to serve as Senior Medical Officer and Chief, Professional Services, 2nd Medical Battalion Forward. His personal leadership, dedication, and emotional maturity spearheaded the establishment of the largest field medical treatment facility in Marine Corps history.... He enjoys my complete trust and confidence. He is, in every respect, ready to assume greater responsibilities and has my strongest possible recommendation for promotion to Rear Admiral."[7]

Despite this high-level vote of confidence, I still had much to ponder. Several colleagues were encouraging me to indicate to the Navy that I was interested in one of their Reserve flag-rank positions. However, I had a bigger dream that might bring the Armed Services and the humanitarian community together in civilian crisis events—other than war. These worldwide occurrences were becoming more commonplace and demanded attention. In the end, I decided that being an admiral was not in the cards and indicated in a letter to the Navy that I was not interested in being considered.

---

7. Letter dated June 27, 1995, from General Charles C. Krulak, USMC, Commandant of the Marine Corps, to President FY96 Rear Admiral, Medical Corps, Selection Board, Bureau of Naval Personnel.

10

On Call in Africa, Southeast Asia, and the Balkans

1990s

> *"My own anger ignited this Croatian doctor's rage, and he arrogantly declared, 'You pay us to treat children with cancer. You said nothing about feeding them!'"*

Physicians are often expected to be on call for their patients at all hours by seeing them in their offices or in a nearby hospital. But being "on call" in the global humanitarian field means traveling to distant, often devastated countries on very short notice. As my career in global health and humanitarian response continued to progress, I experienced the "drop everything and catch the next flight" message many times across the decades.

Humanitarian crises don't just happen overnight, and they certainly don't resolve on their own in any timely manner. Wars without names, which don't warrant enough global attention, can go on without end. If not monitored, refugee camps can range from "uncomfortable" to "deplorable" in quick succession. By the time living conditions have become bad enough for global intervention, the issues causing the crises have likely become so entangled that it's difficult to genuinely understand how the downward spiral began.

Following Operation Provide Comfort in Iraq, I spent many months throughout the 1990s traveling to Somalia, Burma, and the Balkans. My mission for each trip was to observe, assess, inspect, advise, and critique these very different post-conflict, complex environments. Getting the desired results in other countries and working with diverse cultures always demands critically important tactful skills. But sometimes those diplomatic skill sets need to be used in life-threatening situations.

Somalia: February–March 1993

Somalia became mired in a civil war in the late 1980s, a savage, seemingly unrelenting conflict that continued into the early 2000s. In 1991, several clan-based guerrilla groups overthrew dictator Siad Barre, but none of the many armed factions could effectively fill that newly created power vacuum. With no centralized leadership, chaos permeated Somalia with a resulting humanitarian crisis on an untold scale.

In early 1992, the United Nations passed a resolution to provide humanitarian assistance. But the determination to supply food aid, assisted by the United States, led to intense fighting between the warring factions. As the crisis worsened, the UN knew stronger action was needed. By the end of the year, lawlessness and turmoil, especially in the southern region, became catastrophic. The UN then sanctioned the Unified Task Force, a multinational group led by the United States, to try to create a protected environment in which humanitarian operations could function.

President George H.W. Bush authorized the dispatch of 1,800 Marines in December 1992 to assist with famine relief. This military undertaking was part of that larger UN endeavor to restore order in Somalia and to enable food distribution and other humanitarian aid. Code-named "Operation Restore Hope," U.S. forces acted under the authority of Chapter VII of the UN Charter. Chapter VII allowed for the use of force to maintain peace without requiring the consent of the nation involved. Warlord Mohamad Farrah Aidid immediately challenged attempts to protect humanitarian aid deliveries. During the first week of December, those 1,800 Marines landed in Somalia to carry out the UN's mandate.

In February 1993, Monette Melanson was Coordinator for Somalia in the Office of the U.S. Secretary of Defense (DOD). Monette and I were sent by DOD's Office of Global Affairs to Kenya, Somalia, and Ethiopia to discuss Operation Restore Hope in Somalia. The plan was to use the lessons learned from Iraq during Operation Provide Comfort two years earlier in the spring of 1991. We were also charged with looking into continuing requests by other African countries for DOD support for both humanitarian relief and reconstruction.

In adjacent Kenya, from which supplies would first be delivered to Somalia, Monette and I concentrated at the outset on the appalling lack of coordination between Washington-based decision-makers and the U.S. government representatives in Kenya. That mismanagement hampered the initial efforts to deliver food to Somalia. Unfortunately, we saw little direct liaison between local representatives and key personnel back in Washington.

One early morning, the Canadian military escorted us on a flight from Nairobi, Kenya, to Mogadishu, the capital of Somalia. As soon as we landed, our caravan left the airport gates led by armed Marines, a requirement for all vehicle convoys. We soon met up with hungry Somali children of every age swarming around our vehicles begging for food. The first adolescent male I saw, who was trying to grasp my watch, was wearing a University of Hawaii sweatshirt. What an ironic beginning to this inspection tour.

We had our initial meeting in Mogadishu with the Civil-Military Operations Center (CMOC) at which I was introduced to Bob Macpherson, a Marine colonel. Bob would become a fellow humanitarian in the civilian field and be my ally years

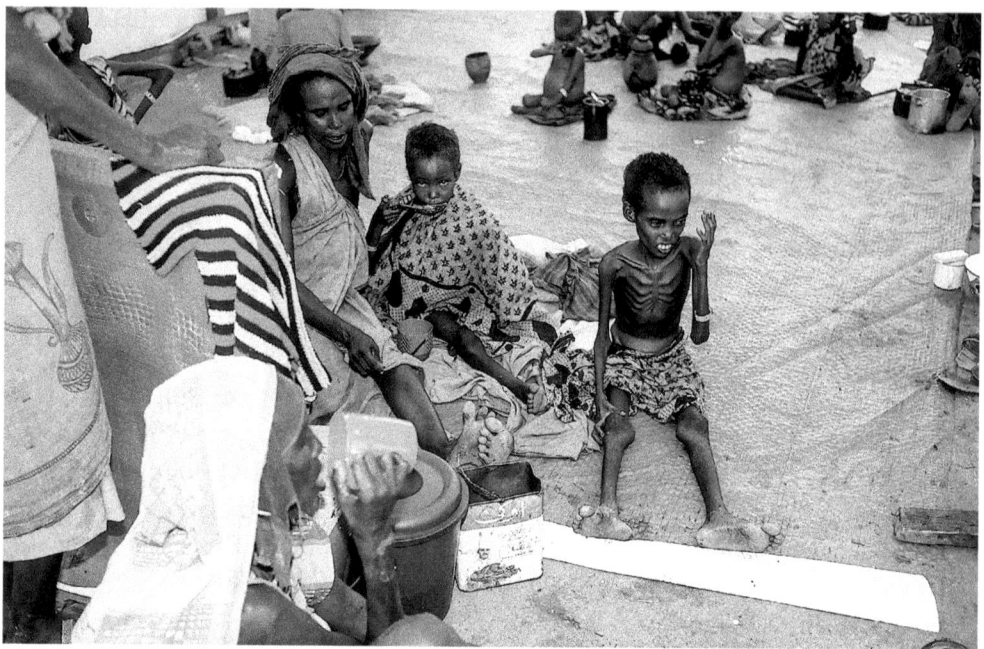

During Operation Restore Hope, which lasted from early December 1992 to early May 1993, UN aid stations were set up to feed starving Somali children (National Archives).

later in Bosnia. While the CMOC was doing an excellent job trying to coordinate all the independent and dependent players in the field, any success was eclipsed by the autonomy of the non-governmental organizations (NGOs) on the ground.

Meeting with Médecins Sans Frontières (MSF) (Doctors Without Borders) and the International Medical Corps, we learned that these two NGOs were planning to be out of the medical treatment business in Somalia within the next few months due to growing security concerns. Most humanitarians in this shattered country felt they were physically threatened even more now than during the previous two years of civil war. They stressed that additional NGO personnel had been killed just since the U.S. Marines arrived in early December 1992. The crimes had shifted from food and vehicle theft to personal threats and deaths.

During this operation, those nations leading these relief efforts repeatedly cried out for Somali leadership to take charge of their own country's destiny. But for the Somalis to take responsibility was easier said than done. First, the Federal Republic of Somalia authorities had to find their way out of a prolonged, relief-directed existence so they could start looking forward to rebuilding their homeland. Second, this desperate country had to reconcile its political differences among the various factions. And third, Somalia had to somehow take responsibility for the security concerns within its borders. Those in power regrettably did not move in any of those directions.

Many countries were offering medical supplies and equipment, resources that were valuable and advanced enough to outfit a 500-bed hospital. But I became concerned with the safety and security of these supplies. I pointed out that these provisions should not be placed impulsively because of the shifting war fronts and unstable areas. This equipment should instead be warehoused, inventoried, and packaged as "second echelon" medical kits to be sent to various health facilities in need. I emphasized that these necessary humanitarian items were too important and too costly to waste.

Since closing in 1991, the U.S. Embassy and residential compounds in Mogadishu were rendered unusable due to the fighting. During our time in this port city on the Indian Ocean, four major U.S. oil companies remained, all salivating to drill in the Horn of Africa.[1] Conoco, however, was the only company to maintain an office in Mogadishu, becoming directly involved in our role in the UN-sponsored humanitarian-military effort. Since the embassy was unusable, the U.S. government rented Conoco's buildings, which were converted into the U.S. administration's home in Mogadishu. One of those buildings also housed us during our stay. But the close relationship between Conoco and the U.S. military force troubled the Somalis, causing many to liken this wartime scenario to a miniature "Operation Desert Storm," namely, an excuse to safeguard oil reserves for future outside exploitation.

One afternoon in one of the Conoco buildings, Monette and I began chatting with the new career Foreign Service Officer. He was now the latest UN Special Envoy to Somalia. Visibly angry, this new Special Envoy invited me into his small office and closed the door. He explained that he now routinely met with the warlord Mohamed Farrah Aidid early each day. After each meeting, he would feel optimistic about the challenges that he and Aidid both agreed upon. But when he listened to Radio Mogadishu at 4 p.m. every afternoon, Aidid reported just the direct opposite from each of their morning discussions. The warlord broadcast anti–UN propaganda, alleging that the UN was purposefully marginalizing him in an attempt to rebuild Somalia. Each of these meetings was incredibly frustrating for the new man on the job because he was just going around in circles and getting nowhere with Aidid.

I asked this new UN Special Envoy to describe Aidid's behavior during their face-to-face meetings. His perception of the warlord was someone who was in complete control of his statements and emotions and he never blinked—even when he was blatantly lying. I defined the similar behaviors of all sociopathic narcissists, citing Saddam Hussein as one example. The U.S. State Department had standard training for negotiations based on a methodology that favored diplomacy, logical thinking, established customs, and non-adversarial bargaining. The instructional sessions were called "Getting to YES: Negotiating Agreement Without Giving In." But these strategies were insufficient and naïve, not designed to work on sociopathic narcissists, and they certainly would never work with Aidid's recognized psychopathology.

---

1. Mark Fineman, "Africa Nation Before Its Civil War Began: They Could Reap Big Rewards If Peace Is Restored," *Los Angeles Times*, January 18, 1993. Available at https://www.latimes.com/archives/la-xpm-1993-01-18-mn-1337-story.html.

In 1991, Operation Provide Comfort in Iraq provided another vital lesson. Measuring a mission's success required a way to determine if progress was being made. The military's task in Somalia was to deliver food and goods that were stacking up in warehouses—and the military's responsibility then ended at that point. The amount of transported food tonnage was used as a way to gauge effectiveness, so with warehouses full of goods, the mission was technically a success.

Realistically, food tonnage was a poor measure of success because once the boxes of food left the warehouse, they were often lost or stolen along the route to the distribution sites. The food that remained was supposedly allocated to the needy people in the villages. But within this civil war framework, the warlords were the dispensers and favored their own tribes almost exclusively, leaving many other Somalis to starve to death.[2]

A more meaningful measure of effectiveness (MOE) in Somalia would have been to check the number of tons of food stored at the time of departure compared to the number of tons delivered. This quantity reflected the actual security goal that the U.S. military was unable to control. Additionally, a less useful MOE employed in Somalia was the number of guns collected. This measure was not significant because the number of arms that required confiscation was unknown, and a steady flow of new weapons kept entering the country. Even if many of these guns were seized, violent acts using modern weaponry still occurred. It would have been better to determine security success by the count of violent attacks against a convoy or at a rural distribution site.[3]

With the problems of food distribution and arms trafficking ever present, we traveled from Mogadishu to Addis Ababa, Ethiopia, to attend the third follow-up UN-sponsored meeting on humanitarian assistance. The talks were billed as the "Conference on National Reconciliation in Somalia." Women's groups from Somalia were significantly represented at the sessions. Having made up more than half of the deaths in this war, they wanted to focus on the rehabilitation of Somali society. But participants wondered just how powerful and capable these groups would be once they returned home.

During this meeting in Addis Ababa, all 15 Somali parties notably agreed to the terms set up to restore peace and democracy. But this accord among the parties, which was signed on March 27, did not last. By May 1993, it became clear that Mohamed Farrah Aidid's faction, although a signatory to the Addis Ababa Agreement, would not cooperate in the pact's implementation.

The overriding concern of our small team, which was shared by the U.S. government, was the obligation of relief and rehabilitation. Security was always on the minds of the NGOs, most of whom felt physically threatened in this highly mercurial

---

2. "Frederick M. Burkle, Jr., et al., "Strategic Disaster Management and Response: Implications for Military Medicine Under Joint Command, *Military Medicine* 161:8, 442–447. Available at https://academic.oup.com/milmed/article/161/8/442/4843392.

3. Frederick M. Burkle et al., "Complex Humanitarian Emergencies: III. Measures of Effectiveness," *Prehospital and Disaster Medicine* 10(1), 48–56. Available at https://pubmed.ncbi.nlm.nih.gov/10155407/.

country. Nevertheless, as we left Somalia on March 15, having spent two weeks on our mission, we were encouraged by new commitments in progress to strengthen the security of personnel, vehicles, and compounds.

Regrettably, the worst of our predictions took place in October 1993 long after we had departed. During the 15-hour Battle of Mogadishu on October 3–4, Aidid's forces shot down two Black Hawk helicopters, which led to the deaths of 18 U.S. soldiers plus hundreds of Somalis killed or wounded. These military losses turned the tide of public opinion in the United States, and President Clinton decided to pull out U.S. troops.

The consequences of this event, unfortunately, reached far beyond U.S. actions in Mogadishu that year. Just six months later, another nearby volatile African nation at the time, Rwanda, began its descent into hell through civil war, which lasted from April to July 1994. After years of unrest beneath the surface, the Hutu majority ethnic group took power and unleashed a brutal campaign of genocide against the Tutsi minority. Before the slaughter ended, an estimated 800,000 people had been killed in just a matter of weeks.[4]

Because of what had happened in Somalia with the killings and graphic images of U.S. military pilots being dragged through the streets of Mogadishu, U.S. leadership at the highest civilian and military levels refused to intervene in Rwanda. Those in power came up with numerous excuses to justify their inaction, haggling over the use of words such as "genocide" and whether or not they were bound to act. Regrettably, the world watched as the United States and other members of the international community did nothing to mitigate one of the most tragic humanitarian crises in modern history.

Thailand-Burma: January 1996

In January 1996, the International Rescue Committee (IRC), the renowned humanitarian aid and relief NGO, asked me to assess its several Thai-Burmese[5] refugee camps before I was to evaluate the progress of IRC teams in Bosnia, Croatia, and Serbia one month later. Thailand, to the southeast, had long sheltered Burmese refugees, including thousands of Karen (Kuh-REN),[6] a large ethnic group traditionally residing along the extensive Thai-Burmese border. For decades, the Karen suffered ethnic and religious persecution, which many still endure today. They have been engaged in conflict with Burma's repressive military government, a struggle that had its origins in the mid–1940s.

---

4. "Rwanda Genocide: 100 Days of Slaughter," BBC News, April 4, 2019. Available at https://www.bbc.com/news/world-africa-26875506.
5. In 1989, the military government officially changed the English translation of the nation, Burma, to Myanmar, but "Burma" is still widely used, often interchangeably with the name "Myanmar."
6. The Karen peoples consist of many distinct ethnic groups, numbering several million in Burma and less than 1 million in Thailand.

By the 1990s, the Karen were confined to a narrow border strip of land inside Thailand. Burmese government officials were protesting at that point that these camps were military staging areas for raids into their country. In 1992, the IRC began providing food, water, health care, sanitation, education, and legal assistance to these refugees in Thailand, many of whom were seeking resettlement in the United States. Even today, in the 2020 decade, occupants are restricted to the camps and are arrested by Thai authorities if they try to leave. Most Karenni have never seen anything of the outside world as they have grown into adulthood.

My assignment was to focus on the malaria program in the camps, which was started in 1996. The project eventually became the long-term WHO Global Malaria Program adopted by the WHO Assembly in 2015. Thailand proper was and still is essentially malaria-free, but those living on the border with Burma were experiencing endemic malaria that is frequently resistant to all medications. The heaviest concentrations of malaria also existed in the highest areas of conflict on both sides of the border. Malaria deaths had risen significantly in the early 1990s, partly due to a chloroquine-resistant strain. The IRC program, using trained village volunteers, independently concentrated on the early detection of multidrug-resistant malaria. Swift discovery has markedly reduced malaria's mortality and morbidity.

The IRC camps I inspected on the border were almost pristine despite the tropical surroundings. I commented that a villager could almost eat off the packed dirt landscape surrounding the thatched buildings because their living environment was seemingly spotless. This attention to cleanliness was likely an important contributing factor to their reduced malaria rates. Sanitation and controlling the female Anopheles mosquito, the insect that is the carrier of malaria, are the major forms of malaria prevention in time of war and its aftermath, especially in Southeast Asia.

During my visit, a team of Burmese men in Thailand prepared to cross the border into Burma to bring supplies to their hidden village deep in the Burmese jungle. We talked about that rainforest site and its malaria surveillance program that brought both early diagnosis and treatment. I was quite curious and wanted to know more about this outreach initiative. The leader offered to take me to the village's malaria laboratory, and, to no one's surprise, I could not resist the invitation. I joined this unauthorized, possibly dangerous expedition across the border into their Burmese homeland.

We couldn't take a direct road into this village since we were in Burma illegally. We therefore had to feel our way through this tangled landscape, a terrain mixed with dense forest growth and steep rock formations. The Burmese trekker ahead of me carried a heavy load of supplies marked "UNICEF" (United Nations International Children's Emergency Fund), yet he started at a relentless trot that never let up. I knew I would be all right as long as I could read that UNICEF sign in front of me. So with great effort, I did my best to keep those large letters in sight as we scrambled along.

The jungle cover I had seen in Vietnam could not compare to this damp, choking foliage. Looking side to side revealed nothing but deep green vegetation, yet I sensed all types of reptilian life nearby. These denizens slinked away through the undergrowth just like the foot of the man directly ahead of me. I kept trying to scrutinize his every move as I clawed for a sure foothold in the slippery brush. This unforgiving morass posed quite a challenge to navigate, and I constantly wondered how my companions knew where they were going.

After a long trek, we came upon a village, its core as impenetrable as the encircling jungle. If I didn't have my guide, I would most likely have missed this site—even from 10 feet away. All the huts blended into the surrounding rainforest, like a perfectly symbiotic relationship between the people and their environment. The village center contained a laboratory with microscopes and a generator—a lab with no walls. The Gram stains used to diagnose malaria were of excellent quality, making an accurate diagnosis possible so a patient could be treated immediately. I was captivated by this setup in this dense green foliage setting.

The Burmese villagers quietly moved among these bamboo structures, which were heavily protected by the thick forest cover. The atmosphere was strangely quiet, the silence taking on a life of its own. Gauging just how many people lived in these conditions was difficult. And yet for the short time I was standing in the middle of nowhere, I saw hundreds of village dwellers come and go in small curious groups. They may have been heading toward a nearby concrete rectangular structure to urinate. Ammonia, a by-product of urea, is a natural snake repellent—and the village certainly needed to keep those snakes at bay. The largest species of snake, the Burmese python, is native to Southeast Asia. They can reach more than 20 feet in length. Even with my task at hand to see this laboratory in the heart of darkness, I was ever watchful for these silent, slithering predators.

The guide explained the area's malaria program, which was modeled after the one employed in the established Thailand border camps. While most of Thailand remained malaria-free, the interactions among the complex landscape, humans, mosquito vectors, and malaria parasites have allowed malaria to thrive along the border as it does nowhere else on earth.

We then made the risky, physically taxing walk back into Thailand. I was exhausted from the heat and exertion, trying to negotiate nonexistent trails and doing battle with insects. But I knew immediately that I would not have made a valid assessment of the camps along the border without knowing firsthand what lay behind them in the thick jungles of Burma.

The next day, I was invited to visit the Médecins Sans Frontières clinic and camp that had recently opened. The physicians ran a type of emergency room setting. They treated the growing health problems of Burmese migrant workers crossing into Thailand, eventually forming mobile medical teams along the border. The clinic had grown over three decades until the organization finally shut down its services in 2011.

Meeting these enthusiastic, young MSF French physicians in the border camps was refreshing. They were just out of med school and probably thinking about where their medical futures might go. I knew the look in their eyes quite well. I had been there myself.

Crossing the middle of their camp was a shallow ravine filled with stagnant water. Loose boards had been placed above the water to form a moveable bridge. As we crossed the wooden planks, the vibration disturbed the water, suddenly engulfing us in a cloud of flies while we balanced ourselves on the boards. This disruption of flies, also carriers of disease, set off alarm bells in my head. But for the moment, I kept these thoughts to myself until I had a chance to see their entire operation.

My hosts then led me to a "meeting room" in an adjacent thatched hut. We sat down to talk about the "research" they were conducting on their patients. Field research was new to them so they were eager for feedback. Unfortunately, I had to tell them that their data were not accurate because they had included just males in their study; females were excluded. Also, their rates of measurement for their research would not be acceptable or recognized by the medical community. But these MSF doctors were early enough in their careers to change their research methodology for more valid results.

When I asked whether the bridge across the stagnant water bothered them, no one spoke. I pointed out that while the emergency medicine they were providing was most helpful to the area population, they were ignoring the malaria-laden area within their camp. Malaria was undoubtedly killing more people than those they saved through their clinic. They admitted they had little experience with malaria, and failed to recognize the significance of a still body of water as a malarial source. This admission surprised me. I then gave them what was probably their first informal lecture on public health and the importance of sanitation in all humanitarian programs.

The young physicians began to talk among themselves as to how they could solve the fly- and mosquito-infested water problem. Given the immaculate camps I visited when I first arrived, I suggested they ask the IRC team to assess their work. The IRC could give them advice about how to clear the camp of other areas of standing water to make sure that those stagnant ponds weren't part of perpetuating the problem.

Since my trip to Burma, MSF has grown into one of the world's most valued NGO humanitarian agencies, along with the International Committee of the Red Cross, in delivering emergency care. I have attended some MSF lectures over the years, and have been relieved to learn about the international organization's focus on emergency care following conflict, natural disasters, and epidemics. Today, MSF proudly talks about ensuring public health protections and programs. These once novice students now saw the importance of public health care and had become teachers themselves.

The Balkans: February 1996

For the entire decade of the 1990s, the republics of the former communist Yugoslavia became embroiled in a separate series of uprisings, some insurgencies even resulting in "ethnic cleansings." Following the death of its autocratic leader, Josip Broz Tito, in May 1980, Yugoslavia broke into six Balkan republics—Slovenia, Croatia, Serbia, Montenegro, Macedonia, and Bosnia-Herzegovina, commonly referred to as "Bosnia." These semi-autonomous republics had been forcefully held together by Marshal Tito for four decades. But with Tito's death, the Bosnian Serb army chief, Ratko Mladić, tore apart the former Yugoslavia, and the population of each republic became divided into the persecutors and the persecuted.

The International Rescue Committee began its work responding to this crisis in the war-stricken city of Sarajevo, the capital of Bosnia, in the cruel winter of 1992–1993. One IRC staff member succinctly stated, "We were seeing a highly industrialized country descend into chaos."

After I was elected to the IRC Board of Directors in the mid–1990s, the Bosnian War finally appeared to be calming down. I evaluated the health situation in three of the beleaguered republics, which once comprised Yugoslavia. My job was to determine how the IRC should respond. The initial review, just a few weeks after my trip to Thailand, was a health security appraisal that would take me first to Bosnia, then east to Serbia, and finally northwest into Croatia.

In February 1996, I linked up with Bob Macpherson once again. I hadn't seen Bob since our collaboration in Somalia in 1993. We met at the airport in the Croatian city of Split on the Adriatic Sea. Bob had arrived earlier that month to do a security evaluation in Bosnia. We then traveled northeast to Zenica, Bosnia, to confer with the director of IRC Services. Bob was already primed with essential information on health security issues, which armed me with data to make accurate assessments of health conditions in Serbia and Croatia.

When I returned to Zenica weeks later, however, Bob was extremely ill with pneumonia, according to my on-the-spot diagnosis. I took him to the Zenica hospital to get an x-ray. The attending physician confirmed that he had pneumonia, but she apologized and bluntly admitted her hospital had no medicines except aspirin. Then Bob and I visited the MSF office of the health team working in Zenica. We found that this highly respected and well-known NGO also had no antibiotics due to an existing blockade by the Serbs. Luckily, Bob's fever finally broke on its own and he recovered. But I added this experience to my review of the problems that reflected all the health care facilities, at least in Bosnia.

Before the Bosnian War began in April 1992, the diverse Bosnian population, comprising 44 percent Muslims, 32 percent Serbs, and 17 percent Croats,[7] had lived in mixed communities. The long-time residents, who were from various cultural and

---

7. Jack Donnelly and Daniel J. Whelan, *International Human Rights* (New York: Routledge, 2018), 12.

religious backgrounds, worked and played together in neighborhoods set against an orange patchwork of tile-roofed homes. Many of these dwellings were now tarnished with one home burned to the ground and the adjacent one, according to the owner's ethnicity, would still be standing and left undamaged. This disturbing pattern now displayed an endless symbol of the hate the Bosnian Serbs had for their Muslim neighbors. Ironically, prior to the conflict, their sons and daughters had played soccer together in the same localities.

In many ways, this war's ethnic insanity played out all across the Balkans, and was tragically similar to what had occurred during the Rwanda genocide in 1994. The Serbs, consisting of paramilitary and former Yugoslavian army units, focused their ethnic cleansing against the Bosniaks, the Muslim Bosnians. But the Croats were both the victims and perpetrators of the madness. And Sarajevo was the site of one of the bloodiest and most prolonged battles of the war. The Bosnian hub of culture was marked by daily sniper attacks and indiscriminate shelling from the Serb national forces. Constant fighting and the mass killing of civilians overwhelmed medical facilities.

I was struck by the near destruction of a once beautiful city. Every park and sports field, including the site of the 1984 Winter Olympics, was turned into crowded graveyards. Even more somber, hundreds of children had been buried in the center of the former Olympics Stadium. Flowers and notices of those looking for their kin covered the key battle sites within the city. A clear consequence of this siege of Sarajevo was a city now laid to waste with a soaring suicide rate.

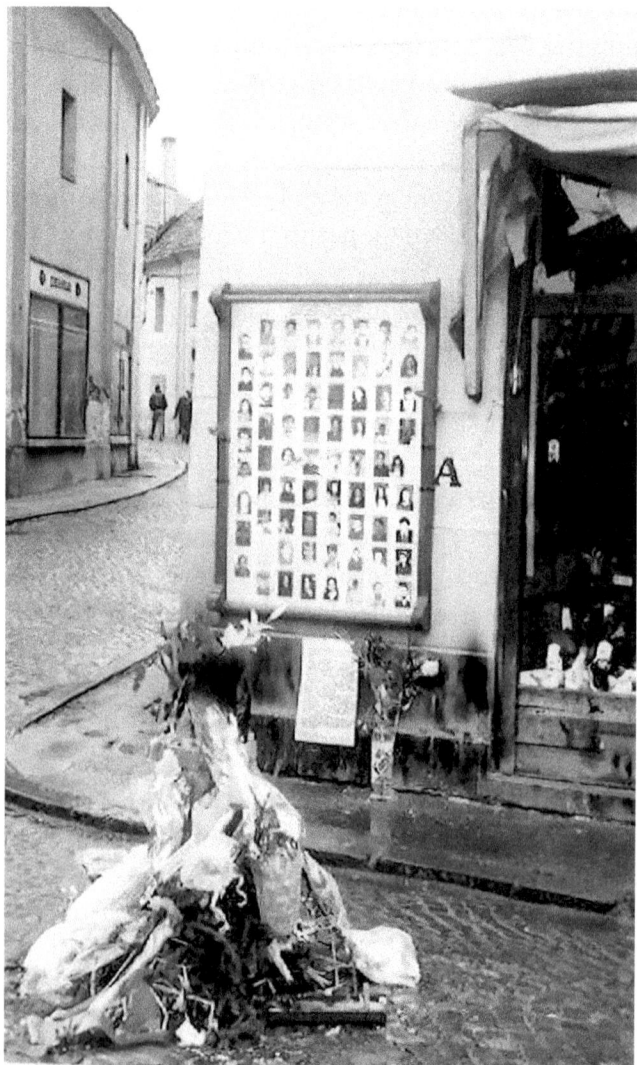

Families posted notices of their missing kin near key battle sites inside Sarajevo during the Bosnian War (author's collection).

In the formerly united Yugoslavia, bound by Tito's iron hand, ethnic and religious rights were protected. With the strongman gone for more than a decade, both Serbs and Croats now claimed the Muslims were not a genuine nationality. In his 1996 book, *Love Thy Neighbor: A Story of War*,[8] Peter Maass writes: "The goal of ethnic cleansing was not simply to get rid of Muslims; it was to destroy all traces that they had ever lived in Bosnia. The goal was to kill history. If you want to do that, then you must rip out history's heart, which in the case of Bosnia's Muslim community meant the destruction of its mosques. Once that was done, you could reinvent the past in whatever distorted form you wanted, like Frankenstein."

The trip across the border from Bosnia into Serbia was very revealing. For the first time, we were seeing increasing numbers of the newly arrived North Atlantic Treaty Organization (NATO) Implementation Force at many border checkpoints. Destroyed tanks had been pushed to the sides of the roads, and I saw no signs of any refugee camps for Muslim Serbs. The few Bosnian Serbs I met were mostly defiant in conversations.

My IRC escort and I stopped at one point for a health appraisal of a small village with a narrow but picturesque main street. I then began walking by myself down the middle of the street, ignored by passing citizens. Suddenly I heard shots ring out in the direction I was heading. Instantly, NATO peacekeeping troops rushed past me, pressing forward down the hill as the gunfire continued. Notably, the locals were oblivious to the commotion and went about their routine because it seemed this deadly turmoil was an everyday occurrence.

I slowly walked back to where I had separated from my IRC guide and continued to observe this village's residents denying or disregarding the existence of the nearby shooting. I was aware that Bosnian Serb soldiers had been placed in refugee camps inside Serbia, refusing to give up their weapons and vowing to return to Bosnia to fight again. These disgruntled soldiers appeared to be the source of the gunfire. Bosnian Serbs did not feel welcome in Serbia.

Outside another Serbian city, we visited several recently built NGO clinics on the city's periphery. They had been operational for more than a week, but I was able to see only a small number of them needing aid. Riding in a vehicle provided by the IRC, we ventured into the city center, which seemed quiet despite the destruction of many homes and important buildings. I asked about public transportation and was advised to go three city blocks farther where we came upon a vast, muddy field. Lined up side by side were 20 wrecked derelict buses.

After returning to the NGO encampment, I advised several officials that they had to move their clinics into the city, preferably to a vacant lot near those buses. That step would display the NGO's willingness to come to the people, who were still anxious and suspicious. The NGO personnel had to convince the citizens that they would stay and only leave the city once local transportation was functioning again.

---

8. Peter Maass, *Love Thy Neighbor: A Story of War* (New York: Vintage, 1997), 85.

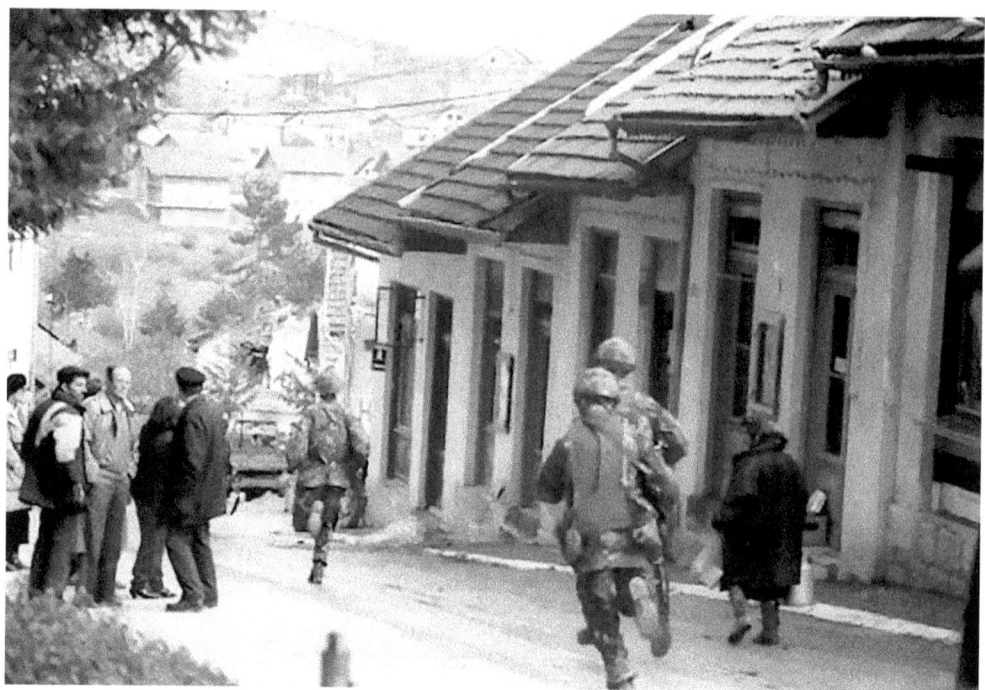

Suddenly Skip heard shots ring out in a small Serbian village. Unconcerned, bystanders went about their business (author's collection).

Our team left Serbia for Croatia which seemed to suffer the least from this prolonged war. My first stop was to listen to NGO workers who had been dealing with the medical rehabilitation of war-related amputees. The NGO rehab programs were ignored by Croatian government medical advisors who had placed all amputees together, separated from their families. To Croatian physicians, "rehabilitation" meant having these amputees live the remainder of their lives playing wheelchair basketball. The doctors did not deal with the physical aspects of amputation, particularly the prevention of contractures.[9] I was amazed by how some outdated views remain in which medical education and advances are lacking. Unfortunately, the NGOs operating in Croatia soon left the country.

I was particularly eager to visit the hospitals in Croatia's capital, Zagreb. Leila Richards, a physician with the International Rescue Committee, had championed several of the medical programs in those Zagreb facilities. One procedure she had managed for three years was a medevac policy that orchestrated hospital treatment and rehabilitation in 10 Croatian hospitals. This setup cared for more than 1,500 Bosnian children and adults with war-related injuries, extensive burns, and amputations, as well as infants and children with leukemia and cancerous tumors. However, the arrangement did not allow the mothers to accompany their children. The IRC

---

9. A contracture is a permanent tightening of the muscles, tendons, skin, and nearby tissues that causes joints to shorten and then stiffen. This condition prevents normal movement of a joint or other body part. Contractures may be caused by injury, scarring, nerve damage, or non-use of the muscles.

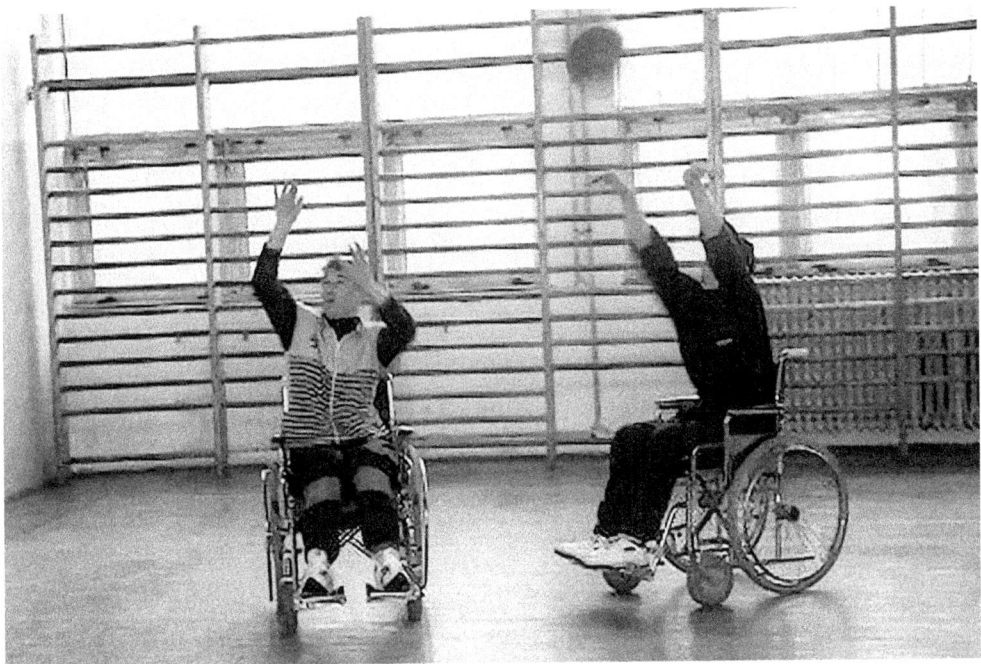

In the limited mindset of Croatian physicians, "rehabilitation" meant having amputees live the remainder of their lives playing wheelchair basketball (author's collection).

financially compensated the hospitals that took care of these Bosnian children and guaranteed their safety.

As a pediatrician, I was eager to observe the care of these infants and children. The program's excellent administration had been well publicized. The head of this particular Zagreb hospital[10] was a physician who was also my tour guide. A massive building with huge wards, this hospital was constructed during World War II. My guide proudly brought me into one of the wards, which was the size of a basketball court and specifically designated for treating children with pneumonia. I found all the children smiling, laughing, and standing in their cribs, a situation not seen even in more developed countries. I learned that these were all Croatian youngsters.

Regardless of their recovery prognosis, this doctor informed me that these children would remain in that hospital ward for three months, even though that antiquated rule of recovery time was unwarranted. When I questioned the physician, he responded that this was hospital regulation, adding that parents were not welcome to visit their children during that period. I found this hospital directive ridiculous. By this time, medical advancements in the U.S. and elsewhere called for antibiotics with minimal hospital stays for this kind of diagnosis.

I was growing impatient because I had repeatedly asked to see the Bosnian Muslim children. Finally, I bluntly insisted that he must stop the tour and take me to see those other young patients. Caving into my persistence, he reluctantly agreed, and I

---

10. University Hospital Center Zagreb is located on the Orebro campus.

followed him out of the ward and down another interminable corridor with empty wards. I didn't see nursing stations or any nurses on duty.

In the distance at the very end of the corridor was a large ward that also appeared empty but for one crib. The strong sun was beating down on a tiny mattress. In the crib was an infant tied down, obviously dehydrated and motionless. His cry was very weak. I examined the skin turgor[11] and the infant's lack of response, quickly asserting that the child was severely dehydrated, malnourished, and desperately in need of intravenous fluids. I was extremely disturbed and disappointed in this hospital guide. He was a physician and had purposely tried to hide these despicable conditions from me. My anger ignited this Croatian doctor's rage, and he arrogantly declared, "You pay us to treat children with cancer. You said nothing about feeding them!"

My indignation was evident and I countered that my visit was over. We were silent as we made our way back through the endless corridors, ending up at the austere entrance to the hospital. During the entire walk, I had the image of that sad and dehydrated infant in my head. My fury intensified as I thought of the number of health care workers in this building, presumably dedicated professionals who allowed this situation to exist. The hospital director then had the nerve to hand me a list of radiological equipment for the International Rescue Committee to purchase for the hospital. Incredulous, I just turned my back on him and walked away. As in many other similarly frustrating situations that I had encountered inspecting such facilities, I could do little to help that unfortunate infant.

This one event did not disparage my feelings for the IRC program, which had saved countless lives. But as with other assessment situations I had made during this particular evaluation process over the years, I came to an important realization: A humanitarian medical aid program must be embedded in a way in which health care assistance interfaces with recipients getting the medical aid. What I had already witnessed was that just under the surface of the smiling faces, projected for my benefit, the intercultural hatreds were still dominant and unforgiving. And they would continue to last for decades, leading to unnecessary and uncounted morbidity and mortality. These kinds of aid programs, in some instances, must have prolonged oversight by a neutral party.

* * * *

On my long flights back to my island home, I would have plenty of time to digest what I had recently witnessed. I concentrated on what I had learned, how this new experience was different from previous ones, or how it was the same. I would always be eager to share the highest highs and the lowest lows with Phyllis.

And how had Phyllis continued to cope with my frequent absences? She often said that our life together had always been, in so many instances, a life apart so

---

11. Skin turgor refers to the elasticity of skin. By pinching the skin, a physician can measure the extent of the patient's dehydration or fluid loss in the body.

adjustment to that reality seemed easier for her. And by now, we had finally settled down in Kailua. The kids were grown and had left.

In 1999, I again headed back to the Balkans, this time to Kosovo. I was part of a NATO and U.S. State Department team assessing the medical aftermath of the war between Albanian and ethnic Serbs in the Serbian southern province of Kosovo.[12] This time, while I looked at the declining public health protections, our IRC team emphasized a new generation of medical leadership that included training in the U.S. and elsewhere.

The humanitarian field is becoming ever more multidisciplinary. Health care has never stood alone in solving the many problems we have faced in the global public health arena.

---

12. The dispute finally ended in February 2008 when Kosovo declared its independence from Serbia.

11

The Center of Excellence

1994–2000

> *"The chief investigator concluded, 'We've never advised this to anyone before, but we strongly recommend that you sue the U.S. Army.'"*

I consider the most important undertaking of my life to also be the most trying, painful period of my life. This chapter of my life ended in failure, great disappointment, and regret during the mid- to late 1990s. For decades, I had a persistent dream of disaster relief and humanitarian agencies effectively cooperating and coordinating their mutual efforts in times of natural and manmade catastrophes. I witnessed both successes and mistakes throughout all of my site visits and evaluations of complex emergencies throughout the last decade of the 20th century. I was determined to help future responses be developed and improved.

That dream came to fruition in 1994 when I founded the Center of Excellence[1] for Disaster Management and Humanitarian Assistance (COE). This COE program in Hawaii was the first of several other COEs being developed across the United States in the 1990s. I remained Director of this COE under three commanding officers of Tripler Army Medical Center until February 2000 when the COE program, as I had envisioned it, ended in tragedy and adversity.

Before 1994, what would eventually be called the "Center of Excellence" was, at that time, designated as a "humanitarian training center" at the University of Hawaii (UH) School of Medicine. I was a faculty member and also Chair of the Division of Emergency Medicine at UH. But I had imagined a more formal structure and home for an all-encompassing center for disaster management. This COE program would promote and host educational and preparatory events concerning civil-military coordination and refugee care in disasters around the world, and the one I was overseeing in Hawaii would specifically serve the Asia-Pacific arena. If the concept worked, a COE would hopefully have a place in each region of the world.

At the time of this appointment, I had recently been involved in complex emergencies in northern Iraq and Somalia as the civil-military liaison. The lack

---

1. In 1994, the Center of Excellence, now called the "Center for Excellence," was mandated by an Act of Congress.

of coordination and preparedness surrounding these joint operations gave me increased cause for worry. The major topic of dispute among the military and all civilian organizations during these experiences was the absence of coordination and collaboration in an efficient and synchronized manner. The Center of Excellence's task would be to expand that harmony.

Enhancing Civil-Military Relationships

From the start of my career to the beginning of the 2020 decade, the one persistent issue, which caused trouble during each deployment, had been trying to augment the working relationship between involved agencies with a stake in humanitarian operations—whether they are related to sudden-onset natural disasters or war and conflict. These parties' disconnects have often been continuous and sometimes detrimental. The bone of contention has primarily been among large non-governmental agencies (NGOs), the U.S. military, the World Health Organization (WHO), and the International Committee of the Red Cross (ICRC).

I often found myself straddling the issues in discussions and also in my lectures. We needed participants and organizations with the best experience, but each expert or group would have a distinct perspective. Admiral Joseph W. Prueher, Commander in Chief, U.S. Pacific Command (PACOM), and future Ambassador to China, was very receptive to the COE concept of coordination. To foster better management and readiness, he encouraged and worked with me to formalize a center to study and train American NGOs, the UN, other international bodies, and military components.

Future COE programs, which were being formed around the country, shared faculty who all provided leadership, research, support, training, and best practices to obtain results. Offering better civil-military coordination and refugee care through training courses would (1) create a framework for adopting change, (2) build a better blueprint for future disaster needs, and (3) offer guidance on how to sustain a humanitarian effort wherever necessary.

Although these centers were different in many ways, they each had much in common, and collaboration seemed promising with the individual COEs to improve an area of need. Every COE concentrated on bringing together disparate groups and agencies that all felt ownership of an issue. No single group acting alone could handle global humanitarian assistance problems. By working together in a COE, organizations could develop joint solutions and hopefully chart a better course of action to work side by side in a crisis.

In most instances, an academic affiliation was key to the COE model because a university could facilitate the necessary research and scholarly approach to real-world problems. These academic links were not an end in themselves, but they were a means to achieve consensus and ensure a measure of success.

Senator Daniel Inouye's Initiative

After several discussions with Hawaii's Senator Daniel Inouye, I found him to be very supportive. His vision was to link the University of Hawaii and the numerous Hawaii-based military resources. That association would be helpful in civil-military conflicts in the Asia-Pacific arena in which humanitarian implications might arise. The Center of Excellence would be headquartered in Honolulu for this Pacific region and form a partnership among these institutions: U.S. Pacific Command, University of Hawaii, Pacific Regional Medical Command, and Centers for Disease Control and Prevention (CDC), which, to date, had no presence in the Asia-Pacific theater. The initial plan was to focus on the neutral campus of the University of Hawaii. The problem remained about how to allocate congressionally approved funds because, as it turned out, Senator Inouye could provide that financial backing only through the military, not through a university.

Senator Inouye sent me a personal letter asking if I would be comfortable having an arrangement with Tripler Army Medical Center in Honolulu. Tripler was the headquarters of the Pacific Regional Medical Command, which encompassed all military branches of the armed forces. Tripler was also home to the Senator's global Telemedicine Program named "Akamai,"[2] which provided health care to multiple remote islands in the Pacific. In the Hawaiian language, "Akamai" means "intelligent." I considered this suggestion as long as COE was accepted as a unique, lateral organization for which independence from the military would be critical to its success.

The mission statement, drafted in Senator Inouye's office in Washington, strongly stated that COE and its collaborators would preserve the separate nature of the Center of Excellence as a priority between partners. These affiliates would reap the success and benefits generated by the flexibility and creativity that COE's autonomy would protect. The "products" produced by COE would be timely and useful for the Department of Defense, U.S. governmental agencies, foreign governments, militaries, and the broad civilian relief community.

Commanding Officer of Tripler No. 1

I had assembled a Board of Advisors, composed of members from the American Red Cross, the Federal Emergency Management Agency, and the Research Corporation of the University of Hawaii. After Senator Inouye briefed the Commanding Officer of Tripler, a general, I set up a meeting with him, the Board of Advisors, and any Tripler staff members who would be working with us. To put it mildly, that first meeting did not go well.

---

2. F. Craig Floro et al., "An Overview of the AKAMAI Telemedicine Project: A Pacific Perspective." In Proceedings of the 32nd Annual Hawaii International Conference on Systems Sciences, Maui, Hawaii, January 5–8, 1999. Available at https://ieeexplore.ieee.org/document/773032?arnumber=773032.

With the representative COE members seated around a large conference table, the General briskly entered the room. Standing at the head of the table with an imposing military bearing, he threw me my first curveball: He would not allow me to introduce myself, let me present the Board members, or even permit me to explain the COE concept. He simply stated that the COE money belonged to Tripler, and therefore he would deal with those congressionally allocated funds as he pleased.

Before he left the room, I tried to remind him of the mission statement that I knew Senator Inouye had previously discussed with him, but my attempt fell flat in mid-sentence. Any further words were curtailed since the General stated he had "no time to go over the details."

The meeting abruptly ended. Left alone in the conference room, the entire Board of Advisors felt insulted and confused as I had not anticipated or warned them of this conflict. Senator Inouye's staff members had assured me that they had briefed the Commanding Officer, and everything COE-related was in order. Not an optimistic or congenial beginning for the Hawaii COE.

Unfortunately, this authoritative power grab by Tripler Army Medical Center resulted in the American Red Cross and the University of Hawaii's School of Public Health's dramatic exit from the Board of Advisors. All the representatives thought they would be participating in a horizontal partnership. The General's comments, however, made short work of that notion. The Board of Advisors had vanished before it had even gotten off the ground. But despite this dramatic setback, I was intent on making the COE's goal come to pass. I felt responsible for what I considered a violation of the congressional language. I shared my discouragement with the Senator's Chief of Staff who was my immediate contact to his office.

Disappointed but not defeated by this turn of events, I was willing to make accommodations with the General to salvage the COE's objective, and he was willing to reconsider the arrangement. Senator Inouye's Chief of Staff agreed to work with the General on the details of the COE's mission. Some semblances of the deal eventually enabled COE to start functioning. We were physically moved several times as I hired more staff. The COE eventually settled into a vacant ward at Tripler, which we shared with the Senator's prized Telemedicine Program.

According to Senator Inouye's office, Tripler was still well aware of the conflict regarding the interpretation of the COE's mission and authority. I asked the Chief of Staff how Tripler would handle a review of the congressional funds if the other partners were not included. Inexplicably, Tripler did not let me see my budget, sign any contracts, or know their contents. Those tasks would be carried out by a business manager, who was formerly military, plus a military officer I had hired for our operational programs, which were financed using delegated COE funds. This policy was a military dictate I could not change. Not knowing where the financial resources were going and how those resources were being allocated caused me great concern.

But I had a safeguard: Funds were negotiated with Senator Inouye's office, and I was constantly assured by Senator Inouye's Chief of Staff that the Senator's team closely monitored these programs. All the same, I suspected that the potential existed for nefarious activities to occur without my oversight, including the use of COE funds for unrelated Tripler purposes. I frequently would console my wife and other COE colleagues that the only benefit to these incomprehensible orders was that I could never be held responsible for any financial blunders. Such a model never existed in the civilian world. In the end, this flawed approach turned out to be fatal to the organization.

On the Same Wavelength

At first, the General's negative attitude did not change, but he made no gesture to impede COE's progress. He began to appreciate the benefits of the COE, openly encouraging its developing programs. My first task was to build a multidisciplinary faculty, all of whom had operational experience. The major contention among the military and the civilian organizations was the lack of effective coordination and not working together smoothly and efficiently, which were two critical missions to advance and improve. The COE needed staff on the same wavelength, subject matter expert (SME) participants, and organizations with the best experience. But each expert or group would have a distinct perspective that represented its views and operational needs.

Being the head of an academic department at the University of Hawaii proved to be no match for Tripler's complicated and often perplexing bureaucracy. A nurse at Tripler warned me that this Army Medical Center was historically considered a place where people's careers were often "cursed." Nonetheless, I was convinced that COE would progress, and I was certain that I could renegotiate some of these issues as the COE's programs succeeded. The Senator's Chief of Staff also reassured me that Senator Inouye respected and admired my program.

Regrettably, I was never able to get the COE's Board of Advisors to reassemble. After that fateful first meeting, every member had resigned on the spot because the General outright dismissed the members' concerns. Annual meetings eventually occurred between the General and the designate from UH's President's office. But my major priority was to fill positions for the required subject matter experts and then have those hired people work on specific assignments. I wanted them all to be significant, undeniable authorities in their respective fields, and also be able to work together in identifying problems in operational communication. Most of all, I encouraged them to seek ways in which interaction could be made better. Tripler and Senator Inouye's office agreed.

Before the General left Tripler as Commanding Officer, he had begun to have confidence in my judgment. He admitted he was educated by my discussions and the programs we sponsored. We became trusted friends. I began to research and hire SMEs who came from the NGO community, the CDC, the UN, and academia.

The General let me run COE but Tripler brought in a civilian business manager. I selected an Army major who was both an osteopathic physician and a nurse, and who was just starting a disaster management career. In combination, the civilian business manager and the Army major were to oversee the budget. Both reported to Tripler, not to me, on financial issues. I was completely excluded from the process, a very uncomfortable personal situation that always left lingering and unsettling feelings.

Commanding Officer of Tripler No. 2

The next Commanding Officer at Tripler, another general, was most helpful in allowing the expansion of partnerships and contributions to NGOs in this country, but to a greater degree, connecting with international organizations. By that time in the mid-1990s, the world was clamoring for the expertise that COE was offering. Funding for the Hawaii COE increased as did the number of staff and programs. An additional COE was being developed with Tulane University and the University of Florida to support the U.S. Southern Command.

The new General championed the Center of Excellence, having a broad understanding of its worth. He felt it was appropriately placed at Tripler as one of the Army Medical Center's operational partners. He proudly talked of COE's contributions, emphasizing that its mission was one that all military medical centers should adopt.

I was required to consult monthly with the Senator's Chief of Staff to keep her updated on our programs. She was always pleased and thought I was managing the relationship with Tripler well—minus the organization's Board of Advisors. But I certainly felt the absence of the protection and solidarity that the Board of Advisors would have provided me.

Under the new General, the COE's programs grew and flourished. He maintained that every major military medical facility should have a COE, which, he declared, was the "future" of military medicine. Despite strong initial opposition to COE by Tripler's preceding Commanding Officer, the Medical Center began receiving kudos for COE's work both nationally and internationally. Many prominent scientists, researchers, and administrators came to Tripler for briefings. In 1997, continued successes resulted in our COE in Hawaii receiving Congress's Federal Program of the Year award.

Tripler, however, refused to distribute congressionally appropriated funds to its academic partner, the University of Hawaii. I was a full professor at UH but my salary with COE, paid by Tripler, not by the University, was only $25,000, which made me the lowest-paid COE employee. That salary discrepancy would likely never be rectified. Instead, I focused on obtaining those researchers who were publishing useful information for the COE mission. I hired Doug Bond from Harvard whose studies focused on identifying Asia-Pacific countries' levels of internal unrest and conflict. His competence and proficiency immediately made him a favorite with Pacific Command leadership, especially with Admiral Prueher.

"If COE Did Not Exist, It Would Have to Be Invented"

In October 1998, Admiral Prueher wrote to Senator Inouye: The COE "has matured to the point of being an indispensable component of operational readiness in the Asia-Pacific area. The COE has helped navigate U.S. Pacific Command through the complexities of humanitarian operations. Its contributors, and especially its interfaces with non-government organizations and international agencies, have bridged a very important gap in our traditional military architecture. If the COE did not exist, it would have to be invented."[3]

That same year, Admiral Prueher personally hosted a workshop at Tripler and gave the keynote speech for representatives of other commanders-in-chief of primary U.S. commands around the world. Admiral Prueher explained the COE model and urged these top officers to adopt the COE mission at their respective regional levels. The Pacific Command was becoming our most consistent customer and Admiral Prueher was its spokesman. His main goal was to support the idea of a likeminded COE program at every combatant command.

To accomplish this goal of civil-military cooperation, we identified and hired the required subject matter experts: a UN communications specialist and well-known academic scholars. Most critically, we established the expertise of the Centers for Disease Control and Prevention for the first time in the Asia-Pacific region. The CDC officials were ecstatic. Before the mid–1990s, their absence had been a major deficiency. The Pacific Command now had ready access to CDC's infectious disease expertise in response to an epidemic or pandemic in the Asia-Pacific region.

Most importantly, I developed a crucial relationship with the International Committee of the Red Cross in Geneva. Many humanitarian issues and the performance of all COE partners focused on working relationships under both the 1949 Geneva Conventions and International Humanitarian Law (IHL). The U.S. military all too often had little knowledge of the structural legalities of IHL or the Geneva Conventions.

In the early 1970s, I was the second American to take the ICRC-sponsored course titled "Health Emergencies in Large Populations" (HELP) in Geneva. As a Navy Reserve officer, I had to resign my commission, take the course, then reapply for the naval commission. This training curriculum was excellent, including learning about the unique differences between the ICRC approach to military combat and that taken by the representatives from Médecins Sans Frontières (Doctors Without Borders).

After coursework completion, I spent an additional two weeks studying more

---

3. Letter dated October 8, 1998, from Admiral Joseph W. Prueher, Commander in Chief, U.S. Pacific Command, to Senator Daniel K. Inouye.

about the Geneva Conventions and International Humanitarian Law at the University of Geneva. Before starting the Asia-Pacific COE, I had taught many HELP courses at the Johns Hopkins School of Public Health, the only venue in the United States that was offering these classes.

Realizing that the HELP courses were essential to the military and COE audience, I began negotiations with Dr. Pierre Perrin, Director of the HELP program at the ICRC in Geneva, to begin this training course through COE.

Because the International Committee of the Red Cross feared possible control of the lesson content by the U.S. military, the talks went to the highest levels of ICRC, taking four years of consultations. The COE program even facilitated funding a translation of the *HELP Manual* from French into English. But ICRC demanded that these classes be given at neutral civilian centers, not offered at military installations and not taught by military instructors. I negotiated with UH's research and education facility, the East-West Center, to become our annual home for the HELP courses, rather than through COE at Tripler.

In April 1997, after many personal discussions with WHO colleagues both in Geneva and at the Pan-American Health Organization (PAHO), our COE was designated as the "PAHO/WHO Collaborating Center for Humanitarian Civil-Military Cooperation." I was asked to head this new organization. The Collaborating Center opened many doors to educate, train, and provide operational research for military forces. In turn, the military would work with civilian counterparts, NGOs, and other participants before and during humanitarian missions.

The Collaborating Center established five directives. First, COE had to identify areas of civil-military cooperation in different types of emergencies: natural disasters or war and conflict. Second, COE had to establish guidelines and recommendations on content, strategy, tactics, and managerial approaches for mutual emergency humanitarian intervention. Third, COE had to formulate recommendations on how civil-military humanitarian cooperation could be integrated into a comprehensive emergency preparedness and response strategy. Fourth, COE had to create Pacific Disaster Electronic Information Networks. Fifth, COE had to develop methodologies for the transfer of disaster response information and skills.

These five guidelines neatly summarized COE's duties. However, one caveat stipulated that if I left COE, the "Collaborating Center" designation would be canceled. The Collaborating Center could not be controlled by the military. The main concern was the ongoing issue: Could COE maintain its autonomy from the U.S. military? During the conferences, several NGO representatives were hostile toward the military, resulting in the proverbial shouting sessions occurring in all our joint conferences. But this rivalry was expected because COE was the only organization that brought all these disparate experts together after many decades of being on opposing sides. Representatives from WHO stated adamantly that no military personnel were to be members. But I explained that this issue needed to be negotiated—yet another one of the many challenges ahead of me and the COE program.

We were making progress, however, at many conferences, and COE was increasingly seen as the place of choice for the Disaster Management and Humanitarian Assistance program. We were making inroads into the cooperation of major international organizations, a singular COE objective. Plaudits came in from Senator Inouye's office and other government groups, as well as academia. In 1998, Robert Seiple, President of World Vision International, a Christian humanitarian NGO, voiced what Admiral Prueher had also asserted: that had COE not already been established, it would have to be created.

Commanding Officer of Tripler No. 3

Shortly after the next Commanding Officer took over, the Command Suite staff organized a meet-and-greet session for this new General. Invitees included department heads and other representative groups to formally present themselves and their programs. When I introduced myself as the Director of COE, the General responded, "I know all about the Center of Excellence and I'm getting rid of it. It doesn't belong in my hospital!"

She then turned and walked away. I was speechless. I had never experienced this kind of disrespect in the civilian or military world. The next day, the General also conveyed that same curt message to those in charge of the long-standing Akamai Telemedicine Program also housed at Tripler.

At the beginning of her tenure, the focus was on removing the Telemedicine Program. The Senator's Chief of Staff was heavily involved in overseeing both the Telemedicine and COE programs. During a brief telephone conversation, she stated that for now "COE was safe." For several weeks I heard nothing about this third General's plans for COE. But in anticipation, I penned a letter that would warn the COE employees of the pending COE program closure.

Suddenly, we found that some of the Telemedicine Program's civilian leaders were being removed, and their office doors were locked to prevent them from gaining access to personal and professional property. This action came uncomfortably close to home since both the Telemedicine Program and COE occupied the same floor. However, the General now envisioned COE as a "primarily military program" not to be under my direction. This abrupt change of control over the program was the antithesis of everything COE had accomplished to date and what the Senator and I had visualized.

Losing Ground

Gradually my authority as Director of COE diminished. At our first University of Hawaii-owned conference regarding the HELP courses, the new Commanding

Officer unexpectedly attended. She welcomed the audience and then took credit for sponsoring the HELP courses. Dr. Pierre Perrin, the Director of the HELP program in Geneva, was present and he became visibly angry. In my previous negotiations with the International Committee of the Red Cross, I had guaranteed that the military would not oversee the HELP program. Perrin was furious with the General's declaration since ICRC had always made it very clear that it would not have any affiliation with the military.

On a positive note, one which I dearly needed, I finally received a phone call I had been eagerly anticipating: Admiral Prueher's strong lobbying with other worldwide combatant commands to adopt a COE program was now a possibility. At the start of the Kosovo operation in 1998, the European Command (EUCOM) requested, through PACOM, that I assist them in the development of their medical response to the Balkan refugee crisis. The recommendation came directly from Admiral Prueher's office at PACOM. These tasks were all new to EUCOM, but recalling the Admiral's conference promoting the COE's talent, the head of EUCOM phoned PACOM and asked for me by name.

I readily accepted but, within minutes, the PACOM General chose to send someone else in my place. I pointed out that I was called specifically because of my special expertise in that field and my history of building this program. I emphasized that the request was promoted by both PACOM's Admiral Prueher and EUCOM. The General was unmoved. When I phoned EUCOM to let them know, the Command's officers strongly objected. They were adamant in stating that they wanted me. I pleaded with the EUCOM Medical Command Director, assuring him that I would also send a UN communications specialist who could guide them in dealing with the other UN health-related agencies they would encounter.

The former UN communications specialist, a British citizen, had tremendous expertise in humanitarian operations and had been awarded the Order of the British Empire for his work. But in this situation, he objected to accompanying someone to EUCOM who lacked proficiency in this area. In the end, he reluctantly agreed to go, realizing the importance of maintaining a liaison with EUCOM for COE's future. He also strongly supported Admiral Prueher's concept of a COE at every combatant command. I crossed my fingers that all would go well, and this cooperation and coordination would be the start of what Admiral Prueher and I had optimistically imagined for COE.

But a successful mission wasn't meant to be. The communications specialist was very helpful, but EUCOM desperately needed medical-humanitarian advice, a service they thought only I could provide. The EUCOM commander angrily stated my COE replacement "just stood there and never said a word." He also phoned Admiral Prueher's office at PACOM and told them the consequences of what had occurred, which reflected poorly on the COE program and also on my reputation. Sadly, to this day, I have been held responsible, even at PACOM, for what transpired on that trip.

No one at PACOM knew that the Commanding Officer of Tripler had prevented me from going even though she knew the significant nature of the mission. Several times I heard the question directed right to me: "You are the COE Director, aren't you?" I knew most people had no idea of the changes being made by the current General, and I wasn't one to publicly complain. Inside, I was denying what was slowly becoming inevitable.

To no one's surprise, the COE never again received a request from EUCOM, and Admiral Prueher's office was finished dealing with our COE for any reason. This regrettable situation seemed to be the beginning of the end of what Senator Inouye and I had conceived for the COE's mission. With COE no longer operating as originally designed as a civil-military program, I was unable to do my job as I felt it should be done.

Death of a Dream

By then a litany of problems had arisen, all going in the wrong direction. First, the dismantling of the Telemedicine Program quickly became mired in lawsuits. I now had to hurriedly formulate contingency plans for COE if I was to remain its Director. I was reassured by Senator Inouye's office that he would work to keep us at Tripler or move us to PACOM. The Senator wanted COE to take the lead in many innovative programs of research and development, as well as training in information technology. But the handwriting was already on the wall.

A few weeks later, the Tripler General phoned me early one morning saying I needed to immediately update the Commander of the U.S. Army, Pacific Command, located at Fort Shafter east of Pearl Harbor. The meeting was to take place within an hour. I had never heard of this particular General and had never participated in any programs or briefings under this Army Command. When I entered his crowded, standing-room-only office, I noted a slide projector set up on his desk facing a blank wall. He sat with a firm face and no greeting. With only the first slide up on the wall, he stopped me and bluntly exclaimed, "I know all about the COE. You are to get rid of every program you have except for the military medical and UN peacekeeping program. That's an order!"

A deafening silence seemed to hang in the room. I distinctly recall seeing broad smiles on several faces of his staff because the General had just fixed this control problem with his terse "That's an order!" edict. I viewed those smiles as the perfect insult. I saw no hope for discussion. I slowly walked to his desk and removed the slide tray. As I quietly marched out of his office and closed the door, muted laughs and applause came from the room. No conversation took place between the Commanding Officer and me in her car on the return trip to Tripler.

I climbed out of her car without saying a word and headed to my office. To gain overall control of the COE program and make it more military-focused, COE was to be converted to a military-led program rather than acceding to its mission of coordination and cooperation equally with civilian agencies, which had been Senator Inouye's initial objective.

11. The Center of Excellence

It had become obvious to me and my colleagues that generals, who had no connection to COE, had ordered me to refuse any programs they found inconsistent with their objectives. I was bluntly told that all programs would cease except for the new UN training program. Also, the HELP and Combined Humanitarian Assistance Response Training (CHART) educational programs, which I had started, would now be managed by the General's appointee, newly titled "Deputy Director." This new control eliminated the ongoing purpose initiated by both PACOM and Senator Inouye. The General's purpose was unmistakable: Redefine the COE as a purely Army military program and have the Deputy use the powerful weight of her superior, the General, to buck PACOM's authority to complete the task. This order changed the original and ongoing purpose of COE that came from Daniel Inouye, United States Senator.

But I was sure the Senator would not let this complete reversal happen. I decided I must keep the programs intact and spend whatever authority I had left to move COE to PACOM, a few miles away at Pearl Harbor. I had three meetings with a senior PACOM general who insisted on my second visit that he could not make any decision until he saw the budget. I explained I had never seen or been allowed to look at the COE budget. I assumed he must have heard of similar legal dictates in the military, but as a civilian, I had never heard of such an arrangement. He was incredulous. He could not believe that this legal arrangement was the case, but, if true, he felt that PACOM could not participate. I was devastated.

I had to advise the Senator's Chief of Staff of the Tripler General's decision, which violated the conditions set up by the Senator himself. She, too, was appalled at this new development and supported COE moving to PACOM. But for this transfer to occur, COE needed to immediately become a nonprofit organization under Internal Revenue Code 501c3. Senator Inouye's Chief of Staff ordered me to seek legal assistance and begin the paperwork.

Unfortunately, nothing came of this attempt to transfer COE to PACOM. When the Tripler General learned of this plan, she ordered an audit of my COE financial transactions, including international travel and the COE's budget. I asserted I was never given the right to view the budget or records of any budgetary transactions. Also, negative accusations had allegedly been made concerning my management style. I modeled my organizational approach after the University of Hawaii's academic programs to ensure constant communication between the varied COE programs. The auditors, of course, found nothing inappropriate, but my tenure at COE was now even more in jeopardy.

Forced Out

Soon after this investigation, the University of Hawaii's President was informed that I would no longer receive a paycheck from COE. Tripler was planning to force me out. Then a senior nurse from the Tripler Command Suite called to say she was sorry I was leaving Tripler. I replied that my departure was news to me and this was the first I was hearing of it. She said plans were in place to fire me and put someone in place more favorable to the General's line of thinking.

The coup moved quickly after that. The next day the General called a meeting of all COE employees announcing that the COE would now have Co-Directors, the Deputy Director of COE, and me. The General gave me this title, knowing that she would soon force me out. This co-directorship came as a total surprise. As the meeting broke up, the new Co-Director told me that Tripler had fired the COE's UN communications specialist, stating that Tripler had received a letter complaining he had made lewd remarks about a former female COE employee. When I asked to see the letter, I was sharply rebuffed. She firmly stated the letter was designated "Top Secret" and I was not permitted to read it.

That evening I told my wife I was resigning before being fired. The next morning, a Saturday, Phyllis and I removed all my books from the small COE library and left the keys on the desk. After several days, just to cool off, I sent a letter of resignation, correctly assuming that with my stepping down, I was in no way taking responsibility for firing the other fine subject matter experts I knew would soon be let go. I left just at the right time.

After I resigned, the new Acting Director of COE turned on other COE staff and their programs, toppling them one by one to keep the General's plan of bringing COE under strict Army control. The liaison to PACOM was informed that his contract would not be renewed. The highly praised CDC program was next.

The Acting Director of COE abruptly announced to the staff members that they were no longer heading the CDC medical program, a violation of the CDC contract. Sadly, both the CDC premier researcher and Director of the CDC program in Hawaii were let go, a major loss to the Pacific region, especially for PACOM. Next, the well-respected Harvard researcher was fired. PACOM had depended on him for conflict assessments within the Asia-Pacific.

The General decided that the next Director of COE had to be a government employee. Meanwhile, the Telemedicine Program sued Tripler, and, after several years, won all three pending cases in litigation. I failed in not joining in the initial lawsuit, but was swayed by the Senator's office that the COE program would survive without one. In April 2000, the Deputy Commander in Chief and Chief of Staff of the U.S. Pacific Command at CINCPAC (Commander in Chief, Pacific Command) wrote me a letter stating that no actions would be taken against me. He thanked me for the "visionary role" I had played in making the COE concept play such a prominent part in humanitarian assistance.

Moving On

I continued to function as a faculty member and Chair of the Division of Emergency Medicine at the University of Hawaii, and then resigned from UH once I took the position of Senior Scholar, Scientist, and Visiting Professor at Johns Hopkins University School of Public Health in Baltimore. While at Hopkins, I also became the Senior Medical Advisor to the Defense Threat Reduction Agency at Fort Belvoir in Virginia, as well as a part-time research scientist at CDC in Atlanta.

Then in 2002, I was asked to become the Deputy Assistant Administrator for the U.S. Agency for International Development Global Health program, which required a new security clearance. I told the two seasoned investigators the entire COE story, including the alleged Top Secret letter containing serious allegations against COE's communications specialist who was fired. I felt all charges were bogus. I gave them names of those at the retitled Center for Excellence (CFE) in Hawaii, as well as other names outside that venue whom they needed to question.

Red Flags

A full year passed before I was presented with the results of my background check. The investigators had, in fact, first contacted the Tripler General, but they were met with an unexpected roadblock. The General stated that the investigators were only allowed to talk to her, the new Director of COE (now CFE), and the new Unit Chief for all military and civilian programs. The investigation team was not permitted to speak to anyone else. This directive sent up a red flag for the investigators. They had never heard of such a demand and would not take orders from the General or abide by her restrictions during their security inquiries.

Early on, the investigators requested to see that so-called "Top Secret" letter. The hesitation in handing over this document became uncomfortably evident because they now knew that federal examiners were aware of the alleged letter. The General later claimed they searched extensively for this ever-elusive letter but could not find it. The investigators asked how a Top Secret document, which had to be housed in a secure safe, could go missing, but they received no response to their simple, straightforward question.

The investigators then showed the General and her staff a Delegation of Authority letter to me dated November 17, 1998, and signed by this General that read in part: "The Commander, Pacific Regional Medical Command, in accordance with AR614–100m and AR 25–50, established the Center as a separate entity/department operating within Pacific Regional Medical Command. As the Center's Director, Dr. Frederick M. Burkle, Jr. is the authorized government representative with decision-making authority in fiscal and operational matters. This includes signatory authority for all support agreements and official correspondence." The General denied ever writing or signing any such letter.

These same security examiners interviewed many others and heard a very different view of my COE performance as its Director. The investigators returned to Honolulu to do a second round of extensive scrutiny, and once more requested to see the mysterious Top Secret letter. Again, that letter could not be found. On a scheduled third investigation trip in 2002, the General was no longer at Tripler, but a new Tripler General openly admitted that the Top Secret letter in question never existed, and the charges against COE's former communications specialist were fabricated.

After their return to Washington, I was invited to the investigators' offices to hear in detail about their year-long probe. I learned for the first time that the major reason for my removal was that I "mismanaged the budget." I was shocked because, once again, I had never seen the budget, had never been briefed on it, and had never managed it in any manner. The investigative team therefore affirmed I could not be held accountable. They even revealed that some COE monies were being used for non–COE Tripler uses.

The investigation confirmed that all contracts were issued through the Deputy Director who had become the Acting Director of COE when I left, as well as through the COE's Financial Officer. Then the contracts were vetted through this route to include the warranted Contract Officer and Comptroller. Any concerns would have been picked up during this process. The investigators confirmed that I never managed the budget during my tenure at COE. They emphasized that their lengthy probes revealed no evidence that any budgetary mishandling was true. They also knew that I was purposefully kept in the dark by Tripler about all fiscal matters. This quickly contrived story of me being responsible for budgets was blatantly false.

I was undeniably eligible, they asserted, for a Top Secret security clearance, and then one of them added, "In our many years of investigating, we have never witnessed a greater violation of the security evaluation process than this one." Given their years of conducting inquiries for other such clearances, they observed that this case involved "criminality" and "severe violation of my rights." The chief investigator concluded, "We've never advised this to anyone before, but we strongly recommend that you sue the U.S. Army."

In April 2020, I had a conversation with the second Tripler General. While he reiterated that he was not involved with COE after he retired, he stated, "The foolishness and intrigue most likely happened an hour after I left Tripler. I just can't believe what happened. I understand from multiple sources how much of what I did and what [the first General] had done simply went away after I left. I was just stunned. If I had known all of this was coming, I would have done something to make the COE damned hard to get rid of. I'm just sorry I wasn't still there to stop it."

I was often questioned about what Tripler was trying to accomplish by destroying both the Telemedicine Program and COE. It seemed that it was all about unmitigated power. With all the rapid firings, leaving only the UN program and two courses intact, it became painfully obvious that the U.S. Army could not tolerate or understand this organization. Neither could it comprehend an arrangement where "strange bedfellows," mimicking the operational reality of various crisis management organizations in the field, were working together in one department, the Center of Excellence. This was the greatest loss. The Army was trained to dominate—and it did.

11. The Center of Excellence

* * * *

As Phyllis noted long after this COE episode had ended that I had my principles intact. I was resolute to see my dream of civil-military cooperation through to the end, but determination just wasn't enough. Power, ego, and personal territorial disputes all played into sabotaging my dream. I compromised to a certain extent but then my principles became more important. Phyllis knew that I always gave 100 percent effort to accomplish my hopes and goals. And she certainly understood that I wanted to always be perceived as a reliable resource to get the job done.

During the past 20 years, I have often wondered where a productive and effective COE civil-military relationship might have headed had the Army left it alone and allowed it to function as originally intended. Unfortunately, the nurse's warning that my career might be cursed became a reality. I devoted six years of my life to the Center of Excellence. But watching helplessly, I saw my one big dream go unfulfilled and destroyed.

12

Baghdad

April 2003

"Our caravan had been fired upon on three separate times, but most of the Iraqi firepower was aimed at my vehicle. I was clearly the target."

Part of me realized that my involvement in the early 1990s with the Kurdish Crisis in northern Iraq might not be the last time I'd see that country. My second participation in Iraq with the federal government in 2003, though somewhat short-lived, was one of the most frustrating and potentially dangerous episodes of my career. But more importantly, our government's failure, even today, has negatively impacted Baghdad and the rest of Iraq. This series of events was not only trying for me but also distressing for the Iraqi people. They warranted better treatment than what the United States and international agencies gave them. The American people also deserved to be better informed than the distorted rationalizations for the invasion of Iraq, justifications repeatedly presented by the George W. Bush Administration.

At the time, I couldn't believe our government's shortsightedness. I didn't understand why we would ignore all the signs demanding a change in our course of action. But in hindsight, I see that my experience was just a microcosm of our larger foreign policy approach: moving away from diplomacy and toward American might. This abrupt change in strategy, unfortunately, would follow us for more than a decade.

On the heels of the horrific 9/11 attack, 2002 was a year that embraced a flurry of activity and accusations, both of which saw a considerable amount of planning for the Iraq War. The more positive, confident term "Operation Iraqi Freedom" would officially replace "Iraq War." I had spent much of the 1990s teaching in Hawaii. I had founded and directed the Center of Excellence in Disaster Management and Humanitarian Assistance, an initiative of Senator Daniel Inouye. I was also periodically conducting occasional medical consultation work in China. But in 2000, I accepted a position as a Senior Scholar at Johns Hopkins University in Baltimore.

Then, in 2001, a friend and trusted colleague, Andrew Natsios, was sworn in as administrator for the U.S. Agency for International Development (USAID). Natsios knew of my expertise in complex humanitarian emergencies and offered me a position on his team. In 2002, I took leave from Johns Hopkins and was honored to be appointed to USAID as Deputy Assistant Administrator for Global Health.

In the aftermath of 9/11, it didn't take long to see that we would be going to war. Having served in Vietnam in 1968, the Persian Gulf War in 1991, and then back for the Kurdish Crisis in Iraq that same year, I recognized that fighting members of the military are not the only ones at risk in time of war. This statement is true of all wars. I couldn't do anything about deaths and civilian casualties due to modern weaponry and military invasion. I did have the ability, however, to try to prevent the cascade of civilian deaths and destruction that would likely follow after 160,000 U.S.-led Coalition forces, also called the Multi-National Force, entered Iraq on March 20, 2003.

All wars destroy crucial public health infrastructure: water, sanitation, food systems, shelter, and immunization programs—the fundamental public services of any advanced society. Without these everyday essentials, social structures begin to fall apart very quickly. In prolonged warfare and conflict, those responsible for humanitarian assistance and recovery also know that preventable mortality and morbidity, that is, illness or spread of disease, can even exceed direct deaths from military action. Public health infrastructure and social protections then rapidly deteriorate. The impact of these services' breakdown is far-reaching.

Then It All Went South

I knew the war could lead to an additional 70 percent to 90 percent of post-war deaths and morbidity, exceeding loss of life from weaponry. But I realized that I had a chance to mitigate some of this impending disaster in my new USAID position. I declared our priority was to restore the public health infrastructure in Iraq after the invasion in 2003. I had the expertise and I now had a mission. Then the Bush Administration blew my objective out of the water.

On January 20, 2003, I was running late to my usual early morning meeting with a small team at the Ronald Reagan Building on Pennsylvania Avenue in which USAID was headquartered. Our colleagues from the State Department would also be attending that gathering. But when I arrived, Ambassador Wendy Chamberlin[1] was pacing back and forth while talking on the phone, looking highly upset. The rest of those present sat in silence surrounding her large desk.

"What's going on?" I whispered to Bernd "Bear" McConnell, head of the Office of Foreign Disaster Assistance (OFDA) at USAID. He slid a piece of paper over to me for my scrutiny. The document had George W. Bush's signature scrawled from one side to the other. The text stated that all humanitarian assistance, which we had been working on for a long time, was being moved from Secretary Colin Powell's

---
1. Wendy Chamberlin had been ambassador to Laos (1996–1999) and Pakistan (2001–2002). In December 2002, she was appointed Assistant Administrator and head of USAID Asia and Near East Bureau.

Department of State—of which USAID was a part—to Secretary Donald Rumsfeld's Department of Defense.

This kind of monumental transfer had never occurred before. I was speechless. Bear and I agreed this reassignment from State to Defense was a mistake, and Congress would never let it happen. To have the Department of Defense conduct its foreign policy would be unprecedented. Though our relationship with the State Department had always been complicated, USAID was intentionally created as part of the Foreign Assistance Act in September 1961. President Kennedy wanted USAID, through this act, to focus on basic human needs and development aid. Having us connected to the U.S. military would mix wildly opposing messages.

Ambassador Chamberlin finally hung up, saying Secretary Powell wasn't in yet but he'd get back to us. Trying to make sense of this situation, the phone suddenly rang, startling us into silence once again. It was Colin Powell. Wendy Chamberlin lit into the Secretary of State and demanded, "Why didn't you tell me this was happening? Why am I just hearing about this now?" Again, total silence as we gave our attention to Ambassador Chamberlin's response, which was one of frustration. "Colin? Colin? Are you there?"

The voice on the other end cleared his throat, paused, then out of seeming uncertainty, cleared it again. He firmly stressed, "I have absolutely no idea what you're talking about." This unparalleled move by President Bush had been done without even Secretary of State Powell's knowledge.

During the next several weeks, as this transfer of responsibility moved forward, we started to see the tug of war on both sides as the leads competed to get certain people into positions of power. Jay Garner, a retired Army lieutenant general, who had been appointed to head the newly named Office of Reconstruction and Humanitarian Assistance, was doing his best to retain many of USAID's Office of Foreign Disaster Assistance people in their former positions. Garner and I had worked together briefly during the Kurdish Crisis 12 years earlier. But apprehension about this move was somewhat tempered by his understanding of the solid model we executed during Operation Provide Comfort, starting in the spring of 1991.

More Military, Less Humanity

The retired general was a quiet, modest, and humane man, but he could also be resolute. Garner wanted us to remain in charge as on-the-scene experts. But Rumsfeld had other ideas. He wanted more military. Rumsfeld and Garner disagreed about who would lead the health task force: Rumsfeld pushed for a military person in Iraq, and Garner argued for me to be on site. I didn't recognize this scenario at the time, but I ended up being the only person from the original list whom Rumsfeld allowed to stay on.[2]

---

2. Bob Woodward, *State of Denial: Bush at War, Part III* (New York: Simon & Schuster, 2006), p. 56.

I was going to continue in my position as Deputy Assistant Administrator for Global Health, be a part of the Disaster Assistance Response Team (DART), and, upon arrival in Iraq, serve as Interim Health Minister. I do not doubt that being a retired Navy captain gave me an extra edge. Though he eventually acquiesced to my presence, the Secretary of Defense put together a medical team under the leadership of a politically connected but inexperienced Navy lieutenant commander. This officer did not know the nature of USAID's responsibilities. The new team then slowly chipped away at our plans.

In this type of situation, a meeting would normally take place with USAID heads and our international counterparts: those from the World Health Organization (WHO), the United Nations High Commissioner for Refugees (UNHCR), and the International Committee of the Red Cross (ICRC). We were all on the same team with identical goals: ensuring health services and mitigating, as much as possible, the devastating effects of war on local populations. These professionals were our respected colleagues. We had previously worked with them on several occasions.

Iraq faced the prospect of waging war in 2003 with an exhausted and inadequate public health infrastructure. This fact was not lost on the Iraqi population and USAID planners. All leaders were unified in the call to lobby for immediately organizing a systematic health data system with international partners. These discussions were enough to draw the attention of decision-makers in the Department of State and USAID to potential opportunities to mitigate preventable public health consequences of an invasion.

The Department of State and USAID's "Future of Iraq Task Force" was organized and eventually led to the signing of multimillion-dollar U.S. contracts with WHO and the UN International Children's Emergency Fund (UNICEF). These two UN organizations were designated to immediately implement and enhance post-invasion countrywide surveillance, training, and decentralized monitoring directed at the most vulnerable populations. Inspection teams in multiple areas would assess the community's access to shelter, food, water, and energy. These teams would also check for illnesses that result from the deterioration or loss of public health protection and prevention programs. Among the Department of State, USAID, and the humanitarian community, this monitoring was universally agreed upon to be our best opportunity to identify and hopefully avert the anticipated war-related, preventable mortality and morbidity we all knew could quickly follow the war.

Rumsfeld Calls the Shots

The meeting to explain this process to the international players was scheduled to take place in Geneva, Switzerland, the location of many international agencies' headquarters. But shortly before the gathering was supposed to take place, the Defense Department canceled the meeting, sending its own crew to the conference. I knew at that point that our team would very likely be replaced by Rumsfeld's lineup of political and military players.

My colleagues in Geneva called me that same day to ask what was going on, questioning the qualifications of these new people and why they lacked so much knowledge about international humanitarian law. To add to all these concerns, my collaborators even asked why we let this problematic situation reach this point. The arriving U.S. teams did not know humanitarian relief. Rumsfeld's new people on the scene demanded to know what every other organization was doing, but they refused to share the intent of the U.S. military. This lack of communication was a violation of the 1949 Geneva Conventions because no humanitarian matters should be kept secret.

Before this transfer of authority occurred, I was working behind the scenes to try to line up resources in Iraq so that when conditions deteriorated, as they surely would, we would be ready to act. This transaction included signing a $100 million contract with WHO. With this operation in place, we could begin immediate countrywide surveillance to see who was sick and dying—and, just as important, why they were dying. But once the sources are identified, of course, a response is needed. A $20 million contract with UNICEF was also put into place, negotiated through USAID-supported International Humanitarian Law requirements. The agreement would have allowed UNICEF to be ready to solve the problems of mortality and morbidity that were sure to appear.

Shortly thereafter, events started to go downhill. After our international meeting was hijacked and our responsibilities were whittled away, I learned that Secretary Rumsfeld had canceled these international contracts. He said that because the war was going to be over in three weeks, the United States did not need to involve these international agencies. Perhaps motivated by the success of the Persian Gulf War, Rumsfeld didn't think we would be in Iraq long enough to justify my requests. He was not alone in holding this conviction. In my initial talks with Jay Garner and other military colleagues, they confidently predicted we would go in, remove Saddam Hussein, give Iraq back to the Iraqis, and hurriedly leave the country. The U.S.-led Coalition forces stayed for the next eight years. So much for Rumsfeld's prophecy of going into Iraq and getting out quickly.

While this scenario was, of course, the ideal setup, these governmental and military officials were grossly oversimplifying what lay ahead of us. I reminded them all that the Iraqi government ministries were being run by Sunni Muslims, a detail that needed to be seriously considered.[3] I was familiar with the personnel in all layers of Iraq's health ministry. In addition, I had already distinguished between those I wanted to keep during my interim leadership and those who needed to go.

---

3. Shia and Sunni are Islam's two major denominations. Mainstream Islam split following the death of the prophet Muhammad in 632 A.D. Sunnis are a majority in most, but not all, Muslim communities. Enmity, based on mutual distrust and differing beliefs, has pitted the two sects against one another for centuries, a history increasingly marked by armed conflict. During the Saddam Hussein era, the Sunni minority in Iraq ran both the Ba'ath Party and all government ministries.

Though many in the top layer were Saddam Hussein loyalists who needed to be removed, I recognized that many Iraqis were in Saddam's Ba'ath Party by force, not by choice. A clean sweep therefore would be very unwise. In Saddam's government, employees had to belong to the Ba'ath Party, whether they liked it or not. If Iraqis wanted a job, a promotion, or research funding, they needed to declare their loyalty to the Ba'ath Party. Understanding this reality would have been very beneficial for U.S. leaders.

Iraq's Interim Minister of Health— in Name Only

Following the rapid fall of Baghdad on April 9, 2003, symbolized by the toppling of the hollow Saddam statue on that date, events quickly unfolded. We received reports from the airport about looting, especially stealing essentials from hospitals and health clinics. The International Committee of the Red Cross, which had continued to function in Baghdad throughout the war, had alerted us that the Iraqi health system was near collapse. As the senior medical officer of the Disaster Assistance Response Team (DART), I was designated "Interim Minister of Health." My mission was simple and critical: I was to proceed to Baghdad to assess the situation and bring emergency medical kits—as many as were needed—to forestall the collapse of the basic health care system and restore it to a functioning system. My presence would signal the beginning of massive external humanitarian assistance.

I was still in Washington at this point, but soon heard from Jay Garner that I was to go to Baghdad and stop the ransacking of hospitals. Nothing more, nothing less. Baghdad is the size of Los Angeles and San Francisco combined, so we knew the pillaging was widespread and would be difficult to address. Journalists were reporting that the 1,000-bed Yarmouk Hospital and other hospitals in Baghdad and elsewhere in the country had been similarly plundered. Widespread theft had stripped these medical facilities of major medications, emergency equipment, supplies, key electronic components of sophisticated diagnostic equipment, dialysis machines, cardiac monitors, and essential wiring for electricity. All these medical centers had either been pilfered or destroyed.

The looters, lacking any shred of morality, went well beyond running off with valuable hospital equipment. Surgical patients were forcibly thrown to the floor as their beds were stolen. Even the motherboard of Yarmouk's CAT scanner had disappeared. Several pregnant women, dressed in Western-style clothing, reported that they were no longer welcomed in the hospitals. In Sadr City, a large Shia suburb of Baghdad, access to two hospitals had been denied by armed, non-uniformed men. This news naturally terrified the Iraqis and prevented them from seeking medical attention. Casualties were not being treated.

Before I arrived in Kuwait City, the jump-off point to Baghdad, the military claimed it was safe to travel through the Iraqi capital in a non-armored or "soft-

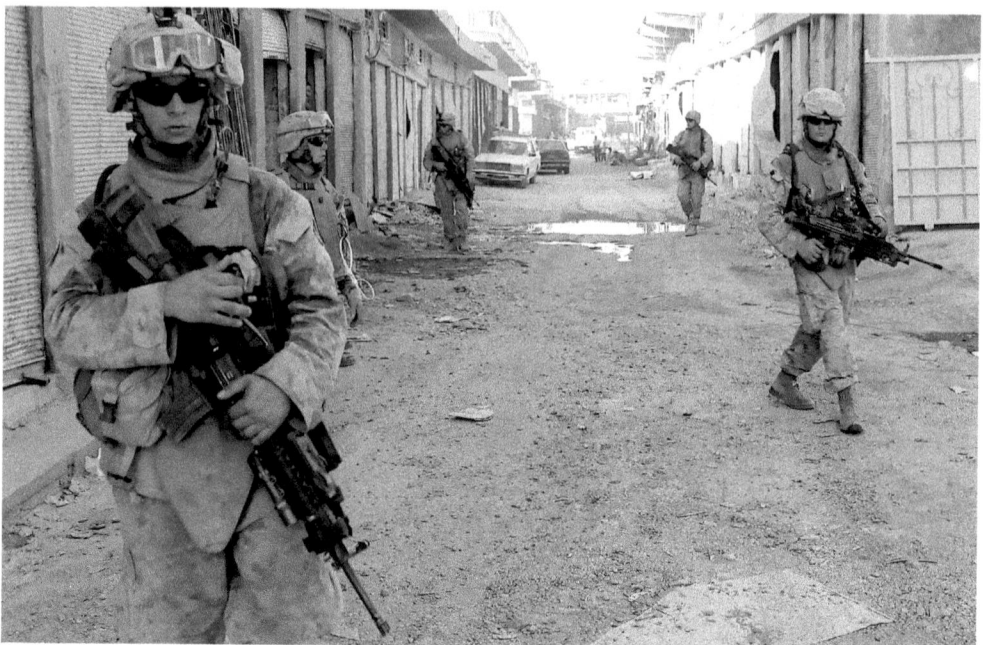

The Marines who had taken Baghdad were assault troops. But the true need on the ground afterward was for military police to keep order in the city (U.S. Marine Corps).

cover" vehicle. Enough armed troops would be on hand for protection. Also, three days had already elapsed without a hostile incident. Despite these claims, our civilian superiors reminded us that it was imperative that any travel to Baghdad be made in armored transport. No exceptions.

I was on the third plane to land at the recently renamed Baghdad International Airport, about 10 miles west of the center of Baghdad. Before April 4, the airport was Saddam International Airport. It was nighttime but the crew used no landing lights. Once on the ground, I immediately met Marines with infrared gear and we sped off to the hangar. I said I needed to go into Baghdad the next day, but due to much confusion about whether or not it was safe to travel in an unarmored vehicle, it took us three days before we could get into the city.

Just noon the following day, April 13, a convoy of five Humvees finally arrived at the airport—and their spelled-out designation—"High Mobility Multipurpose Wheeled Vehicles"—certainly lived up to their "multipurpose" name. Two of them, equipped with .50 caliber turret guns, took up positions at the front and rear of the caravan. The second and fourth Humvees were open in which four Marines were armed with automatic rifles. The third, a bullet-proof Humvee, was assigned for me and the Army Civil Affairs officers who would accompany me to an emergency meeting with hospital administrators desperate to reopen their hospitals, particularly Yarmouk Hospital. The meeting would take place in central Baghdad at the Palestine Hotel. However, I had made it a priority to meet first with the International Committee of the Red Cross at another location to clarify our responsibilities.

12. Baghdad

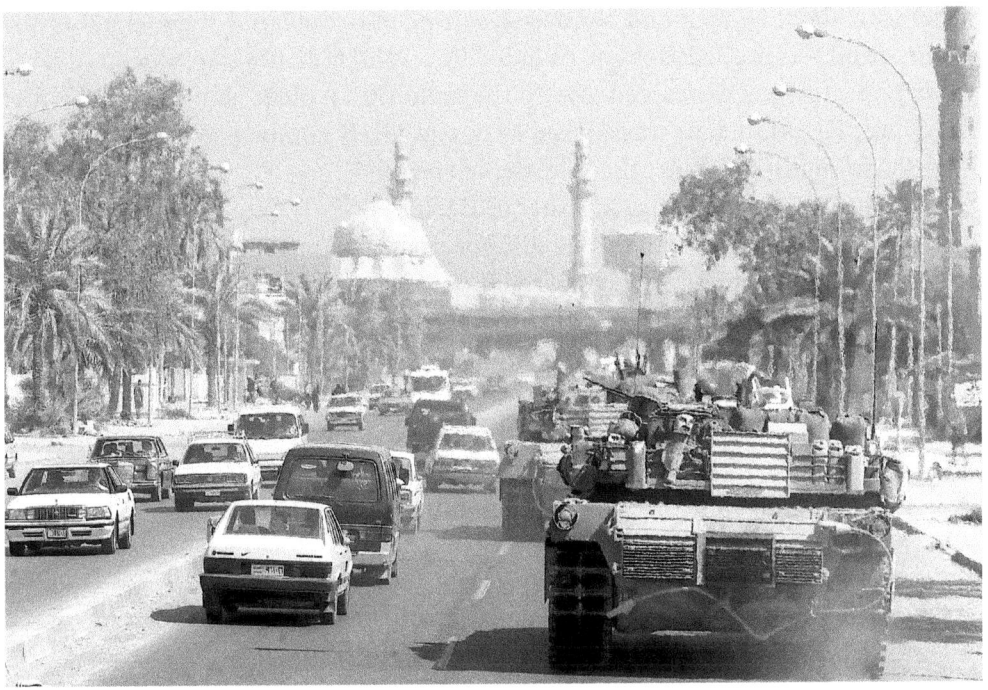

Two Marine Corps M1 tanks patrol Baghdad's streets on April 14, 2003, just five days after the city fell (U.S. Marine Corps).

At this point, only one remaining radio station was operational in Baghdad. We heard the radio announcer broadcast my name as the Interim Minister of Health, along with details of the time and location of our emergency meeting. Large crowds were anticipated adding yet another challenge to this effort. So much for security in a city that had just surrendered to U.S. troops days before.

As we began our trip, a sandstorm hovered over Baghdad, blurring buildings and streets and making the landscape indistinguishable from the skyline. Even though it was barely 2 p.m., the darkened sky made it appear as though dusk was falling. The drab, bleak city looked even more somber. It was eerily quiet as our convoy moved eastward, cautiously and alone toward the Fourteenth of July Bridge,[4] which crosses the Tigris River. Battle debris still littered the span. Once we entered east Baghdad, we witnessed empty streets, except for small gatherings of about two dozen young men gathered on various corners, eyeing us suspiciously as we drove by. I was becoming increasingly concerned and agitated.

We drove for what seemed many miles without any hint of Coalition forces. No signs marked the street names and Google Maps wouldn't come into existence until 2005. A few U.S. Marine tanks were the only evidence of a military presence. We then found the entrance to the sandbagged ICRC building at the end of a dead-end

---

4. The only suspension bridge in Baghdad, it connects the center of the city south to the Karrada Peninsula. The bridge is named for the day in 1958 when the Hashemite monarchy was toppled. On November 13, 2003, a bombing in Baghdad would close the bridge for nearly a year as a precautionary measure.

street with about 20 men and children awaiting our caravan. I stepped out of the Humvee and was immediately surrounded by several Marines stepping up to serve as my protectors. As we walked toward the building, an older man appeared out of the crowd. His white hair was slicked back and nicely combed. With near-perfect English, he inquired, "Who's the Minister of Health?"

I replied, "I'm the Interim Minister of Health."

Before I could ask his name, he disappeared back into the crowd. As I turned around, I saw the person in charge of the ICRC delegation come to meet me. He and a small cadre of ICRC expatriates had remained in Baghdad during the invasion to ensure, under the Geneva Conventions, that civilian casualties were cared for and shielded. No one with weapons was allowed inside so my Marine protection stood guard outside. I entered the building with the three Army Civilian Affairs personnel who had accompanied me in the convoy.

"I wasn't sure you realized I was the Interim Minister of Health," I said to the ICRC official who had greeted me.

"No," he replied. "I didn't know your title."

"Well, I just met one of your guys outside."

The man stopped in his tracks. "Who?"

"It must be an Iraqi who works for you," I answered and described his appearance.

The ICRC official just shook his head and stated, "I have no one who fits that description."

I brushed off those words and proceeded to take part in the ICRC session. But the outside incident remained in the back of my mind, as well as recalling those crowds, friendly or unfriendly, awaiting our appearance. As the three-hour meeting ticked on, the gravity of Iraq's medical crisis sank in. The Coalition forces, as the occupying power, had an obligation under international law to control looting and restore essential health services as quickly as possible—an acknowledgment of our purpose for being in Iraq. I admitted that humanitarian agencies remained far behind the Civil Affairs units in terms of their ability to respond.

On the drive to the ICRC compound, I noticed that security would have to be increased considerably in Baghdad before any sizable humanitarian effort could be realized. We were also informed that the water and sewage systems had been destroyed, and the wastewater was backing up in Sadr City. I knew that trying to get those systems back into working condition would be met with a huge safety issue.

Delivering emergency medical kits, each containing essential supplies for a population of 10,000 for three months, would also have to take a back seat to security requirements. A rush to provide assistance would only lead to more looting. Until formally permitted to enter Baghdad, the Disaster Assistance Response Team would coordinate with Civil Affairs units to restore, as much as possible, essential health services based on assessments carried out during the past few days.

We concluded that safety measures should be concentrated at 10 public hospitals, a plan that would guarantee that everyone in the city would have access to emergency care. As if to punctuate the gravity of the health emergency being discussed, we received word that a 12-year-old girl had been shot in the chest immediately outside the ICRC building. With the aid of an ICRC ambulance, she was driven to the nearest hospital but no one thought she would survive.

Finally, I had to give these ICRC authorities the bad news. In a briefing on April 11, less than 48 hours after the fall of Baghdad, Rumsfeld had proclaimed that U.S. forces were not actually "occupiers" but were instead "liberators." If the U.S. government stood by Rumsfeld's declaration, this was an entirely new ballgame.

While "occupiers" versus "liberators" sounds like simple wordsmithing, the consequences were enormous. By altering this declaration, we were no longer required by the Geneva Conventions and International Humanitarian Law to complete any of the humanitarian requirements, such as restoring public health protections required under the Geneva Conventions' Articles 55 and 56.[5] The ICRC officials looked at me in disbelief, as if they didn't hear what I had just said. I added meekly, "Today, I'm just the messenger. I am as disappointed as you."

But the head ICRC official was livid. What could I possibly say in return? I tried my best to assuage the situation by saying, "Let's try to do everything we can to mitigate this public health tragedy, and I'll do my best to change the mind of the U.S. government."

A Bullseye on My Back

With some weak agreement in exchange, we said our goodbyes and walked outside to the caravan. I got into the passenger seat of the armored Humvee, the third vehicle, and we headed for the exit. We drove toward a long thoroughfare that would lead to one of the many bridges crossing the Tigris. But as soon as we turned onto the main road, I heard a sound on the roof, similar to gravel hitting the underside of a metal fender. We quizzically looked at one another. In the second vehicle ahead of us, a Marine, wearing only a sleeveless flak jacket, stood up, yelled, and pointed his rifle. He fired right over our Humvee toward the back of the convoy.

Chaos followed. Shots were coming from the rear and right. Pop! Pop! Pop!

---

5. Article 55 states: "To the fullest extent of the means available to it, the Occupying Power has the duty of ensuring the food and medical supplies of the population; it should, in particular, bring in the necessary foodstuffs, medical stores and other articles if the resources of the occupied territory are inadequate." Available at https://ihl-databases.icrc.org/en/ihl-treaties/gciv-1949/article-55.

Article 56 states: "To the fullest extent of the means available to it, the Occupying Power has the duty of ensuring and maintaining, with the cooperation of national and local authorities, the medical and hospital establishments and services, public health and hygiene in the occupied territory, with particular reference to the adoption and application of the prophylactic and preventive measures necessary to combat the spread of contagious diseases and epidemics. Medical personnel of all categories shall be allowed to carry out their duties." Available at https://ihl-databases.icrc.org/en/ihl-treaties/gciv-1949/article-56?activeTab=

Some slugs pinged off my Humvee's heavy steel armor. The vehicles in our procession immediately rushed ahead, disjointed at first, then together as our ponderous armored Humvee slowly gained speed. Several hundred yards later, automatic fire rang out from both sides of the street with my armored Humvee again the target. Marines in the second vehicle emptied their magazines in all directions. The racket was deafening. Our driver struggled to force his 9mm pistol out of the narrow side window to fire at a man who was shooting from a nearby rooftop.

"Turn right! Turn right!" I shouted above the din. "The main route is covered by snipers!"

We could talk by radio to each of the other vehicles in the convoy, but we couldn't reach the Marines at the airport. Our heavy Humvee seemingly stood still as the two lead ones sped away. The occupants waved frantically and beckoned us to catch up and to follow as they made that all-important right turn at the next intersection. We needed to stay off the predicted five-mile route and go by another road. To catch up with them, our driver slammed on the gas, and we managed to close the distance before turning right.

A welcome silence was broken by nervous radio checks and hearing orders to tighten up the column. But frustration ensued because both turret guns on the open Humvee had jammed. Only wide empty streets loomed ahead. Suddenly, the second Humvee opened up with automatic fire, shooting at invisible targets thought to be on the edge of a bridge overhang.

Heading west again, we slowed as the column moved cautiously around a major traffic circle and entered a wide street with a median. I knew that this road would lead to one of the bridges across the river and onto a main road in the direction of the airport. We could only see women and some children milling around. Our vehicles abruptly slowed down behind two buses parked in tandem on the right side. As our driver tried to negotiate around the buses, both of the buses moved and were now parked side by side, partially blocking our path. Then, yet again, AK-47 bullets began raining down on us. The source was a blown-out window on a building's upper floor. More destructive machine gun rounds were trained on us from the front of the convoy.

My vehicle again seemed to be the primary target. Then the radio crackled and our last Humvee in the line reported, "Man in combat boots on the corner we just passed. He has a radio in hand!"

Out of the blue, we heard a whoosh sound similar to a rocket-propelled grenade launch between the second and third vehicles—but no explosion. The civilian Iraqis started screaming and running for cover, or they sprawled flat on the pavement as our vehicles swerved and hurried ahead to maneuver around the buses. With the two jammed turret guns useless, the open vehicle, which carried the exposed Marines in front, was the only source of firepower to protect our group. Visibility was poor in the Humvees, especially to the rear, which made it difficult to check the whereabouts of the two transports coming up behind.

12. Baghdad 177

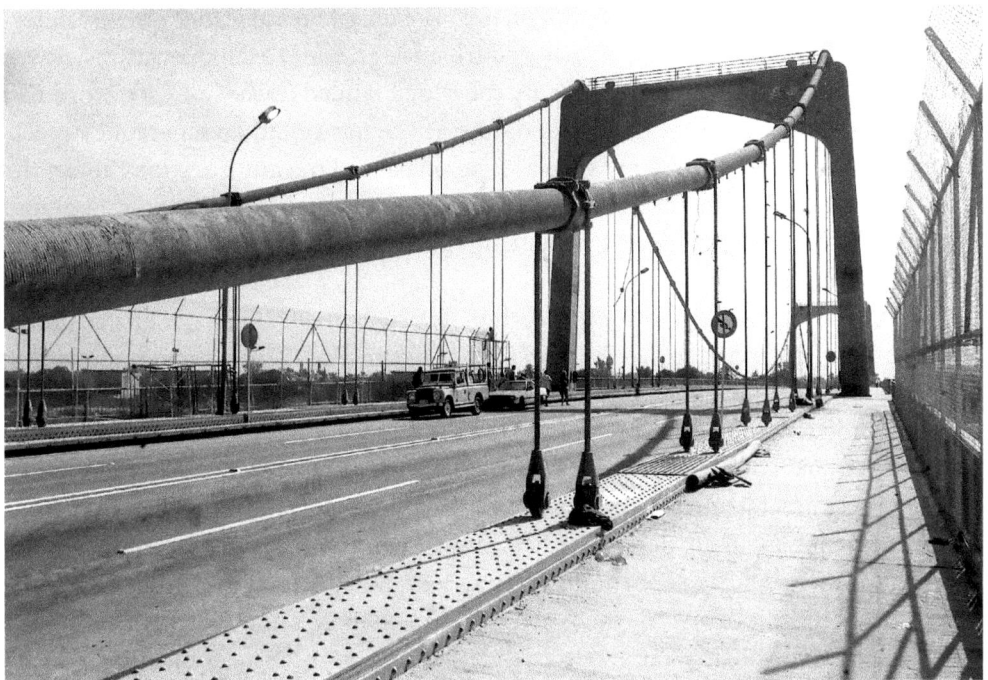

Baghdad's famed Fourteenth of July Bridge, which spanned the Tigris River, served as the perilous escape route for Skip's convoy on April 13, 2003 (U.S. Army).

After we made it past the bus obstacles onto a wider road, our convoy stopped two blocks down the street beside two Marine tanks with their occupants straining their necks to see what was causing all the commotion. The Fourteenth of July Bridge was not far away. The convoy then moved across the bridge to the west. We were all astonished that the shooters had concentrated their fire only on the third and fourth vehicles.

Stopping quickly to assess the situation, I asked if anyone had been wounded. I didn't have my medical kit with me, but my instincts were one step ahead of this unexpected calamity because I could help any wounded if needed. Miraculously, the blizzard of hostile fire produced no casualties. No one in the unarmored vehicles even suffered a scratch. We realized my Humvee, fortunately heavily reinforced, seemed to be the only one that was hit. The on-the-spot damage assessment included a dented armored Humvee and a shattered window in the last Humvee.

Our caravan had been fired upon three separate times, but most of the Iraqi firepower was aimed at my Humvee. I was the target. I was certain that the Iraqis' specific sniping focus was ordered by that inquisitive gentleman, the one who had asked me at the ICRC for the name of the Minister of Health.

I learned much later that Muqtada al-Sadr, a Shia cleric, had issued a "fatwa," in Western terms, a death sentence against me. He had wanted the position of Minister of Health for himself. I was the only obstacle standing in his way. If his followers had killed me, then they could join Allah and he could become Health Minister.

After returning to the airport, I reported the ambush to the Disaster Assistance

Response Team in Kuwait by satellite phone. The on-site team leader quickly determined that Baghdad was not nearly secure enough for DART operations. I was ordered back to Kuwait immediately. By the time I landed in Kuwait City, word had spread those plans had not gone well. General Garner called an emergency meeting at a nearby hotel. But, to my surprise, no one asked me any questions about the Iraqi ambush. Everyone thought my perilous ride through the streets of Baghdad had been a fluke and it wouldn't happen again. They didn't seem to grasp the danger—or maybe they didn't want to know.

When Garner walked into the meeting, he proclaimed, "I just got off the phone with the Boss," referring to Secretary of Defense Rumsfeld. "The whole team is going into Baghdad the day after tomorrow. But I'll need someone to make the arrangements for me to meet certain people." He then turned to me. "Skip, you know the city and you just got back. I'll need you to go back to Baghdad tomorrow and make some of these arrangements. Let's start with Yarmouk Hospital as a meeting place."

Was General Garner serious? I had almost been killed! As I sat in that meeting room, my mind raced through the day's events, anticipating what new dangers awaited me tomorrow. Garner then made a few more announcements. I looked around at the crowd. This was a well-attended, standing-room-only meeting. I didn't recognize the majority of the people, but I think some were transportation specialists and others were oil experts. Garner wrapped up his talk and I quickly came back to reality when he asked, "Any questions?"

My hand shot up. "General, you know we have a security issue in Baghdad. You have no armored vehicles. No one even has email to communicate." Remembering the frustration of the Marines and the lack of military police personnel, I then added, "We also have no security people. Are you at all concerned?"

Because I was seated in the first row, he walked up to me, put his hand on my shoulder and affirmed, "Skip, the only security problem you're going to have is that you'll be surrounded by Iraqi citizens kissing you and giving you gifts."

Everyone laughed—but it was an uncomfortable laughter. I looked like a fool.

Garner turned around and walked toward the contingent in the room, reminding them that the original plan was to be out of Iraq entirely in three months. "But," he added, "Secretary Rumsfeld told me just a few minutes ago that we'll be out of Iraq in three weeks!"

Everybody clapped, let out a few whoops, slapped each other on the back, and got up to go finish packing. I sat in that room dumbfounded by the lack of understanding of the chaos at hand. I'd spent enough time in the military, however, to know this situation was not up for discussion.

A One-Person Team

I then made preparations to be back on the plane the following day. The next night, lying on the cement floor of a Baghdad airport hangar, I stared at an old jet

12. Baghdad

engine as I replayed the events of the day in my mind, trying to make sense of any of them. I realized I was still wearing the same clothes from our harrowing escape through the city—khakis, a shirt and tie, and a blue blazer. I was committed to making this mission work, but I started wondering if I was on a team all by myself.

When our complete group finally landed back in Baghdad, we rode through the city in big, open trucks as if we were construction workers headed for a job—with no security whatsoever. My first meeting was at the administrator's office at Yarmouk Hospital, which was packed with supervisors from hospitals all over the city. The former Sunni administrators were gone, and the new personnel were all Shia, none of whom had ever had any managerial experience. I began presenting our plans, highlighting that we had to work together to minimize the number of indirect deaths. I did my best to address everyone's concerns.

All of a sudden, the door flew open and people in front of it were shoved aside. Muqtada al-Sadr, the Shia cleric, strode assertively into our meeting room at Yarmouk Hospital. He walked along the wall until he stood about 10 feet from me. Black-turbaned and bearded, the young man's dark, hooded eyes locked on me with a menacing scowl, thinking his glare could intimidate me. Whenever his angry lips parted, I noted his crooked and discolored teeth. I had heard of Sadr but didn't know much about him or what he looked like. His father had been assassinated by Saddam Hussein. Muqtada al-Sadr was the man who had issued the fatwa against me. He left the room, the meeting finally ended, and my Marine guards escorted me outside. I never saw Sadr again.

Regrettably, not much came of this gathering with the hospital staff. The military, however, did translate our emergency plans into operational orders. An Army Civil Affairs lieutenant colonel agreed to be my eyes and ears on the ground in Baghdad until I could return. We learned that the Iraqi Ministry of Health, unlike other government offices, had not been burned or looted. The colonel found that small numbers of dedicated health workers had returned to work, but they were frightened by two rogue Iraqi groups who had occupied the ministry building and were intent on its destruction.

Three weeks later, at which time the war was decidedly not over, Rumsfeld removed three people: Jay Garner, Ambassador Barbara Bodine who was set to be Interim Interior Minister, and me. Paul Bremer was brought in on May 11, 2003, to succeed Garner and lead the entire operation. Bremer was chosen to lead the Coalition Provisional Authority (CPA), knowing very little about the history or culture of the country. Astoundingly, he believed that Sunnis and Shia all got along well together. A former diplomat, Bremer had also held domestic posts in the Department of State before leaving the Foreign Service to eventually head several consulting firms.

In late April, after several months of planning for the restoration of Iraq's health care system, I told Jay Garner that I was through. My departure was already a fait accompli since Rumsfeld had recently indicated that Garner, Bodine, and I were being replaced. Nevertheless, my own decision to resign was based on two reasons: I could not violate the Geneva Conventions, and I had no use for Cheney and Rumsfeld's uninformed, counterproductive policies. Their course of action had very severe, long-range consequences that would result in deaths—preventable deaths.

Declaring "a Public Health Emergency"

I also learned that I was being replaced as the principal health official by James Haveman, who had formerly been involved in human services management. Haveman did not have a medical degree, and he had never worked in a post-conflict environment. He refused to collect data on existing clinics and did not include the private health care system in his planning, even though it had been serving half the country's needs. Haveman was not the man for the job.

I left Iraq as Interim Health Minister in 2003—a minister who had no voice. But, as a last duty, I intentionally declared to several reporters and to my colleagues, loud and clear, that Baghdad had to be seen as a "public health emergency." This designation meant the United States would be under some pressure to act on that pronouncement. The Bush Administration would have to make considerable effort to reverse this deteriorating situation. Rumsfeld and Cheney were angered by my declaration, not wanting to hear or admit that a health crisis existed. As a physician and humanitarian, I felt I had a moral and ethical obligation to speak out.

To recruit and interview Americans for CPA positions during "Iraq's reconstruction," Bremer used methods eerily similar to those used by Saddam's Ba'ath Party. Iraqis had to pledge allegiance to the Ba'ath Party to get jobs, receive promotions, or maintain stature. In May 2003, Bremer's recruiting team members passed over well-qualified, seasoned professionals for those CPA positions due to the uncertainty of their "adherence to the President's vision for Iraq."[6] Instead, Bremer's team chose young, inexperienced people who had to be seen as loyal to the Republican Party. During job interviews, candidates were asked politically loaded questions: "Who did you vote for in the 2000 election?" and "Do you support Roe v. Wade?" The irony was inescapable: Rumsfeld's team used a pointedly discriminating hiring process in Iraq on the heels of removing Saddam just as Saddam's high-ranking officials used the same selective hiring techniques.

All about Oil

Throughout Operation Iraqi Freedom, many involved had to wrestle with their presence in Iraq after learning that the pretext for the invasion was false. In 2002,

---

6. Rajiv Chandrasekaran, *Imperial Life in the Emerald City: Inside Iraq's Green Zone* (New York: Penguin Random House, 2007), p. 91.

12. Baghdad

the argument by Secretary of Defense Donald Rumsfeld and Vice President Dick Cheney was that Saddam was responsible for the 9/11 attacks. Rumsfeld and Cheney declared this alleged Iraqi complicity as "fact" and therefore a terrorist situation, distinguishing it from a regular cross-border war. They also believed that the 1949 Geneva Conventions did not apply. But no one from Iraq was ever implicated in 9/11. The Saudis quietly walked away. The Bush Administration even sent home the Saudi family members of Osama Bin Laden, who were living in the United States at the time.

As with many other circumstances of this kind, the invasion was tied to economics. When I went to Iraq as the Interim Minister of Health, one of my goals was to stop the looting. I lived with just a small group of military personnel, including Army and Navy medical staff who assisted me. They all knew why I was in Iraq, but three other civilians from the oil industry were also present. We all wondered why they were here.

The ransacking occurring in Baghdad and the rest of Iraq might have been stopped, but priority wasn't given to raiding the hospitals or museums. All security was focused on the oil ministry. From the beginning, oil was backing this invasion, but for the longest time, that argument was denied by those in power. The Bush Administration and supporters used the pretext of "weapons of mass destruction" being present, but, of course, no such weapons were ever found.

In all my experiences, I have repeatedly learned the critical significance of cultural competence and ethnic understanding. To make any progress in global health or humanitarian efforts, we cannot overstate the importance of having an understanding of a country's history and customs. We need to integrate our teams with efforts made on a local basis. In the case of Iraq in 2003, unfortunately, I don't feel we needed to be in that country in the first place. Through our actions, we made the situation much worse for the United States and elsewhere in the world.

Everyone with international experience was stunned when Paul Bremer announced that he was demobilizing the Iraqi army shortly after he arrived in Iraq. The majority of those troops were Sunni and they would no longer be paid. I knew the real trouble was just beginning. Within two weeks, a large majority of these soldiers were joining resistance groups they probably didn't know much about at the time. A few weeks later, they linked up to a growing insurgency.

I'm sure Paul Bremer was motivated by good intentions. But then he eliminated every Ba'athist member from the Iraqi government and dissolved the Iraqi Army in its entirety. By making these two moves, he unknowingly signed up the United States, as well as many military service members and contractors, for more than a decade of war. Suddenly, thousands of Iraqis found themselves without a job, without an income, and without a purpose. I think Bremer's decree to disband the Iraqi army was perhaps the biggest mistake we made in the Iraq War. We created the insurgency by bringing it on ourselves.

As I watched the situation unfold, the most frustrating part was that we *could have* done something about the health emergency. The Bush Administration-induced chaos was now beyond my control. I knew the World Health Organization and UN International Children's Emergency Fund grants, which were abruptly canceled upon the successful invasion of Iraq, would have at least eased some of the burgeoning crisis. Since U.S. troops began withdrawing from Iraq in December 2007, the number of deaths continued to increase and the statistics were staggering.

Had we admitted our role as an "occupying force" and followed through with our duty to restore public health protections, we absolutely could have mitigated the consequences of the invasion and occupation. The U.S. lost the capacity to identify populations at risk and to understand their needs for two reasons: We stopped the international health response and recovery contracts, and we did not have any strategic recovery or surveillance plan in place. A shortage of baseline data led to an ad hoc response to health system recovery, which concentrated more on structural repair than on actual system failures. Morbidity and mortality outcomes were never even measured.

* * * *

Since the U.S. invasion of Iraq in 2003, Donald Rumsfeld's argument that we came as "liberators and not occupiers" has been turned on its head. The Secretary of Defense's admission not only came too late but also was buried and unnoticed in the news cycle. The war led to a long, bloody occupation that at times spun completely out of control, which kept U.S. troops in Iraq for years. The Iraq War resulted in hundreds of thousands of war-related deaths—about 300,000 Iraqis, approximately 4,500 U.S. troops, and almost 400 Coalition troops.

Twenty years after the United States "liberated" Iraq, that nation remains a fragile and unsteady "democracy." Throughout the ordeal, the rest of the world was unaware of any humanitarian consequences. Due to the lack of humanitarian aid, the number of deaths will never be known.

13

Sleuthing in Liberia
August 2003

"The child soldier approached the car window where I was sitting. With a menacing smile, he wielded his machete. Once again, we all froze in fear."

After my disconcerting and perilous experience in Iraq, I left my concurrent positions at Johns Hopkins and the U.S. Agency for International Development in the summer of 2003. With much relief and ready to head home, Phyllis and I returned to Oahu. At age 63, I seriously contemplated retirement and let others assume the mantle of medical crisis management for international disaster scenes.

Withdrawing to paradise, nevertheless, wasn't meant to be, at least not at this point. As in so many instances, life happens while you're busy making other plans. Late in August, I received a call from the Executive Director for Emergency Services of the World Health Organization (WHO) in Geneva. He asked if I could do an immediate assessment in Liberia, a nation in West Africa wracked by civil war among multiple factions.

But his subtext was calling for some detective work into a very sensitive personnel issue that had arisen. The UN Special Humanitarian Coordinator wanted to fire the WHO Representative (WR) in Liberia. The Executive Director said he would go himself, but he was medically unable to leave Geneva. He had just returned from Baghdad and was dealing with wounds suffered in the horrific truck bombing of the UN Headquarters housed in the Canal Hotel. That brazen terrorist attack on August 19 had killed Brazilian Sérgio Vieira de Mello, at that time the UN High Commissioner for Human Rights and UN Special Representative for Iraq, as well as 22 of his colleagues.[1] I had left my position as Iraq's Interim Minister of Health just four months before. Had I still held that title, I would certainly have attended that ill-fated hotel meeting.

During our conversation, the Executive Director stated that the World Health Organization needed someone to go to Liberia without delay during this critical

---

1. Eight months after the attack, Abu Musab al-Zarqawi, a leader of al-Qaeda, declared responsibility for the bloodiest attack that had ever targeted UN personnel. Available at https://en.wikipedia.org/wiki/Canal_Hotel_bombing.

time of a many-factioned civil war. That person had to have experience in both public health and international medical crisis management services. The Executive Director said I was that person. We briefly discussed my views on providing urgent care aid to augment the ongoing non-emergency services provided by the WR in Liberia. The Representatives from the World Health Organization supervise that agency's offices under the WHO Regional Office for Africa (WHO-AFRO). The WRs manage WHO's core functions at the national level, and they also provide direction in the key functional areas of advocacy, partnership, policy, and administration. For the most part, WRs are proficient in public health and diplomacy, but they are not necessarily tuned into emergency responses.

The Executive Director's follow-up email to our phone call was very diplomatic. "Although WHO assets have been expanded and accelerated to meet emergency requirements, the UN Emergency System and its leadership, as well as some NGOs [non-governmental organizations] and donors, have raised serious concerns about the capabilities of existing WHO resources during the emergency phase."

I realized, however, that this situation was even more complicated. His discerning language was a cover for something more current. In addition to evaluating the medical situation in a shattered Liberia, he wanted me to check into the discord in Liberia among the NGOs, the UN Coordinator, and WHO's WR, all on the scene in Monrovia, the capital. And that was the subtle aspect of this request. I would have to conduct this second task skillfully and discreetly. The Executive Director quoted the UN Coordinator for Liberia, who strongly asserted that "health had become a serious issue and that a strong emergency capacity within the WR's office was seriously lacking,"

This current WR had served in Liberia for some time, but the UN Coordinator made his demands known. He wanted the Executive Director to fly immediately to Monrovia, despite his significant injuries, to "fire the WR." His request, though, completely oversimplified the structure and organization of these international governance bodies. The World Health Organization is operationally separate from the UN, and the UN Coordinator had no such jurisdiction to oust the WR.

Into Volatile Liberia

And so I went to Liberia. I would somehow do an evaluation, expedite the emergency services component from WHO-AFRO, and, most importantly, appease the UN Coordinator. Accompanied by several WHO colleagues, all these objectives were to be undertaken during a raging civil war. I suspected I would have to use some of my professional analytical skills as a psychiatrist in addition to gauging humanitarian needs. At the time of that unexpected phone call in 2003, I had previously served in the African nations of Nigeria, Kenya, Somalia, and Ethiopia. I had never been to Liberia, but that gap in my worldwide travels was about to change. I arrived in Monrovia on August 29, 2003.

13. Sleuthing in Liberia

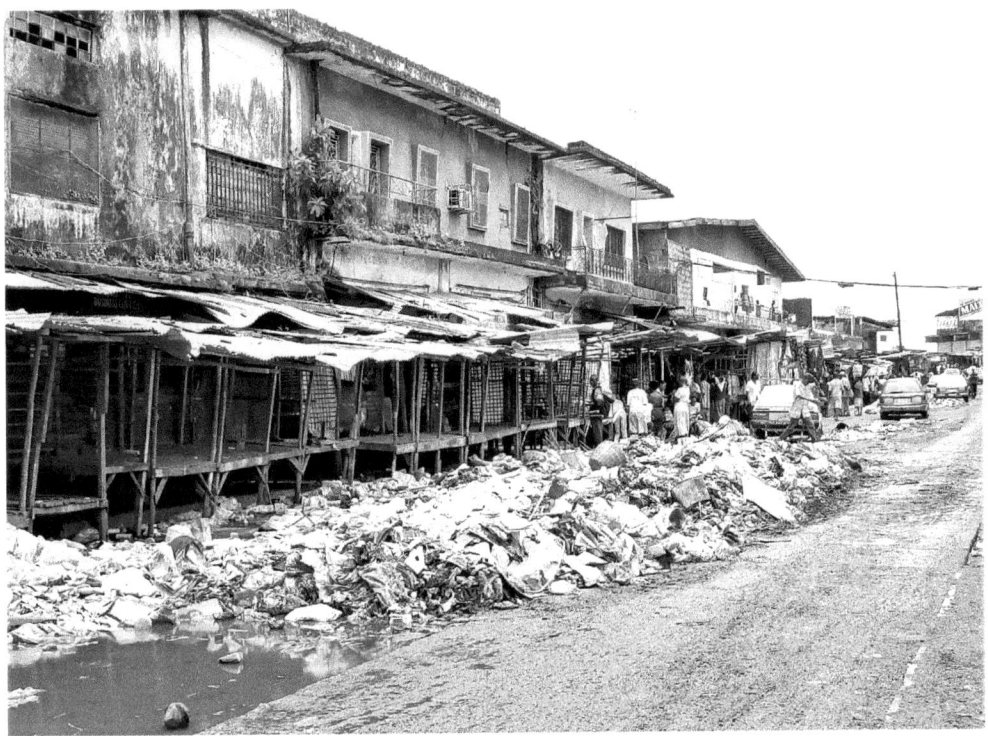

Utter devastation from years of civil war was a common sight in Liberia (author's collection).

Liberia's 19th century history is unique among African nations, especially the meanings behind the country's name and the capital's name. Liberia came from "liberty" and "Monrovia" was named for President James Monroe. Between 1821 and 1847, just a few thousand free people of color and former slaves from the United States were transported and resettled in the region that would be called "Liberia" in 1824. This project was sponsored by the American Colonization Society. The United States oversaw the colony, giving it a "moral protectorate" status throughout the 19th century to prevent European nations from seizing Liberia to add to their growing African colonial empires. The United States eventually supported the establishment of the Republic of Liberia in 1847 and continued to keep close ties with that new nation.

Liberia spent much of the 19th and 20th centuries ruled by Americo-Liberians, descendants of the original settlers born in the United States. But following a coup d'état in April 1980, the country became much more unstable. In 1989, Liberia was plunged into more than a decade of civil wars, exploited by warlord Charles Taylor.[2] This most recent civil war would end in 2003,[3] not too long after our team left. Taylor,

---

2. Charles Taylor served as Liberian president from August 1997 to August 2003. He was convicted in 2012 of war crimes and crimes against humanity, among many other charges, and was sentenced by an international tribunal to 50 years.

3. The First Liberian Civil War was from December 1989 to August 1997. The Second Liberian Civil War was from April 1999 to August 2003. Hundreds of thousands died in these conflicts.

an accused war criminal, would eventually be sentenced to 50 years in prison. After 14 years of conflict, he left behind a country completely in shambles with near-total eradication of its infrastructure.

The cost of the internal war had long-term effects on the health of the population. Beyond the direct outcomes of mortality, I knew I would find consequences on the looming horizon. For example, the electrical grid operated only in Monrovia, essentially leaving the rest of the country without power. And while 293 public health facilities existed before this second civil war, as many as 242 sites were deemed nonfunctional due to destruction and looting afterward. The Liberian population was left with very few authorities keeping track of their health needs and protections.

In the Time of Cholera

Health professionals well versed in global and humanitarian work know that fewer than 10 percent of deaths in war and conflict are actual casualties of war. The remaining 90 percent of deaths result from disasters or failed public health protections. In the case of many African countries, an overwhelming majority of mortalities are caused by preventable but untreated malaria, diarrheal disease, and malnutrition. Tragically, most of these deaths are children under the age of 2. In Liberia, I noted that the leading health issue was cholera.

Even though the port at Monrovia on the Atlantic Ocean had been opened only one week, victims felt it was safe to visit the cholera treatment facilities in the capital when they felt ill. But at least 250 new cases occurred each week. To try and get ahead of this outbreak, WHO was carrying out a chlorination program throughout Monrovia focusing on the 5,000 wells destroyed or intentionally polluted.

Outside Monrovia, where humanitarian agencies provided some services, much of the population had little or no access to health care. Most, if not all, physicians had fled the country by the time we arrived. This professional medical void left a health and hospital system maintained by an estimated 300 nurses, along with paramedics who filled in as physicians and former medical aides who often acted as midwives.

The World Health Organization and its WR worked out of the aging but adequate offices in the center of Monrovia. The WR and I had known each other from attending the same international medical society meetings. I always thought of him as sincere and well informed. However, as the days progressed, I realized he had little knowledge of emergency service needs.

Shortly after arriving in Monrovia, I attended one major conference led by the UN Coordinator. The WR spoke at length on chronic health issues, all very important but decidedly not what the UN Coordinator needed to hear. This UN Coordinator was becoming more irritable and restless as the session time slipped by. Because

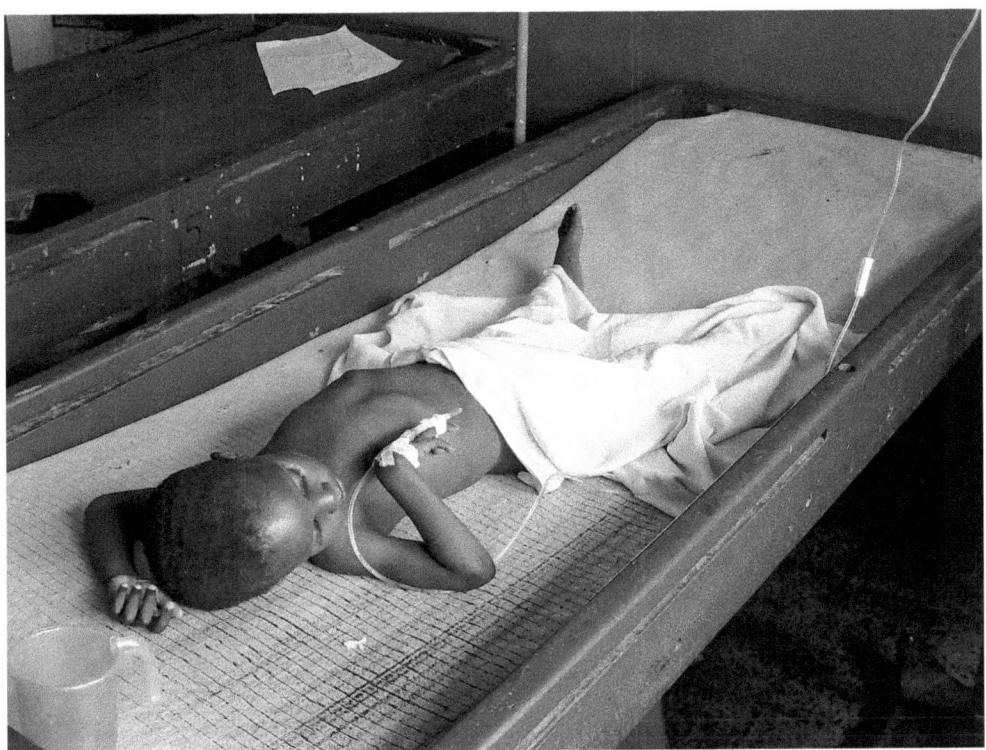

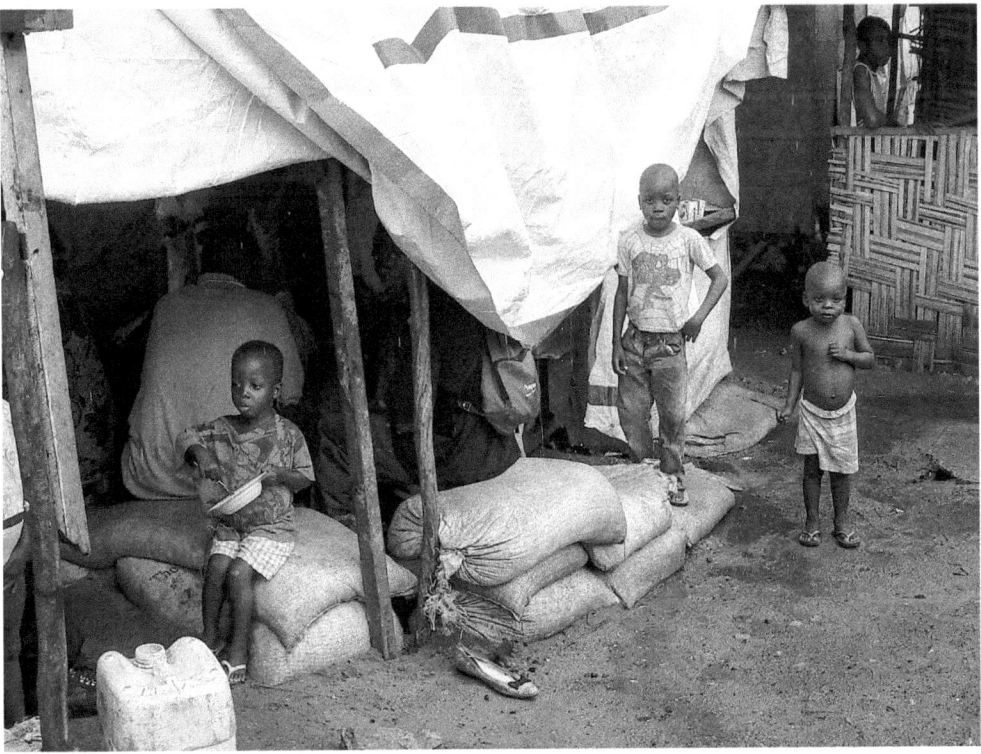

Top: In the few hospitals still operating in Liberia, most beds were reserved for cholera patients. A child is being rehydrated intravenously in this bed. *Above:* Children from families displaced by war find shelter wherever they can (both photographs author's collection).

it was too late in the day for any NGO presentations about emergency health issues, I observed several people walk out once they realized that the WR's talk focused only on non-emergency matters.

The Child Soldiers

Outside the walls of this well-organized meeting of international stakeholders, the reality on the ground was far more alarming and complex than chronic health conditions. For more than 14 years of civil war, Charles Taylor had become notorious for creating armies of "child soldiers"[4] as he pillaged the country. He used and abused these children. He resigned from the presidency, went into exile in Nigeria, then was subjected to detention by UN authorities. But many of his armed child soldiers still remained at large. They had no interest in returning to their former lives. With Taylor gone from the scene, an absurd situation existed. All negotiations for Liberia's future would take place between these immature and mostly leaderless child soldiers and the caretaker government.

Many of these youths had never been to school. They were severely traumatized by the horrors of war, even if they put on faces of toughness and brutality. They had no means of supporting themselves outside their two existing rebel groups known as either "Liberians United for Reconciliation and Democracy" or the "Movement for Democracy in Liberia." Beneath their ragged jungle uniforms, they were just children who had been groomed and brainwashed by unforgiving members of a well-armed militia. Unfortunately, these child soldiers still dominated and controlled the three population areas surrounding Buchanan, Lofa Bridge, and Tubmanburg. Our task was to visit each of these regions to get a true sense of the emergency health needs' scope.

Due to poor roads, the trips to each of these towns took a full day. Lawlessness remained a major problem across Liberia. Rebel groups and child soldiers frequently stopped us, flaunting their automatic weapons. Despite this intimidating behavior, they followed the agreement to allow UN and NGO vehicles to go through their so-called "checkpoints."

Three Crisis Hotbeds

The first fact-finding destination for our group was Tubmanburg. A WHO team had reported major health issues in this area, such as malnutrition in 75 percent of

---

4. Charles Taylor recruited an unknown number of young children, perhaps as many as 38,000 to 40,000 children and adolescents, to become part of his rebel militia called the "National Patriotic Front of Liberia." These "child soldiers" comprised the Small Boys Unit. They became soldiers and given guns, but they also served as sex slaves, cooks, and even as transporters of dangerous ammunition. Available at: https://www.newsweek.com/2013/07/31/when-liberian-child-soldiers-grow-237780.html.

the population, as well as malaria, diarrhea of unknown origin, acute respiratory illnesses, measles, and scabies. But even before these serious health problems could be tackled, security was the priority. The weekend before we arrived, the soldiers, who were serving with Liberians United for Reconciliation and Democracy, had burned homes and churches in the area, forcing 11,000 victims to move back to camps.

Our second information-gathering trip was to Lofa Bridge on a one-lane dirt road rife with washouts. Every village along the road was deserted, destroyed, or abandoned. I saw a devastated countryside with few people left. All health facilities had been recently plundered and demolished. No health workers were present because most had moved out due to a lack of security. Everyone our team had met warned us that even without a clear adult leader, child soldiers were still recruiting new children. Yet the people we encountered on the trip were planning to bring their families back home from Monrovia. With an almost complete breakdown in communications, they had fled to the capital not knowing how dangerous the city had become.

Lofa Bridge boasted one "doctor," a previous paramedic, who now called himself a "black bag MD." To feel personally safer, he would venture out to treat these victims of war, especially children who were chronically malnourished. Traveling to see patients reduced the risk to him and to those under his care. He also had no choice but to venture out because rebels had trashed his clinic. They also had been on the prowl, kidnapping and arming children.

But the urgency was apparent as soon as we arrived: Medical personnel needed to begin immunizations, organize a basic health care delivery system, and jump-start sanitation activities with an emphasis on clean water. Looking down several wells, we found animals rotting at the bottom. One deep well tragically contained a child's remains, an image I've never been able to erase from my heart or mind.

The third and last investigative trip was to Buchanan, a fishing town and an Atlantic trading port. We went through multiple rebel checkpoints before being delayed at the Saint John River bridge entrance to the town. With an AK-47 slung across his chest and exerting power with his machete, a young soldier pressed us for cigarettes and money. We slowly drove away without honoring his demands, but our team was justifiably on edge.

The day we arrived, Buchanan had just reopened its market. Many young women were cautiously navigating the bridge and small paths with food balanced on their heads. I noticed that the young men with Movement for Democracy in Liberia appeared less disciplined than the soldiers operating with the Liberians United for Reconciliation and Democracy we had seen on our trips to Tubmanburg and Lofa Bridge. These combatants in the Movement for Democracy in Liberia faction were more outspoken, threatening, and aggressive.

Our first stop was the local hospital, and I immediately noted that most beds were assigned to cholera victims. Then our group toured the former operating room in which everything but the surgery table had been ransacked. Straddling the hospital grounds was the internally displaced persons camp.

"I Do Not Want to Live by the Muzzle of a Gun"

We met a tall, thin rebel commander identifying himself as "Jerry Kowell." This seemingly affable "officer" told us he was originally from the Ivory Coast, just to the east of Liberia. We all sat down together and I recounted the forced stops and looting we had just witnessed on our way to Buchanan.

Kowell then surveyed the scene around the table. To enhance his status, he proudly stated that he was a "colonel." I sat directly across from him and sensed his penchant for titles. Leaning forward, I announced that I, too, was a "colonel," the Navy captain equivalent rank in the U.S. military. The young "colonel" quickly jumped up, stood at attention, and saluted me, a move which certainly startled my colleagues.

Kowell remained in this military stance in deference to my declared rank, and I took advantage of his admiration for the military. Using psychology, I faced Jerry, as a captain to a colonel, and decided to speak with a decisive military tone and sense of purpose regarding our inspection tours. I methodically itemized a list of grievances and needs, including security guarantees and access to warehouses for food and medicines. I complained about our group being detained at multiple checkpoints. I stressed the need for wells to be chlorinated. And to remain focused on those poisoned wells, I insisted on the removal of at least 30 decaying bodies from several contaminated wells. My WHO colleagues became increasingly nervous as I spoke, their eyes widening at my audacious requests. They wondered if my resolute demands would lead to anger or backlash from Jerry Kowell.

Referring to his version of a "military code of justice," Kowell repeated that he would personally deal with any soldier who abused a Liberian citizen, though I wasn't sure if he and I agreed on the meaning of "abused." He then stated that he was 18 years old and emphatically pleaded that he wanted peace. Still standing at attention, he dropped his head, which, I believe, was to hide tears. Kowell quietly added that he hoped to return to school, openly lamenting, "I do not want to live by the muzzle of a gun."

Acknowledging everyone at the table, he smiled and said that he aspired to be a sociologist. I nodded in support, saying that kind of respected career would be a wonderful profession for his country. I then looked around the table for my colleagues' reactions. Some of the team may have approved my firm stance on our needs. Sometimes tactful assertiveness pays off.

The meeting ended and we silently returned to our WHO vehicles. Slowly driving back across the bridge over the Saint John River, we left Buchanan behind us. We were immediately stopped by the same adolescent who delayed us coming across the

13. Sleuthing in Liberia

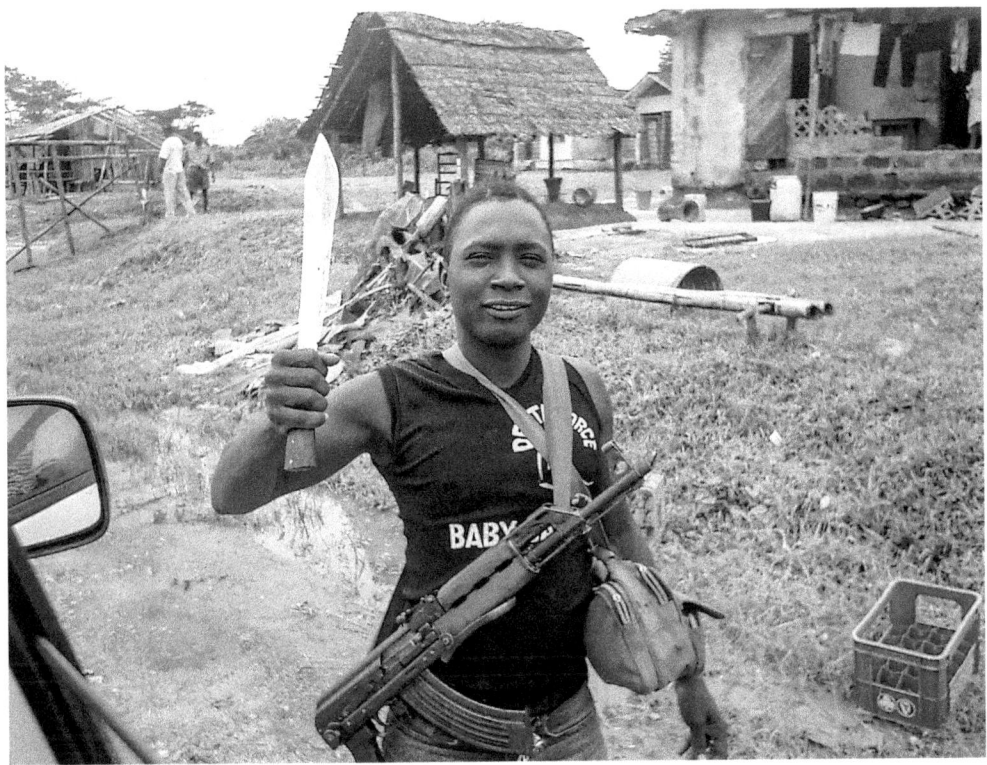

A Liberian "child soldier" approached Skip's car window near Buchanan, wielding his machete and carrying an AK-47 (author's collection).

bridge from the other direction. The child soldier approached the car window where I was sitting. With a menacing smile, he wielded his machete. Once again, we all froze in fear.

To my team members' shock, I rolled down the window and asked his age. He responded that he was 16. I then questioned at what age he became a child soldier. He proudly replied that he was 6 years old when he joined this rebel group. This adolescent established his dominance by brandishing this razor-sharp blade, then requested that I take his picture. I obliged in order to dispel the tension, and then I thanked this teenager. He smiled, I smiled, and then we sped away.

Everyone in the car collectively exhaled as we pulled away unscathed. But just a short distance up the road, we noticed some young women, their wares carefully poised on their heads. Before our eyes, we watched in horror as they were accosted by the young soldier's comrades. The women were dragged behind a building kicking and screaming in panic. We could hear their cries for help but were powerless to come to their aid.

That scene tormented me in the days afterward. To witness such a violent act leaves an indelible memory, though it paled in comparison to what those young women endured. Regardless of my perceived stature on the Liberian scene, I was helpless to confront these adolescent "soldiers" without jeopardizing my safety.

Looking back, this scenario seems like a microcosm of the power dynamics at play in many complex and protracted conflicts that occur around the world.

Not a word was spoken during our trip back to Monrovia as each of us tried to process what we had witnessed and experienced that day. And I'm quite certain a few of my new colleagues thought I might have been too reckless in the way I dealt with "Colonel" Jerry Kowell and the young soldier raising his machete. But under these circumstances, I didn't have the luxury of time to think through the best responses. I had to rely completely on my intuition, which, thankfully, had been honed since my early days in Vietnam and further refined with many other deployments in later years.

Back in Monrovia, I went through an exhaustive four days of interviews not only with multiple NGOs, but also with the World Food Program, World Bank, and UN operational personnel. The WR and the WHO team were unaware of these meetings. In such conflict situations, WHO holds a unique position in the wider health-related humanitarian community. The organization is expected to immediately identify the disease and conduct injury surveillance, note vulnerable populations and their locations, and oversee both curative and preventive programs. The World Health Organization then provides countrywide monitoring and coordination of health services. In addition, WHO aids in the recovery and rehabilitation of ministries of health and health care systems.

I scheduled individual meetings with many health service NGOs: Medical Emergency Relief International, Operation Mercy, Liberian Red Cross Society, International Committee of the Red Cross, Médecins Sans Frontières, Christian Health Association of Liberia, and the Lutheran World Federation. All those international NGOs expressed appreciation for the interest and easy-going working relationship with WHO and the WR. They all strongly felt, however, that WHO personnel lacked sufficient staff and leadership to work effectively in an emergency. The health problems and need for direction were massive and would last for years, but WHO and its WR were incapable of taking the lead. Although they did not want the UN Coordinator to take over the health services, they recognized he was losing patience.

The NGO representatives I questioned independently were puzzled. They each wanted to know why the WR had not immediately requested an emergency team to be sent by WHO's Regional Office for Africa (WHO-AFRO). This new lineup of players from WHO-AFRO, who were familiar with this area of Africa, could supplement emergency professionals.

The "UN Syndrome"

These representatives were insightful and impressively realistic. They pleaded for those with emergency services experience to start working with the WR, stressing that the WHO directorship was not prepared to face this crisis properly. The UN Coordinator, they thought, knew of WHO's incompetent dealings in Liberia.

I perceived the underlying problem to be centered on the definition of "emergency," and also whether or not WHO realized that Liberia was now facing a true emergency. Every NGO representative expressed the same opinion. For whatever reason, WHO was locked into a "no emergency mindset" with no sense of urgency. These representative agents felt that WHO was not up to the job, and the organization did not show any operational capability and capacity. In other words, WHO seemed to be only "talking shop" and unable to take action, thus becoming ineffective in emergency management.

This failure to act was just one of their worries. Collectively, almost to an agency, organization, or person, these NGO representatives had a vision of WHO's expected and assumed participation in Liberia during the emergency relief and recovery phase. They were not needlessly complaining or being petty with the WHO office in Liberia. These delegates were putting serious thought behind their concerns and answers, and desperation was now overcoming their increasing unease. Most felt WHO, as a whole, was not committed to implementing its valuable resources, which were necessary to work successfully as a major participant in a much-needed emergency response. The NGO agents all wondered if WHO's lack of action at this point might change in the future.

The most knowledgeable and perceptive representative I met was an American nun-missionary who had worked in Liberia since 1977. She supported the World Health Organization despite all the agency's problems, but advised me not to provide them with funds. With great firmness, she declared, "Give them a car if they need it—but not the money!"

I felt I had to extract more information from this missionary. She was honest and thoughtful, seeing potential in the WR but that the UN, being so weak, had fallen into what she called the "UN Syndrome." This very knowledgeable woman said the UN was running everything and ignoring all the local people with talent. Many had underlined this point in our meetings, and I was not sure how WHO should handle that problem in the long run.

I went back to the WR's office and asked him if we could meet privately the next day. I had to consider how I would present my deep anxieties and press him to start making urgent demands. The time had long passed for making soft recommendations.

At that agreed-upon meeting, I first asked if I might give him some advice, and tactfully praised the job and reputation he had acquired before the crisis. Without mentioning names or organizations, I stated that I was reflecting the direct apprehensions of interviewed professionals. Emphasizing that the NGO delegates all wanted his leadership, I underscored that they were losing patience with WHO's inaction. The NGO reps still trusted the WR but time was running out. These agents wanted an immediate emergency services response from WHO-AFRO and also from the Geneva offices. Calling for assistance, I added, would never reflect on him as overreacting. His feelings were not important now but his guidance was essential.

I identified the type of crisis personnel who needed to come without delay: two epidemiologists, a statistician, a health information professional, a sanitation engineer, a health administrator, and an additional clinically oriented medical officer. All those medically related human resources I spoke to had experience working as a team. The WR related that the Regional Office for Africa was sending a few reinforcements, but I interrupted him and stated they were not enough. He must request these specialists himself.

I pointed out that the first sign of leadership, which everyone was seeking, should come at once. He had to change the nature of his presentations at the UN coordinating meetings. The information he had previously provided, I contended, was not relevant to the crisis at hand. I tried to convey the gravity of the situation in which Liberia now found itself. At the next day's meeting, he needed to simply acknowledge that WHO had no new information on the developing emergency. He had to then introduce the NGOs one by one to provide their respective assessments. The following day, the WR received kudos from the NGO audience for his talk, which was a definite sign of taking positive command. But unfortunately, his biggest critic, the UN Coordinator was not present.

I was planning to leave in two days and the last item on my agenda was to see the UN Coordinator behind closed doors. The WR was not informed of this prospective meeting when he requested that I remain for three more days. For those next few days, we therefore talked of nothing but synchronizing operational-level emergency services.

On my last day in Monrovia, I was scheduled to fly to Geneva in the evening. That morning I went to the WHO bureau early, hid my bag in a closet, and set out alone on Monrovia's main thoroughfare to head to the UN headquarters. I had never been to this head office and had not made an appointment. I sensed many eyes following me along the way but encountered no trouble. The campus that housed the UN offices was beautifully manicured, a distinct contrast to the rest of Monrovia, much of which was in ruins from this ongoing civil war.

I entered a large marble-staired gothic building where the UN Coordinator had his office. I introduced myself to his secretary, apologizing for not having called beforehand. I wanted to keep this meeting secret from WHO personnel who might have been perplexed as to the nature of my actual role in Liberia.

Suddenly, from a room behind the secretary's desk, I heard a deep authoritative voice shout, "It's about time! Where have you been?"

As I entered his office, and even before I sat down in a large chair in front of his desk, he inquired about the WR. "Have you fired him yet?"

I then politely introduced myself and simply said, "No, I did not fire him." I told him I was leaving that night and would meet with WHO's Executive Director for Emergency Services the next morning in Geneva.

He sat up straight, red in the face, and screamed, "You are not to leave the country until he is fired!"

Maintaining my composure, which was critically important, I calmly replied, "No, you don't want me to do that." Firing the WR, I explained, would be unnecessary. I added with some insistence, "It would also be an embarrassment in the international community if you tried to enforce it." Stating the problem in a confident voice, I also acknowledged that he was certainly entitled to be upset. And using more skillsets from my diplomatic toolbox, I said that I, too, was disturbed and understood his concerns.

This kind of trouble has often happened, however, when crises occurred and professionals in charge were unfamiliar with how to deal with them. The WR, I continued, had remarkably changed his presentations so he wouldn't humiliate himself in future morning meetings. Most importantly, I pointed out that emergency personnel were on their way from Geneva and also from WHO-AFRO to support the needs on the ground.

Twenty years later, I am still amazed at Liberia's dire conditions at that time in mid-2003. I reviewed the brief notes I had made in which I outlined the UN Coordinator's closing comments. He wanted me to immediately address the emergency issues with WHO-AFRO saying, "Now, no time to wait. Need to get the emergency team in with leadership skills."

Trying to Make a Difference

I returned to Geneva that night and met with WHO's Executive Director who had originally called me. His painful facial wounds from the Baghdad terrorist attack cast a visual reminder of that bombing just two weeks earlier. But we had business to discuss. The Executive Director admitted that we agreed on the summary I had written. After making some tweaks, he affixed his signature to make my report final and official.

A month later, a senior member from the WHO Regional Office for Africa sent an email to all WHO personnel. He wrote, "What's your opinion of the man from the USA sent to Liberia from WHO Headquarters to help you? Did he make a difference? Is he still in Liberia?"

Maybe those simple questions mirrored my thoughts after I returned home. I hope I had made a difference. But many moving pieces were involved and Liberians had to process so much trauma. Trying to assess if I had any effect is a challenging task. And now, two decades after my short visit to Liberia, I would like to say that the country, among some of the poorest in the world, has rebounded and is turning itself around on the world stage.

* * * *

In mid–2014, however, just 10 years into the rebuilding and recovery following the last brutal civil war, the worst Ebola[5] epidemic in recent history began in nearby Guinea, hitting Liberia and neighboring Sierra Leone extremely hard. Thousands died and their fledgling health system was completely overrun. By the end of December 2014, Liberia experienced the most deaths. Four months later, no deaths were reported.[6] And on another positive note, maybe Jerry Kowell did become a sociologist and is doing his part to make Liberia a better place. I can always hope.

---

5. The Ebola virus disease (EVD) is named for the Ebola River, located in the Democratic Republic of Congo. Ebola's symptoms include fever, aching, loss of appetite, diarrhea, vomiting, hemorrhaging. Available at https://www.cdc.gov/ebola/signs-symptoms/.

6. Almost 5,000 Liberians died from the Ebola virus. On May 9, 2015, WHO reported Liberia free from the Ebola virus. Available at https://ebolaresponse.un.org/liberia.

PART IV

Bringing It All Home

14

A Wound Forever

> *"But all was not as it seemed. I found myself fighting a lonely, secret war, as did many other veterans from Vietnam and from conflicts before and since."*

"A Wound Forever" recounts my 1968 Vietnam traumatic brain injury (TBI). Blast injuries in the Vietnam War were relatively unusual. During that 20-year war, 12 percent to 14 percent of combat casualties had a TBI, based on evidence of massive head trauma and a lethal wound of the chest or abdomen, compared to 35 percent of gunshot and fragment wounds, mortars, grenades, and mines. The Iraq War (2003–2011) numbered about 19 percent gunshot and fragment wounds, whereas blast injuries in that war and the war in Afghanistan accounted for about 22 percent of all injuries. Mines and improvised explosive devices (IEDs) have supplemented small arms and artillery.

In today's wars, we rarely see the bullet wounds that dominated my time in Vietnam. Instead, the major wounds to civilians and military personnel have resulted from blasts, which are now more powerful and more indiscriminate. While blast waves generated from these explosions may not cause visible injuries at the time of the impact, they most likely inflict great physical and mental pain on the victims. Those combatants with TBIs are "often faced with physical, cognitive, and social limitations that may persist for a lifetime."[1] TBIs not only challenge the wounded, but also they deeply affect family members.

Most combat-related TBIs are classified as "mild." About 15 percent of the cases exhibit physical disabilities and symptoms that persist beyond three months, resulting in chronic conditions. In my case, I never reported any symptoms beyond the initial blast event, and I registered that blast incident only to my fellow physicians at Delta Med.

I have witnessed the myriad of chronic physical, cognitive, and behavioral issues across the decades. The most common form of TBI, that is, an acute or mild concussion, has multiple definitions that have currently led to mild TBIs known as the "invisible injury" of these conflicts.

---

1. Andrea Guevara et al., "Association Between Long-Term Cognitive Decline in Vietnam Veterans with TBI and Caregiver Attachment Style," *Journal of Head Trauma Rehabilitation*, 2015 January-February 30(1); E26–33. Available at https://pubmed.ncbi.nlm.nih.gov/24695269/.

Regrettably, since my service in the Vietnam War, the traumatic consequences have never left me, and those aftereffects have worsened during the past six decades. My TBI became a major factor in deciding that I could no longer spend the time and energy on global conflicts and humanitarian work that took me to faraway lands. I was getting older, as much as I tried to deny it. This period of realization also became a time when my life and Phyllis's life became "one again." This chapter re-experiences a transformational moment in time.

That fateful day in Vietnam was Friday, November 1, 1968. In an instant, my world had turned upside down. A 130mm artillery shell exploded above and behind me, and I would never be the same again. The blast wave impacted the base of my neck and the back of my head, hurtling through my ears, nasal openings, sinuses, mouth, and down my throat. In a microsecond, my brain violently slammed against the rear of the bony cranium, then my brain ricocheted off the inside front of my skull. Brain tissue bled, the delicate bones of my inner ear were jolted, and both eardrums and nerve sheaths were traumatized.

A rebound pressure wave instantly hit my face as the initial blast echoed from the cement floor beneath me. Then blood vessels in my left eye ruptured, clouding the vitreous humor, that is, the gel tissue behind the lens, with red blood cells. The wave rattled through my teeth and silver amalgam restorations, emerging at different rates—slower through tooth structure than through metal. Many of my fillings loosened at that instant. Knocked senseless, I have not felt "normal" since that terrifying moment 55 years ago.

When I look back over a half-century career as a physician, naval officer, global health professional, academic, and, of course, husband and father, I often marvel at how I pulled off all these daily challenges in life as symptoms of my injury worsened over time. To colleagues, students, patients, and even to myself, I always seemed to carry out my duties with efficiency and enthusiasm. But all was not as it seemed. I found myself fighting a lonely, secret war, as did many other veterans from Vietnam and conflicts before and since. In my 30s and 40s, I held the warning signs at bay, learning to live and function with my handicap—and it was a handicap. But as I advanced through middle age, my infirmities intensified and became more difficult to manage. Cursed with an invisible wound, I had no choice but to carry on, even though my brain and nervous system had been seriously damaged. My big takeaway from Vietnam was a TBI.

Close Encounter with Death

This violent, split-second event at Delta Med was a life-changing episode for me. But the medical personnel at this forward casualty field hospital, where I had been serving for only four months, did not know the full extent of my injury at that time. My symptoms were not immediately evident. I crawled into the safety of the triage bunker and then somehow found the strength to stand up. I remained confused and disoriented. Corpsmen and physicians, who were rapidly mobilizing to resuscitate gravely wounded casualties, were talking all around me. But I heard nothing other than an overwhelming rushing sound in my ears. Profound nausea engulfed me, a strong physical sensation recalled long after the impact. And even to this day, I have never been free of the loud ringing called "tinnitus" in my right ear.

Once back inside the bunker, a corpsman motioned to me that he wanted an IV bottle from a nearby shelf. As I weakly clasped the bottle, my body stiffened in horror upon seeing a large snake with narrow white stripes suddenly making its black undulating presence known. The serpent then slithered to the back of the shelf seeking refuge among medicine bottles. Within minutes of each other, I experienced a concussion and stood in front of a highly venomous banded krait. Even in time of war, November 1, 1968, was a day to forever remember.

The corpsman took the IV bottle from my hand, immediately realizing something wasn't right. He gently sat me down in a corner of the bunker where, in a haze, I watched the triage teams do their work. After a time, I was finally led to my hooch where I lapsed into a 20-hour dreamless sleep.

When I awoke, I felt a terrible pain on the right side of my head and in the back of my throat, and I also noticed decreased vision in my left eye. I walked under my own power to sick bay where a fellow physician, Dr. Robert Farkas, examined me. He found fresh blood behind my right eardrum, but he couldn't determine if the tympanic membrane had been perforated. My left ear appeared normal. With no sophisticated ocular diagnostic instruments in a war zone, he was unable to analyze the condition of my eyes. Nevertheless, all his findings were consistent with the symptoms of a severe concussion.

The hearing in my left ear returned a few weeks later, but the tinnitus persisted in the right ear. The initial pain that I felt in the roof of my mouth, along with added difficulty in swallowing, diminished over the next several weeks. The soreness I felt in my teeth lasted two more days until five amalgam restorations fell out spontaneously. For the remainder of my Vietnam tour, only the acute tinnitus, right-sided deafness, and cloudiness in my left eye lingered. Shrugging off the remnants of my momentary encounter with death, I returned to triage duties. During this same period, I also tried to deal with the outbreak of bubonic plague among the civilian children. I gave little thought to any possible long-term effects of my blast injury.

However, as the years passed, the ever-distracting tinnitus and moderate hearing loss in my right ear continued. I also began noticing hyperacusis, a state in which very quiet sounds are comfortable, but ordinary sounds, such as voices at conversational volume, seemed too blaring or distorted. Even a refrigerator compressor would sometimes seem too loud. A sudden harsh noise, for instance, a barking dog, caused discomfort or pain. Never having had significant motion sickness, I now faced the rapid onset of seasickness that prematurely ended my enjoyment of sailing.

Keeping My TBI Under Wraps

As a physician, I often self-diagnosed and self-medicated. Even while working in emergency rooms or traveling extensively to Africa, Asia, and the Middle East, I managed my illnesses. While serving in the Persian Gulf War in early 1991, I carried valium in my pocket as insurance to keep possible recurring symptoms under control. But I never allowed my traumatic brain injury to stop me from performing my duties. And not wanting to be thrown out of the Navy, I did not let anyone know my secret, except, of course, Phyllis. I conducted physical exams on everyone else, but in the years ahead I avoided having my annual hearing checkup.

As I approached my late 60s and early 70s, I began noticing increased bouts of vertigo, nausea, and anxiety when lying on my side. Trying to focus on small details displayed on a television screen was often the trigger. Then the "drop attacks" began—sudden, spontaneous falls while walking or standing. Recovering quickly after the events, I didn't note any loss of consciousness and could call to mind what had just occurred.

These spells grew more frequent and increasingly serious. They started with a feeling of heaviness in the right side of my head and then resulted in numbness in my right face, nose, and upper lip. These symptoms were accompanied by diarrhea and projectile vomiting and an immediate need for sleep. On one occasion, without warning, I was overcome by dizziness and rapid movement of my eyes. I distinctly recall lying on the bathroom floor for nearly 10 hours enduring uncontrolled vomiting and diarrhea. If ever I needed a wake-up call, that unsettling incident was it. I could no longer self-manage my TBI.

In 2009, I went to the Mayo Clinic in Rochester, Minnesota, for an extensive evaluation, which included a brain MRI (magnetic resonance imaging). The scan showed changes to the frontal lobe white matter, as well as the right-sided 9th and 10th cranial nerve tumors stemming from the 1968 blast to the back of my head. The MRI indicated that the blast wave entered my head through the foramen magnum, the opening in my skull. The foramen magnum is known to produce deep brain bleeding and shearing of the brain's nerve fibers due to brain injury. At the time of the blast, my brain shifted and rotated within the bony skull.

For my drop attack seizures, I received Gentamicin antibiotic injections into and through my right eardrum, a procedure called "ablation."[2] But within 24 hours, I developed a severe imbalance. My physicians assumed that the left-sided function of my inner ear, which controls balance, did not compensate for what was lost on the right side causing chronic imbalance. This condition has permanently affected my gait, and I need a cane to stabilize myself. I have gotten a total of eight such injections to control recurrent seizures, and have since been outwardly seizure-free.

---

2. Ablation is a chemical destruction of the involved tissue. In this case, the goal was to inactivate the right-side hearing-balance system.

In 2019, audiometric testing not only revealed a substantial decline in my right ear's high-frequency hearing, but the examination also indicated a profound hearing loss with very poor speech discrimination. The right ear is now chemically treated and the inner ear balance (vestibular system) on that side no longer functions. My seizures aren't related to inner ear dysfunction anymore, making it likely that the right-sided symptoms are also linked to my TBI.

An additional neurological and neurophysiological evaluation also exposed a significant decline in my memory function. The lowest scores came from the right brain hemisphere affected by the blast wave. Also, the brain MRI showed mild cerebral atrophy and changes to small blood vessels, which probably caused some harm to the white matter in my cerebrum.

Despite lasting vision problems with my left eye, a standard ophthalmoscopic examination did not disclose any pathology. However, retinal coherence tomography, that is, sectional imaging, disclosed a thin layer of old blood across the face of the retina, resulting in chronic granular blurriness. Reading is very difficult because I see words as if I were looking at them through gauze.

The layer of old blood obscuring my retina was the result of the blast wave, which caused bleeding within the fluid part of the globe of the eye. This symptom has remained with me as a daily reminder of so long ago. These blood cells have since turned into a waxy, fat-like substance similar to cholesterol. During my frequent flyer days, I usually took a window seat so I could nap uninterrupted. As I often looked out into the brightness through my left eye, I saw distinct clumps of red blood cells, the source of blurred vision in that eye. Those long-dead cells still linger, as with the other signals of my TBI. They are souvenirs that are forever frozen in time from Vietnam.

Falling Through the Diagnostic Cracks

I have been suffering for more than five decades from the damage caused by the blast wave. That previously undiagnosed injury now has a long-winded-sounding name for this specific TBI condition. This syndrome is called a "foramen magnum and occipital crest focused-associated blast injury." During the Vietnam War, other types of brain damage may have been widespread due to mine explosions and enemy shelling. My brain trauma was not common. But it was also not unique

We are now learning much more about how a blast wave can affect the brain in many wide-ranging ways. Almost six decades after Vietnam, neurological research suggests how a TBI can harm the central nervous system, as well as showing that damage is more complex than originally perceived. For both the Department of Defense and the Department of Veterans Affairs, the previous regular basis for determining if a TBI was "mild," "moderate," or "severe" was the length of time the victim had lost consciousness. This criterion applied only to cerebral hemisphere-focused blasts—those blast waves that strike the skull from the sides and commonly initiate the loss of consciousness. Casualties who didn't fit into this common TBI category usually fell through the cracks of diagnosis due to a lack of awareness of the deep-rooted and debilitating effects of this particular TBI.[3]

Researchers are now investigating the role of blast waves and their impact on biophysical, neurobiological, physiological, and cognitive impairment that may get worse in a matter of hours, days, and weeks—sometimes lasting for life.[4] Unfortunately, military decision-makers have concentrated only on the duration of loss of consciousness to define "mild," "moderate," and "severe" TBIs. In my case, the so-called "TBI" that I sustained would not have qualified then or even now as anything more consequential than being considered as a "mild TBI." The military's criterion of duration of being unconscious was unclear in my case. I blacked out briefly, but whether or not I lost consciousness is debatable.

Animal research has shown that head position relating to the blast is critical. Rats' craniums were subjected to a blast wave, which struck the posterior cranium in the region of the occipital crest and foramen magnum. The rats then developed persistent, ongoing signs of damage three weeks later.[5] Because those blast waves didn't directly involve the cerebral hemispheres or lead to prolonged unconsciousness, meaningful evidence of central nervous system impairment was not ruled out. Similar symptoms, which were revealed in many of my medical evaluations, paralleled the findings in the animal studies. Neurological research now implies that the way blast waves impact the central nervous system may be more complex than initially assumed.[6]

These discoveries have important implications not only in my case but also for the military and the Department of Veterans Affairs. Many years after my blast wave repercussions, I received a diagnosis of a "mild TBI" because the blast focus on my head was not on the side of my skull, but in the very back and then in the face and forehead. I experienced only a brief loss of consciousness post-impact that may have lasted a mere few moments. That rigid diagnosis alone, which has lasted for decades, has limited any understanding of the depth of my injury. Nevertheless, the extent of my traumatic brain injury, as well as a delayed onset of symptoms, should place me in a more significant category than simply a "mild TBI." Based on the last 50-plus

---

3. Chol D. Kim, "Traumatic Brain Injury Screening for the Armed Forces Military and Veterans," *McGeorge Law Review* 2008 (40), 449. Available at https://scholarlycommons.pacific.edu/greensheet/53/.
4. Frederick M. Burkle et al., "Delayed-Onset Neuropathological Complications from a Foramen Magnum and Occipital Crest-Focused Traumatic Brain Injury (TBI) During the Vietnam War," Parts 1–3, *Military Medicine* October 2021. Available at https://academic.oup.com/milmed/article/187/7-8/938/6386460.
5. Olivia Uddin et al., "Chronic Pain After Blast-induced Traumatic Brain Injury in Awake Rats," *Neurobiology of Pain* 2019 August–December (6),100030. Available at https://www.sciencedirect.com/science/article/pii/S2452073X18300278.
6. Geoffrey Ling et al., "Explosive Blast Neurotrauma," *Journal of Neurotrauma* 2009 (26), 815–825. Available at https://pubmed.ncbi.nlm.nih.gov/19397423/.

years of my progressively incapacitating symptoms, I can confidently state that my experience has been anything but "mild." Those injury classifications should not be based solely on loss of consciousness.

Definitions and Decorations

A mild TBI is the most common type of brain disability affecting military personnel, even though this condition is the most difficult to diagnose and the least understood. Results from animal studies indicate that veterans, who have had the type of damage I incurred, may have long-lasting and sometimes progressive, long-term disabling effects. A growing body of evidence suggests that a single TBI can (1) produce ongoing brain gray and white matter atrophy, (2) precipitate or accelerate age-related neurodegeneration, and (3) increase the risk of developing Alzheimer's disease.[7] Yet many of these developments never reach the veteran, or they are not recognized by the Department of Defense through updated TBI criteria. The military bureaucracy rules by definitions. If a military member didn't lose consciousness following an explosion, he could not have suffered a critical TBI. This explanation was as true during the Vietnam War as it is today, even though the science says otherwise.

Traumatic brain injuries have become a more common occurrence during wars in the last few decades. And the definitions and parameters for categorizing them and determining appropriate decorations have continued to change—though not always in a logical manner. In 2011, the Secretary of the Army, John McHugh, approved a policy allowing soldiers to receive the Purple Heart—the military's oldest award—for concussions and mild TBIs that did not result in loss of consciousness.

Also in 2011, the Secretary of the Navy, Ray Mabus, discussed updates to the standards and procedures for awarding the Purple Heart after receiving a diagnosis of a TBI. He pointed out that military neurologists had discovered that mild TBIs were more prevalent than previously disclosed. Secretary Mabus rightly stated, "Wounds suffered while defending our nation, whether seen or unseen, deserve our utmost gratitude and respect."[8]

Jim Nierle, head of the Navy Department's Board of Decorations and Medals, sowed further confusion in 2011 on this brain damage issue. He said that sailors and Marines may be awarded the Purple Heart for certain mild TBIs that were caused by enemy action, a statement which narrowed the indicators.

Nierle noted, "If they suffered a loss of consciousness or had to be given the

---

7. Ann C. McKee and Meghan E. Robinson, "Military-related Traumatic Brain Injury and Neurodegeneration," *Alzheimer's & Dementia Journal* June 2014 (10), S242–253. Available at https://pubmed.ncbi.nlm.nih.gov/24924675/.

8. Press release, Secretary of the Navy Public Affairs, January 4, 2012, as cited in *The Flagship*. Available at https://www.militarynews.com/norfolk-navy-flagship/news/quarterdeck/navy-updates-purple-heart-award-policy/article_de1f41b3-3437-5ab5-a9c4-08047c66dca8.html.

disposition of 'not fit for full duty' by a medical officer for a period greater than 48 hours after a concussive event, they may qualify for the Purple Heart."[9]

Then in April 2015, the Office of the Secretary of Defense sent to all service assistant secretaries an updated definition and reports on TBIs. But the classifications did not include clinical updates that clarified the current controversies and inadequacies regarding TBIs.

Fast-forward five years to January 2020: Traumatic brain injury became international news following an Iranian missile attack on the Al Asad Airbase in western Iraq. Responding to the assassination by a U.S. drone strike of prominent military leader Qasem Soleimani, Iran launched more than a dozen ballistic missiles at the base on January 8, each carrying an estimated 1,000-pound warhead. The consequences were devastating.

Even though no fatalities occurred, that statistic belied the unseen human toll, waved off by Donald Trump, the U.S. Commander in Chief, who proclaimed, "I am pleased to inform you, the American people should be extremely grateful and happy no Americans were harmed in last night's attack by the Iranian regime. We suffered no casualties—all our soldiers are safe and only minimal damage was sustained at our military bases."[10]

Several days later, President Trump further downplayed the situation by stating at a news conference in Davos, Switzerland, "I heard they had headaches. No, I don't consider them very serious injuries, relative to other injuries that I've seen."[11]

Those pronouncements were premature, dismissive, and inaccurate. Despite the confusion in definitions and lack of clarity about which specific TBIs "deserve" a medal, survivors tell their own stories, not unlike my experience more than a half-century earlier. For example, Army intelligence officer Major Alan Johnson said the missiles sounded like freight trains roaring by. He was knocked temporarily unconscious by the first blast.

Johnson vividly remembered, "There [were] people throwing up; everybody had headaches. [I have] headaches every day, horrible tinnitus or ringing in the ears. PTSD [post-traumatic stress disorder]. You know, I'll be willing to admit that. I still have nightmares."[12]

Army Sergeant Kimo Keltz was stationed in a guard tower on the exposed perimeter of the base when one salvo hit just 30 yards away. Keltz had curled into a fetal position to protect his vital organs, but the blast wave lifted him two inches

---

9. Shawn Snow and Meghann Myers, "Heart Following Iran Ballistic Missile Attack, *Yahoo News*, February 5, 2020. Available athttps://www.militarytimes.com/flashpoints/2020/02/04/nearly-60-service-members-could-be-eligible-for-the-the-purple-heart-following-iran-ballistic-missile-attack/.

10. Cory Dickstein and Caitlin M. Kenney, "Trump: No Americans Harmed in Attack by Iran," *Stars and Stripes*, January 8, 2020. Available at https://www.cnas.org/press/in-the-news/trump-no-americans-harmed-in-attack-by-iran-which-appears-to-be-standing-down.

11. Helene Cooper and Eric Schmitt, "Trump Dismisses Troops' Possible Brain Injuries as Headaches," *The New York Times*, January 29, 2020. Available at https://www.nytimes.com/2020/01/22/world/middleeast/trump-iraq-brain-injuries.html.

12. David Martin, "Inside the Attack That Almost Sent the U.S. to War with Iran," *60 Minutes*. Available at https://www.cbsnews.com/news/iran-missle-strike-al-asad-airbase-60-minutes-2021-02-28/.

off the tower's floor. When the attack was all over and he and his comrades emerged from their positions, they were much relieved. These men had survived Iran's retaliation. Nevertheless, it would take hours, even days before they realized that more than 100 soldiers and airmen had suffered TBIs—with Keltz being one of those victims.

Keltz later stated, "Because of how many blasts I took within such a close radius of me, it felt like someone hitting me over the head with a hammer over and over and over."[13]

Doctors told him he had "concussive syndrome," a condition that may afflict him for the rest of his life. If that's the case, similar to mine, Kimo Keltz and many of his comrades are in for a rough ride.[14]

In wars today, we rarely see the bullet wounds that often dominated my time in Vietnam. Instead, the major wounds to civilians and military personnel arise from blasts, which are now more powerful and more indiscriminate. While these blast waves may not cause visible injuries at the time of the actual event, they inflict great physical and mental pain on many who were close enough to feel the impact. Between 2000 and 2019, the Defense and Veterans Brain Injury Center reported nearly 414,000 TBIs among American service members around the world.[15]

Invisible Wounds of War

While many others have deeply felt the physical effects of brain injuries, as I have, countless more have been faced with their shadowy wounds. Wars cannot be fought, no less won, without those in the ranks. But the impact of the trials of war on a person has never been truly appreciated by those not involved in the fighting. Military leadership has always maintained an element of disdain and reproach for psychological victims, labeling them as "cowards," "malingerers," or "lacking in moral fiber." Ignorance and unpreparedness in caring for the military and civilian population's psychosocial needs during wartime have remained as pervasive, denial-driven subjects. Not much has changed since the end of World War I in 1918.

Civilian and military leadership will always do what is necessary to keep their armies intact and invincible. Yet the individuals who are compelled to go to war,

---

13. *Ibid.*
14. Four months following the Iranian ballistic missile attack on January 8, 2020, the Army announced that it would award the Purple Heart to 23 soldiers for their injuries, troops who had been medevacked to hospitals for treatment. However, the Army declared that 56 other service members suffering from TBI symptoms did not automatically qualify them to receive the award. Although paperwork was submitted for these troops, no further Purple Heart awards were forthcoming. Current evidence indicates that "politics" played a role in the Army's decision. Unfavorable publicity has caused the Army to reconsider Purple Heart applications for more than 30 additional troops. Available at https://www.cbsnews.com/news/purple-heart-us-soldiers-iran-al-assad-air-base-attack-traumatic-brain-injury/ .
15. VA Research on Traumatic Brain Injury (TBI), Office of Research & Development, U.S. Department of Veterans Affairs. Available at https://www.research.va.gov/topics/tbi.cfm#:~:text=The%20Defense%20and%20Veterans%20Brain,TBIs%20were%20classified%20as%20mild.

that is, those serving on the front lines, plus their families and their communities, are the ones left to navigate the psychological battles that continue long after a war ends.

This plight has sadly not changed in the last century. From "shell shock" in World War I to "breakdown" or "combat fatigue" in World War II, physicians scrambled to understand how to screen for this tendency or how to quickly treat it so the soldier could return to the battlefront. Fifteen years after the Vietnam War, studies concluded that 15 percent of those Americans who served in that war were experiencing post-traumatic stress disorder (PTSD).[16] This syndrome first appeared as an analytic category in the 1980 *Diagnostic and Statistical Manual of Mental Disorders*. Unfortunately, as the incidence of PTSD in Vietnam veterans fluctuated anywhere from 3 percent to 50 percent, many debates ensued around the validity of diagnoses and symptoms that continue even today.

* * * *

Although the majority of TBIs may be "mild" and allow the person to work and have a seemingly normal existence, I can testify that this type of injury, sorry to say, is a lifelong partner. In the time of Vietnam, only vague information was available to my peers and to me regarding diagnosis, accompanied by a lack of recognition. I would like to see more emphasis placed on brain health and treatment research. Studies may facilitate additional options for those recently diagnosed with traumatic brain damage. Society needs to be more supportive to help manage these hidden wounds in the years to come.

The past 55-plus years haven't been easy for Phyllis in seeing how my TBI has impacted our everyday life together. My TBI has affected both of us with periodic rough patches. She found it difficult to witness what I was going through at times, as I often couldn't hide my symptoms. But she also knew that I persevered and would do whatever it took to do my job wherever my assignments took me. Phyllis has always been by my side when I experienced this lonely, secret war dating from November 1, 1968.

A 2023 study recognized TBI as a "chronic condition" that can affect multiple "domains of health and function, some of which might deteriorate over time with patients becoming more disabled."[17] We now understand that TBI can be a chronic and unrelenting disease. For me, that one blast injury decades ago has become my chronic curse. I will live with my invisible wound for the rest of my life. And I hope Sergeant Kimo Keltz and Major Alan Johnson's journey through life with a so-called "mild" form of TBI won't be as distressing as mine has been.

---

16. "PTSD and Vietnam Veterans: A Lasting Issue 40 Years Later," U.S. Department of Veterans Affairs, Summer 2015. Available at https://www.publichealth.va.gov/exposures/publications/agent-orange/agent-orange-summer-2015/nvvls.asp.

17. Kristen Dams-O'Connor et al., "Traumatic Brain Injury as a Chronic Disease: Insights from the United States Traumatic Brain Injury Model Systems Research Program," *The Lancet Neurology* 2023 June 22(6):517–528. Available at https://www.sciencedirect.com/science/article/abs/pii/S1474442223000650.

15

Hard-Earned Lessons

"I feel so fortunate to have had some part in this new field, although it came with many hard-fought and hard-earned lessons, none of which I regret."

My medical career took many twists and turns following my return home from Liberia in the late summer of 2003. And while I had to adjust to not being deployed to the front lines of humanitarian crises, I was at least no longer being shot at—a most welcome change to my life. I had learned so much in my journeys to distant locales, observing many similarities throughout those years. But I became frustrated in watching the same mistakes being made repeatedly—even decades apart—whether in war or crisis response. The blunders we had made in Vietnam had been quickly forgotten by the time we became involved in the Persian Gulf War in 1991 and then in the Iraq War in 2003.

War and its tragic consequences jarred me out of complacency early in life, but, unfortunately, we seem to have learned nothing in the aftermath of wars. I was therefore determined for others to benefit from the lessons that I had gained in the field of humanitarian assistance and disaster medicine. We had to be better equipped to make a true difference. In addition, we had to avoid the duplication and missteps that my generation had encountered as this fledgling field of disaster medicine began to come together as a profession in the last quarter of the 20th century.

Passing the Torch

More than ever, I wanted to pass on my experiences, successes, and failures, all of which I had acquired in the field, to those who were taking up the mantle of humanitarian assistance in times of crisis. An entire new group of professionals stated that they worked in disaster medicine, but what did that mean? I did see an incredible influx in the development of academic courses and programs. During the past several decades, I noted competitiveness among new institutions and international NGOs. Each organization sought to prove it was the best at what it did, respectively. But I grew very exasperated because I could see that the world offered more than enough humanitarian crises to go around.

I became more involved in policy writing, giving speeches about frameworks and organization, and teaching whenever and wherever I could. In 2012, for example, I had the prestigious honor to give the annual Joseph Leiter National Library of Medicine Lecture at the National Institutes of Health in Washington. My presentation was titled "Future Humanitarian Crises: Challenges to Practice, Policy, and Public Health" in which I summarized what I was hoping to do on a broader scale in this new phase of my life.

During this time, I was also granted an academic appointment at the Center for Humanitarian Health, which is part of the Johns Hopkins Bloomberg School of Public Health. I was later named a professor and a Senior Fellow and Scientist at the Harvard Humanitarian Initiative, which gives attention to humanitarian crises and leadership. The goals of the Center for Humanitarian Health and the Harvard Humanitarian Initiative are three-fold: (1) to develop both the multidisciplinary competencies needed for every health care worker who would become involved in humanitarian public health crises around the world; (2) to document and to learn from health care workers' achievements and failures; and (3) to see the new directions that those challenges might bring.

After years of pushing against the ocean as an individual, I was ready to take a few steps back to see what was needed to reduce the futility of working solo within a failing crisis-mode system. I was fortunate to be associated with talented colleagues to improve the system, that is, change how disaster medicine was practiced in the field. I also wanted to see how a trained, formalized workforce could be built.

My colleagues and I labored tirelessly to create competencies, such as emphasis on emergency medicine, mental health, nursing, and prehospital medicine. In addition, we made every effort to generate other health-related specialties for those who would be part of this medical sector. But we also had to formulate programs and develop faculty for teaching humanitarian assistance and disaster medicine—both encompassing critical components of public health. Multiple certifying courses were created around the world.

Decoding Vital Signs

Health professionals deployed to disaster settings have to be able to speak the same crisis management language, count on one another to perform set tasks, and be able to work in new and challenging environments. They also need to be able to think creatively, use on-site available tools, and find resourceful ways to obtain important data. For example, an Australian aid worker proved it could be as simple as climbing the nearest tree to get a better view of the crowd if the uncertain situation called for how many people were in line or required assistance.

While numerous specialties were within the field of competencies, I was often called on to teach triage management, given my time and experiences at Delta Med in Vietnam. I frequently had people calling me after their deployments to say how helpless they felt by not having the right tools or training to be able to provide the necessary aid and support. Too many professionals from high-income countries were being sent to humanitarian emergencies in low-resource settings. They did not have the physical examination skills to assess patients, or they relied too much on imaging or other tests that were in short supply in those environments. In the United States, physicians are often not even the ones taking vital signs anymore. Our health care system has now become so fragmented that those duties are delegated to medical assistants or other staff who use modern monitoring devices to take patients' vitals at the outset of the exam.

In triage, it is the injury to the body that is critical. Many of these physiologically interpretive-based skills have been lost over time, and may not even be taught anymore because we have shifted to more dependence on technology. Due to waning skillsets and their ever-present need in crisis environments, I have become passionate about bringing these triage vital signs skills back to more mainstream use. It is not just about measuring and reporting the pulse rate, body temperature, blood pressure, and oxygen level. We need to obtain a true assessment of the patient followed by a potential prognosis. To do this evaluation, physicians must "decode" these vital signs. They must also understand how these critical medical indicators inform a diagnosis.[1] The focus of many of my teachings during this period was attaining valuable information from those all-important vital signs.

Honored Down Under

Our collective efforts slowly gained traction throughout the United States, Canada, Europe, Asia, and Australia. But in Australia's health services, I noted the lack of extensive public health training, which is an essential component of all crisis management. I visited Australia nine times as a lecturer at Monash University in Melbourne, but I also made myself available as a consultant. My advice was to expand public health training beyond physicians by opening up public health courses and degrees to nurses, paramedics, administrators, and every other future public health expert. This increase in training would reflect the multidisciplinary nature of the challenges this specialty area of crisis management demanded.

The Australian capacity for preparedness and response capacity is currently rated among the best in the world. For more than 15 years, I have been extremely proud that Monash University has hosted the annual "Burkle Lecture," featuring a

---

1. Frederick M. Burkle, Jr., "Triage and the Lost Art of Decoding Vital Signs: Restoring Physiologically Based Triage Skills in Complex Humanitarian Emergencies," *Disaster Medicine and Public Health Preparedness*, February 2018, 76–85. Available at https://www.cambridge.org/core/journals/disaster-medicine-and-public-health-preparedness/article/abs/triage-and-the-lost-art-of-decoding-vital-signs-restoring-physiologically-based-triage-skills-in-complex-humanitarian-emergencies/22506C65C3D34B6-35730D7ED5A85EFB8

prominent individual in the medical field who speaks on a variety of subjects related to international disaster medicine.

On other fronts, my close relationships with both Japan and China continued, trips to those countries made more accessible from my home in the middle of the Pacific Ocean. My textbook, *Disaster Medicine: Application for the Immediate Management and Triage of Civil and Military Disaster Victims*, was first published in 1987. The book was translated into Japanese and turned out to be a bestseller in Japanese medical circles. The book was even more popular in Japan than in the United States.

Disaster Medicine became a precursor to a host of articles and expanded book volumes, which are now published worldwide. More emerging disaster medical setups were also appearing in China. With my former participation in building those programs, I was invited in 2018 to be the lead speaker during the opening of the University of Tianjin medical complex in northern China. My talk concentrated on crisis management. I was excited to watch these advances happening simultaneously across so many countries.

In the publishing field, I encouraged the development of what became two respected medical journals. The first journal, *Prehospital and Disaster Medicine,* is now the official publication of the World Association for Disaster and Emergency Medicine. The second journal, *Disaster Medicine and Public Health Preparedness*, was first sponsored by the American Medical Association. This periodical presented new research and knowledge across disciplines and locales shared by the growing number of experts in the field.

Impact of Climate Change on Refugees

While academic progress and workforce development were ongoing, my colleagues and I watched populations grow denser. The effects of climate change became clearer, and rapid urbanization took over cities at an unprecedented pace. Too many people were living in crowded environments, an alarming scenario because infectious disease then becomes much more difficult to stop. Also, rising incidents of food, water, and energy scarcity in countries around the world have been contributing to the worsening refugee crisis.

As I wrote in the foreword of a book by Tener Veenema, *Disaster Nursing and Emergency Preparedness: For Chemical, Biological, and Radiological Terrorism and Other Hazards* (2018), the consequences of climate-related disasters have increased by more than 50 percent in the last decade. This surge in calamities is caused by the loss of essential aquifers and viable land, as well as the onset of major droughts. These catastrophes, which leave countries unable to survive or participate in any adaptation to climate change, further exacerbate internal migration, urban warfare, and domestic civil unrest.[2]

---

2. More on these issues can be found in the essay "Politics and Global Public Health: An Explosive Combination" at the end of the book in, "Four Perspectives on the World's Challenges and Concerns."

A 2009 study found that from 1950 to 2000, 80 percent of major wars occurred in the existing 34 most biologically diverse and threatened areas of the world.[3] As these areas become smaller and disappear, the number of conflicts can be expected to increase alongside the competition for resources. People were also starting to relocate. These populations on the move led to so many being internally displaced, thus worsening the refugee situation overall. Dire circumstances resulted that created a huge civilian mortality burden.

Around this time, my colleagues and I also witnessed a rise in antibiotic-resistant infections in several disaster settings. In 2014, *The Atlantic* profiled this problem of invincible bacteria in Jordan, highlighting the drastic reduction in the effectiveness of available antibiotics for historically routine infections.[4] The author noted that the ability to treat the *E. coli* bacteria in 2000 with available antibiotics was effective 80 percent of the time, but by 2014, this percentage had dropped to just 37 percent.

All these issues propelled me to continue teaching courses, evaluating programs, and publishing as many articles as possible. These challenges are critical for our planet, and I was committed to getting the medical community on board to understand these concerns. The threats of the 21st century would be both demanding and increasing—and we needed to be ready.

The Embolus

Unfortunately, cumulative personal health issues began to curtail my ambitious teaching schedule. In 2010, while flying across the Pacific to Japan to speak at a major medical congress on an island north of Tokyo, I suffered what I immediately knew was a pulmonary embolus. This blockage involved a blood clot that had traveled from my leg to my lung. Fully recognizing this life-threatening emergency, I remained immobile in my seat for nine hours, counting the minutes before the plane would touch down in Tokyo. I dreaded getting off the plane because what lay before me—in one of the biggest airports in the world—was the longest walk to customs and immigration.

Although I knew that my Japanese medical contacts were already at the meeting, I convinced the ticketing agents to let me back on the very same plane to return to Honolulu. For the duration of that second journey, I willed myself to be calm and motionless. I hoped I would go unnoticed in my single window seat. I was not as successful as I had hoped. My obvious distress was noticed by the crew members, but they are trained to be observant. Flight attendants continued to offer me oxygen throughout the nine-hour ordeal.

---

3. "Study Finds Most Wars Occur in Earth's Richest Biological Regions," Conservation International, February 20, 2009. Available at https://phys.org/news/2009-02-wars-earth-richest-biological-regions.html.
4. Elizabeth Whitman, "Invincible Bacteria in the Middle East," *The Atlantic*, October 28, 2014. Available at https://www.theatlantic.com/health/archive/2014/10/invincible-bacteria-in-the-middle-east/381671/.

When I arrived in Honolulu, I struggled through security to ensure that my physical agony was not obvious. I met Phyllis at the curb outside immigration, and she rushed me to a major medical center where I informed the triage nurse that I had a pulmonary embolus. Despite my own evaluation, ER personnel initially disputed my self-diagnosis, mistaking the embolus for a heart attack. Thankfully, the embolus was finally detected two days later while I was in a critical care unit.

I used that diagnosis in future lectures to emphasize the point: "Always listen to the chief complaint!" And more broadly, focus on what the patient is saying. Hearing the patient's specific medical problem is an ongoing issue in the power dynamics of health care that physicians still struggle with today. I was fortunate that I was able to recover from this embolus, but physically, this event came as quite a shock to my body. Leading up to the onset of this blood clot, despite my youthful vigor on the inside, my hair had slowly turned white to remind me of my age. But after the pulmonary embolus occurrence had ended, my hair gradually began to turn back to brown and gray.

Phyllis vividly remembered my embolus because what affected me impacted her. She immediately realized that something was very wrong when she picked me up in Honolulu. But knowing me as she did, she understood that it would prove pointless to even discuss slowing down considerably on my travel obligations. I had to go wherever I was sent to get the job done—even with "some bumps and bruises," in her words, along the way.

The Tale of a Filter

I wish that this embolus was the extent of my wild stories to tell at parties, but my recovery from this episode became even more bizarre. Before leaving the hospital, I had a filter inserted into my inferior vena cava, which is the large vein transporting blood from the lower body to the heart. The blood from my legs would go through the filter, catching any clots before they reached my heart or lungs. After three months, a physician was supposed to remove the filter. But while I was under anesthesia, the doctor realized the filter was inserted horizontally and not vertically, so he couldn't take it out.

These filters are intended to have a limited lifespan and will ultimately begin to break up, which was a frightening prospect. Time passed while I tried to figure out what to do about this dangerous situation. Some colleagues eventually connected me with the surgeon in Boston who had invented that filter. I made arrangements for her to extract it. At this point, it had been in my body for nearly two years, so I was ecstatic to get this unwelcome device out of me.

But just before the surgery, the doctor came in to see me. She unexpectedly said, "You should know that after it's been in this long, it cannot be removed." And that was that. After coming to Boston from Hawaii, I regrettably had to fly 5,000 miles back home with my filter still intact.

Many articles began to appear at that time on the complications of using these filters, stating they were often put into patients who didn't need them. Tragically, they could lead to deaths. But a few of these publications mentioned a surgeon at the Mayo Clinic in Rochester, Minnesota, who took on more dangerous cases. Coincidentally and luckily, our son Christopher, who had become a physician himself, was working at the Mayo Clinic. He was able to set up an appointment with that surgeon who agreed to remove it.

The surgery was performed under conscious sedation because I had to be a willing participant in this process to respond to commands to assist with its removal. The procedure was long but the surgical team finally pulled out the filter. The surgeon held up the filter to show me the shards of my inferior vena cava hanging from it. At that point, I didn't care. It was out. I may have set the record for the longest time of having an internal filter in place—quite a dubious achievement.

In Decline

As my health continued to get worse during the early decades of the 21st century, I had one hobby that I would not relinquish—writing. I persevered and encouraged others to do the same, offering research project ideas that needed to be explored and shared. I continued to lecture and accept some speaking engagements. But I began refusing many invitations and instead recommended some trusted colleagues to give those addresses in my place. I noted the gradual development of a positive and expanding process. Disaster medicine and awareness of global public health were becoming more mainstream. And those two issues kept me going, intellectually and physically, even as my health waned.

The writings of this new generation of disaster medicine experts would fortify the burgeoning specialty requirements for the field, which, by that time, had become a recognized global reality. As of now, an army of health professionals in so many countries can call themselves "disaster medicine and crisis management experts." We can all confidently use the same professional jargon. This accomplishment is a great improvement from my earlier deployments in the 1980s and 1990s, as well as being more effective in responding to global health disasters and humanitarian crises.

I am now losing my former stamina and becoming progressively indisposed. But staying connected to the younger generation coming up in the field of disaster medicine is one of my greatest delights. I enjoy being an active mentor, consulting with students, and even reviewing their papers. On many occasions, I have seen some of those scholarly papers appear as published journal articles, which has been most gratifying.

I have been able to shift from a crisis response mindset to more introspective thinking and considerations for the future. And in keeping with this reflective thinking in my later years, I once asked Phyllis if she had anything to say to me but never dared to voice.

She simply replied, "No." But she added, "I only worried that you might give up your dream of coordinated humanitarian assistance before you were finished."

Phyllis understood that I longed for the day when health itself was more globalized, not managed across the country—and certainly not across state lines. She knew me so well.

Some of my dreams, unfortunately, will remain just that, castles in the air that will likely never become true realities, at least in my lifetime. The Center of Excellence is one prime example. Every day I lament the lost potential of bringing together the military and civilian worlds to combine their assistance efforts in the field of disaster medicine. So much good could have been realized if egos, hierarchy, and entrenchment had not been factors.

Having cross-collaboration between military and civilian disaster medicine has become increasingly needed and useful in war and disasters, both abroad and at home. I first noticed this cooperation during my deployment to Iraq responding to the Kurdish crisis. When all sectors can work together, synergize their strengths, and make up for one another's weaknesses, the response is so much more effective. Mortality and morbidity can be reduced and we can optimize available resources.

More civilians are becoming casualties of wars and conflicts. Since February 2022, the world has watched the tragic devastation and murders that have unfolded in Ukraine as that country has been decimated by its neighboring dictator. The number of Ukrainian residents Putin has intentionally targeted is front page news. Civilian fatalities in wartime have risen from 5 percent at the turn of the 19th century into the 20th century, to 15 percent during World War I, to 65 percent by the end of World War II, to a jarring 90 percent in the wars of the 1990s in which more children were killed than soldiers.[5] Putin has killed and injured thousands of Ukrainian noncombatants, and the official number will never be known.

This unsettling trajectory should compel us to bring all sectors together to reduce these numbers by any method possible. The military has learned an incredible number of lifesaving strategies during the past decades that can help civilian disaster medicine. Even the STOP THE BLEED® campaign,[6] launched in 2015, has resulted in lower mortalities following tragedies. The world we live in today unfortunately has no "front lines." The horrors of terrorism and rampant shootings can now be experienced at any movie theater, marathon finish line, church, synagogue, mosque, entertainment venue, or subway train. We cannot see borders between violence and peace.

Blast injuries, gunshot wounds, and mass casualty events were previously seen

---

5. https://childrenandarmedconflict.un.org/wp-content/uploads/2018/07/Children-Armed-Conflict-Annual-Report-Summary-2017-web.pdf.
6. The American College of Surgeons, as licensed by the Department of Defense, instigated the worldwide STOP THE BLEED® campaign in 2015 by sending medical kits, which included tourniquets, to instruct several million people how to stop bleeding due to a critical injury. Available at https://www.stopthebleed.org/.

just from one sovereign state at war with another sovereign state. Only military responders needed this training. Foreign and domestic violent extremism toward civilian targets has brought these destructive consequences home to neighborhoods in all countries. This concept was also seen in the Boston Marathon bombing on April 15, 2013. Although nearly 200 runners and bystanders were sent to area hospitals, all survived largely because the military surgeons and nurses who had worked in Iraq and Afghanistan and were now employed in area hospitals. Their lessons spread throughout the trauma care sector.

Understanding the consequences of this new state of the world, a 2009 conference in Boston brought together doctors from Israel, Pakistan, India, and other individuals who were familiar with terrorist attack injuries and needed triage systems. They willingly shared their valuable knowledge with local responders.[7] We have to coordinate more of these military medical lessons with the civilian world. We must have an organized humanitarian response to any disaster or terrorist attack to ensure that most lives can be saved.

In the wake of the COVID-19 pandemic, what especially concerns me is that we have massive, existential issues right in front of us that no one with the power to make changes seems to be talking about. No one is adequately talking about climate change. No one is talking about the importance of public health protections and how they can contribute to true global health security. Issues have become so politically polarized in recent years, and nationalism has taken a new seat in the spotlight. We must have a shift in how we view and respond to global health.

I've long considered myself a global citizen, pushing for public health worldwide. In the early 2000s, globalizing health was becoming a major topic of discussion, an issue catching my interest. On several occasions when organizers sat down to discuss the initiative to emphasize the importance of global health, the meetings were led by economists. No health professionals were in the room. Economists were much more organized worldwide at that time than health professionals, and they decided the health of a country couldn't be improved until the economy had improved. While we successfully and rapidly globalized communications and travel, economic power groups frustrated the opportunities to globalize public health.

One country cannot get an abundance of public health care and public health elements, such as vaccines, a trained workforce, and needed supplies, and another country be limited to access to any vaccines, medical supplies, and professional health care workers. This contrast was especially true when considering epidemics and pandemics. We must have equity in global public health requiring a multidisciplinary, population-based management approach.

The training and expertise to truly prevent, mitigate, and respond to ever-increasing crises also need to change. Narrow focuses on health outcomes are no longer sufficient. Multidisciplinary skillsets and diverse areas of knowledge should

---

7. Arthur L. Kellermann and Kobi Peleg, "Perspective: Lessons from Boston," *The New England Journal of Medicine*, May 23, 2013, 1956–1957. Available at https://www.nejm.org/doi/full/10.1056/NEJMp1305304.

be emphasized. If we are ever to outrun the cascade of global crises, critical medicine and nursing expertise must be augmented to better understand worldwide public health epidemiology.

What has been keeping me up at night since late 2019 is watching hundreds of public health professionals either retire early, get fired, or leave the field. This depressing state of affairs is due to misinformation, political pressure, or other threats concerning their safety throughout the Covid pandemic. The loss of public health professionals is happening right before our eyes. I won't be here much longer to see the effects of their departure, but I'm afraid that we will not be able to recover.

This unfinished work has to be passed to future generations of humanitarians and disaster medical experts. But change does not happen overnight, and I am lucky to have observed the formalization and recognition of global disaster medicine and public health within my lifetime. I feel so fortunate to have had some part in this new field, but the success of this up-and-coming field came with many hard-fought and hard-earned lessons, none of which I regret.

* * * *

As the writing of this book winds down, I am now 83. In my current physical state, I am more forgetful, permanently walk with a cane, and spend countless hours in the bathroom. Nevertheless, I could never give up research and writing on issues that remain unsolved or express themselves as new and demanding crises. "Perspectives" in a following appendix address concerns that remain mystifying, tragic, and unresolved. What energy I have left has been focused on those subjects near and dear to me.

But I am now facing terminal cancer. I have experienced every negative feeling and complication that both the disease and therapy can offer. In my case, the cancer was directly related to Agent Orange[8] exposure in Vietnam. Delta Med, just a few miles south of the DMZ, registered the highest levels of Agent Orange saturation in South Vietnam. While serving at Delta Med, I often observed that few plants seemed to grow in what historically was a major agricultural industry for the local population.

In a bizarre twist of irony, after spending decades on the other side of the theoretical "table," I was now experiencing, with prolonged and agonizing chemotherapy and sleepless nights, a deep and enduring depression. I contemplated suicide for the first and only time in my life. But I was not ready to leave Phyllis.

I remember psychiatric sessions with patients who experienced mental illness. I am relieved that I never made light of their expressions of despair, even though

---

8. Agent Orange was an herbicide used by U.S. forces in Vietnam to defoliate the landscape and make it more difficult for the enemy to find cover. Agent Orange was stored in barrels with an orange band on the outside. Among the herbicide's components was dioxin, a highly toxic contaminant. Available at https://www.aspeninstitute.org/programs/agent-orange-in-vietnam-program/what-is-agent-orange/.

15. Hard-Earned Lessons

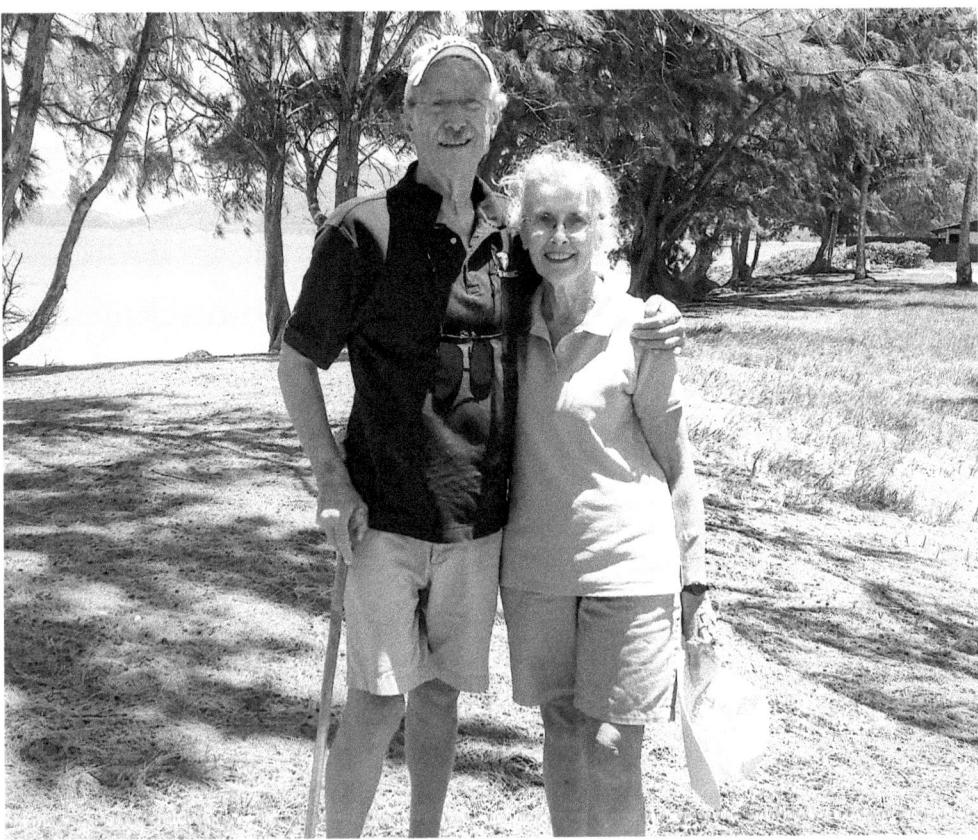

Skip and Phyllis, still by his side after more than 60 years, near their home on the windward side of Oahu (photograph by Jan Herman).

I admitted to them that I really didn't know or truly understand the intensity of their distress. They opened up, and, more often than not, our relationship in therapy changed for the best. I learned so much about life from them and what the last days of a person's life can be—moving from torture to relief. And I have tried to channel those lessons and insights as I now walk that path myself.

Phyllis and I have talked many times over the years about my ongoing dream of synchronizing aid in times of disaster. She recalled many crucial events and conversations I had forgotten, or I was too busy or too thoughtless to remember. I was ready to give up so many times, but Phyllis always gave me the strength to keep going.

My wife is the most unselfish person I know. The example Phyllis and her parents set for me so many years ago was perhaps more than I deserved. Yet they saved me and gave me hope. Immature as I was, I didn't know how to thank my wife who has played so many roles in my life—wife, teacher, lover, best friend, parent, and role model for our three children.

But what I do know, without the lingering doubts that I might have in myself, is that I love and admire Phyllis with every fiber of my being. Her actual name, Philomena, derived from the Irish, means "strongly loved," and from Greek mythology, "powerful love." Phyllis' name could not have been more appropriate. There is no question that I love and admire Phyllis with every fiber of my being. Phyllis's love has sustained me throughout our years together. And the many hard-earned lessons I experienced in my career—both near and far—were tempered by our enduring love.

Epilogue

The Vietnamese I worked with at Delta Med strongly believe the soul's final destination is the moon, a sacred place where the spiritual essence may find ample refreshment. In contrast, for those living in a Western culture, Earth's nearest neighbor has always appeared barren, lifeless, and inhospitable.

Astronauts on the six Apollo missions that landed on the lunar surface found no evidence of water on the moon a half-century ago. The existence of water seemed far-fetched. With temperatures ranging from 260°F to −280°F, water cannot persist. Any water vapor is broken down into hydrogen and oxygen by sunlight.

Nevertheless, unmanned satellites and lunar landers have been scrutinizing the moon's surface ever since, probing every nook and cranny, to unlock more lunar secrets. In 2009, the upper stage of a NASA rocket impacted Cabeus Crater, sending up a plume of debris. Immediately following that contact, the Lunar Crater Observation and Sensing Satellite flew through that cloud of powdery fragments ejected by the rocket's impact. The satellite detected what appeared to be pure crystalline ice mixed in the lunar soil. Scientists have hypothesized that any ice that remains on the moon today was likely deposited over eons by the regular bombardment of water-bearing comets, asteroids, and meteoroids.[1]

In August 2018, NASA's Moon Mineralogy Mapper instrument detected surface ice at the moon's north and south poles.[2] Appearing to be more abundant at its south pole, ice has been found principally at the bottom of deep craters where the sun never shines.

In 2020, a special infrared camera, located aboard NASA's 747 high-flying Stratospheric Observatory for Infrared Astronomy (SOFIA), confirmed the presence of water molecules on the moon's sunlit surface. These molecules are not water in a liquid state, but rather water molecules so spread apart that they do not form ice or liquid water. Scientists now hypothesize that more water may be distributed on the moon's surface than has previously been found as ice in deep, cold, sunless craters.[3]

In 2023, Chinese lunar scientists detected water trapped in glass beads from

---

1. Abigail Tabor, editor, "What Is LCROSS, the Lunar Crater Observation and Sensing Satellite?" NASA, March 8, 2019. Available at https://www.nasa.gov/ames/lcross.
2. Frank Tavares, "Ice Confirmed at the Moon's Poles," *NASA Science News*, August 20, 2018. Available at https://www.sciencedaily.com/releases/2018/08/180820203638.htm.
3. Sean Potter, editor, "NASA's SOPHIA Discovers Water on Sunlit Surface of Moon," NASA, October 26, 2020. Available at https://www.nasa.gov/press-release/nasa-s-sofia-discovers-water-on-sunlit-surface-of-moon.

soil samples returned to Earth from the Chang'e-5 mission, the fifth Chinese lunar exploration, to the far side of the moon. These scientists estimate that the tiny glass spheres may contain billions of tons of water buried in soils beneath the lunar surface.[4] Future lunar explorers, such as Vietnamese souls, may indeed be refreshed by water on the moon.

---

4. Genelle Weule, "Water on the Moon Stored in Glass Beads: Chang'e-5 Samples Reveal," ABC News, March 28, 2023. Available at https://www.abc.net.au/news/science/2023-03-28/glass-beads-moon-change5-china-water-apollo-.soil-hydrogen-impact/102142150.

Appendix 1: Tributes

A Legacy: Honored by Saint Michael's College,
the United States Congress, and a Vietnam Veteran

> "As your volunteerism matures, use whatever bully pulpit you have to expose
> and change those inequities that you see in the world. The risk is worth it."

In the spring of 2016, Saint Michael's College, my alma mater, honored me with an invitation to give the commencement address to its 109th class. I eagerly accepted this offer with much enthusiasm. I titled my talk "Challenging the Next Generation: Service to Others." A few weeks later, Senator Patrick J. Leahy of Vermont, who was also a graduate of Saint Michael's—and from my Class of 1961—presented me with a tribute beyond my wildest imagination. On June 7, 2016, he had my commencement speech inserted into the 114th Congress's *Congressional Record*.[1]

I deeply appreciate these two very high levels of recognition late in life: an opportunity to speak to a new, promising generation and my commencement talk being recorded in the *Congressional Record*. And at the end of this chapter, my friend and colleague Bob Macpherson has written admiringly about my career in his glowing tribute "Listening to the Heartbeat of Humanity."

So to Saint Michael's, Patrick Leahy, and Bob Macpherson, I am deeply humbled and grateful for your generous and heartfelt words. They are gifts to be forever treasured.

Senator Leahy's Tribute

Mr. LEAHY. Mr. President [President pro tempore Orrin Hatch], one of the formative parts of my life was being a student at Saint Michael's College in Vermont. It was especially so because of the people I met there. One of my most memorable classmates is Dr. Frederick Burkle.

Skip Burkle was one who cared greatly about what he was learning and showed moral leadership even then. As students, we both lived in dorms that resembled World War II-era barracks. Fortunately, the living conditions for students at Saint Michael's have improved since then.

---

1. Commencement speech given on May 15, 2016, at Saint Michael's College. Transcript appears in the 114th Congress's *Congressional Record-Senate*, June 7, 2016, Vol. 162, No. 89, 103–105. Available at https://www.govinfo.gov/content/pkg/CREC-2016-06-07/pdf/CREC-2016-06-07-senate.pdf.

Last month [May 15, 2016], now–Dr. Burkle spoke at Saint Michael's College giving the commencement address. Everyone who was there actually listened to a man who spoke of his own background. He spoke also to the moral compass he has developed both in school and since in the military and in his scientific work.

So much could be said about his career. I agree when he said, "My humanitarian work was the most meaningful I've ever done." That makes so much sense because few people I have ever known have begun to approach his life as a humanitarian.

Mr. President, I ask unanimous consent that his speech to the graduating class [of 2016] be printed in the *Record* because I want those beyond Saint Michael's College to read what an outstanding person has said.

"Challenging the Next Generation: Service to Others"
CONGRESSIONAL POINT OF ORDER

There being no objection, the material was ordered to be printed in the *Record*, as follows:

Saint Michael's College Commencement Address
Colchester, Vermont: May 15, 2016
Frederick M. Burkle, Jr., M.D., M.P.H.
Physician, Scholar, Humanitarian

"Challenging the Next Generation: Service to Others"
COMMENCEMENT SPEECH GIVEN BY FREDERICK M. BURKLE, JR.

Greetings to you all!

There are many reasons to celebrate this day. This graduation is a milestone for you and your entire family.

Saint Michael's also needs to be celebrated and commended. As an academic, I do not know of any other college or university this year, or in recent memory, that has shown both the insight and courage to declare "Service to Others" as the theme of graduation. Only at St. Mike's!

I'm not surprised! The implications of this decision are many and must be applauded. Most importantly, it brings great hope and wisdom for the future of this generation and those that follow.

I have been asked to speak to you on what in my life and college experiences influenced my humanitarian career. My first concern when asked was: How does someone who graduated in 1961, 55 years ago, tell his story to the class of 2016? Let's give it a try.

In truth, if you knew me in high school, you would have voted me the "least likely graduate to ever give a commencement address."

I attended an all-male Catholic high school in southern Connecticut. I was painfully shy, occasionally stuttered, was easily embarrassed, struggled to be an average student, and was hopelessly burdened by what is known today as "severe dyslexia." I only began to read in the fifth grade.

My father, emphatically and loudly, said "no" to the idea of college. He had labeled me a "lazy dreamer." So to him, college was a waste of good money. You would agree I was certainly not a prize academic prospect!

So here I am and now I've got to explain to you how I got onto this stage as a commencement speaker.

I would not be here today without the help of some very unselfish people. I call them my "own personal humanitarians." We all have them.

Not going to college was a serious blow I could not live with. For years I had held on to an otherwise quite impossible and secret dream of being a physician—a dream which simply arose many years before from viewing very early *Life* magazine photos of doctors treating starving children in an African jungle hospital.

Having been born two years before World War II, all my life was one war after another with equally dire photos of both World War II and Korean War casualties. And soon after, during high school, emerged my generation's war in a strange and unheard of country named Vietnam, a war which actually began to build up as early as 1954.

My story, in great part, is a love story. I met an equally shy girl when she was 13 and I was the older man of 14. We went steady during high school and secretly dreamed of our future together. With college off the table, the military draft seemed inevitable. She urged me to plead my case to the High School Academic Dean, a stern gray-haired Brother of Holy Cross, to both loan me the application fee and forward a decent recommendation. I was shaking in my boots. He silently pondered the circumstances yet nodded his head and agreed to accept the personal risk despite the potential anger of my father.

The very next day there was a check waiting for me!

There were others. While working as an orderly in a local hospital, I met two very caring physicians. They embodied everything I wanted to be. They introduced me to a small French Catholic Liberal Arts College named Saint Michael's in rural Vermont that I never heard of. Both were World War II veterans who attended St. Mike's and then medical school on the GI Bill. Despite their busy schedules, they took time to counsel and encourage, spoke highly of the quality of the education, but also cautioned that the academic experience would demand much more.

St. Mike's was the only place I applied. With luck, I was accepted. My girlfriend's parents, not my own, took me to campus. There was no turning back!

Falling in love with St. Mike's was a little slower and not nearly as romantic! Matriculation at St. Mike's was a shock and, at first, a disappointment. Maybe my father was right. Will I fail and embarrass myself once again?

From the outset, the St. Mike's academic faculty made it clear that everyone on campus was required to take four years of liberal arts. This included a long list of the world's literature, history, arts, and philosophy from the beginning of written time. This included a comparative study of all religions, and a compelling semester of logic that forced us to deliberate the philosophical "how" and "why" problems that stressed the minds of every adolescent, like me, whose brain had not yet matured.

It took me three trips to the bookstore to carry all the required reading back to the small shared room in a former World War II poorly heated, wooden barracks that once stood where we are today.

We desperately asked why such torture was necessary. I'm to be a scientist. Why did I have to study the liberal arts? I pleaded. Something must be wrong! With my reading disability, my anxiety level was palpable to everyone.

The science faculty made it quite clear that to pass the rigorous requirements for recommendation to graduate school required excellent marks in both the sciences and the liberal arts. They offered us multiple examples of notable statesmen and Nobel laureates alike who, empowered by incorporating the lessons learned from the liberal arts, made major breakthroughs for mankind, such as human rights, freedom of speech, the splitting of the atom, penicillin, the Magna Carta, the Geneva Conventions, and the U.S. Constitution itself.

Slowly, St. Mike's, without my knowledge, began to hone, tame, and humble me by introducing new ways of thinking and reasoning.

I, like all my classmates, had to give up that concrete black and white thinking of youth to meet the demands of the outside world.

Most students incorporated those new concepts to one degree or another over the next four years. Confidence was built through testy debates on what our increasingly complex world demanded of us. The process reintroduced me to the academic world I thought was unfriendly, and gave me a new love for books which were once the enemy of every dyslexic child.

Less than a month into my freshman year, a profound geopolitical event occurred that no one had anticipated or was ready for. On October 4, 1957, we huddled around the one radio available in the barracks to listen to the faint battery-powered beeps of the Russian satellite Sputnik. The following day, the faculty held an "all-student assembly" to discuss the impact of the satellite launch on mankind and openly asked if any students would consider changing their major to the sciences. The "Space War" had begun in earnest. Everyone's sense of security suddenly changed and with it many Cold War humanitarian crises sprang up around the world, many of which, in a short decade, I became mired in myself.

Every generation has their own "Sputnik" moments. Your generation already has more than your share.

The liberal arts and the comparative religion courses prepared me for my life as a humanitarian more than I ever realized at the time.

Yes, we all read the Bible and debated its meaning, but we also found a certain solace in understanding that similar beliefs were universal among many other religions and the cultures they were tied to.

All religions that have survived over the centuries collectively teach "social justice," a language all its own that defines the fair and just relationship between the individual and society. It is that shared social justice that I have in common with my humanitarian and volunteer colleagues on every continent, might they be Muslims,

Hindus, Christians, Jews, Buddhists, agnostics, or atheists, and whether they live in the Middle East or rural Vermont.

All the major wars and multiple conflicts that I became engulfed in over my lifetime were all fought over "whose god was the true god!" Unfortunately, these wars continue today.

Admittedly, and probably somewhat selfishly, I fell in love with the challenges of global health and humanitarian assistance.

And yes, that shy girlfriend who supported my application to St. Mike's and I were married my first year of medical school and we had three children by the time I finished my residency at the Yale University Medical Center.

Service to one's country was mandatory then, and the government obliged by drafting me into the military. In 1968, I was rapidly trained and rushed, within 20 days, into the madness of the Vietnam War as a combat physician with the Marines.

Subsequently I was recalled to active duty as a combat physician in five major wars, and over the years moved up the invisible ladder of leadership in managing conflicts in over 40 countries. I've worked for and with the World Health Organization, the International Red Cross, and multiple global humanitarian organizations. I found myself negotiating with numerous African warlords and despots, including Saddam Hussein in Iraq.

I set up refugee camps, treated horrific war wounds, severe malnutrition, scurvy, the death throes of starvation, and cholera, malaria and blackwater fever, to name but a few. When I was only a few years older than you, I had to manage the largest Bubonic Plague epidemic of the last century.

Eventually, in 2003, I served the State Department as the Senior Health Diplomat and first Interim Minister of Health in Iraq where I was the target of three assassination attempts by the same Sunni military that now, more than a decade later, make up today's ISIS forces in Iraq and Syria. Yes, it is madness.

Obviously, my work was often quite dangerous. Making uncomfortable but real decisions over who survives and who doesn't, simply because there are scant resources, is always a nightmare. Over 1,000 fellow humanitarian aid workers have been killed during my time, many, many more than any United Nations Peace-keepers.

I have seen more senseless death and suffering than anyone my age should be allowed to witness. The same "how" and "why" issues that I first struggled with in Logic class at St. Mike's were now reframed in very basic daily struggles of both ethics and morality.

As such, I moved more and more to care for the most vulnerable—the children, women, the elderly and disabled who make up 90 percent or more of those who flee or become ill, injured, or die in every war. This became my calling.

While some of this may impress the budding health care professionals in the audience, everything I experienced in war was preventable. It need not have happened. War is not the answer.

But my humanitarian work was the most meaningful I have ever done. I have no regrets. The saving of lives when the victims themselves have given up and working with some of the most selfless people in the world is addictive, and for a physician the adrenaline rush, intensity of the work, and the diagnostic challenges are comparable to nothing else.

As Medical Director of the last Orphan Lift out of Saigon in 1975, I was secretly slipped into a refugee-crowded, already surrounded and hostile Saigon during its last days to find abandoned and ill infants, many alone and starving in dank and dirty orphanages. We airlifted out 310 nameless infants in file boxes. Twenty years later, by chance, I met an attractive and ebullient Asian woman, now a graduate student who had been the valedictorian of her college class. She was one of the infants I rescued. Life comes full circle. It was a really good day.

The scientific research that defines my academic career has me closely working with like-minded colleagues in Iran, Israel, Iraq, China, the European Union, and many others. And yes, another example of life taking full circle: The Nobel laureates, once touted in 1957 as examples for us to emulate by the St. Mike's science professors, selected a 2013 research study I co-authored to be presented and debated at their World Summit in Spain last year. Good people are listening and reading your work. So for the future academics and scientists in the audience: Never give up!

Hopefully, my now fading career allows me to reflect and offer some parting Grand-Fatherly advice: The essence of volunteerism is found in understanding the culture of the people we engage with, even within our own communities. In my experience, we did not understand the culture of Vietnam or Iraq, and when General [David] Petraeus was asked at the 10-year mark in Afghanistan what he would have done differently, he said, "I would have learned more about the culture!"

Graduation marks your movement from the protective culture of the campus to a culture that is more complex, unforgiving at times, but also very exciting and worthwhile.

Most young volunteers are understandably burdened by the non-action they have reluctantly inherited from my generation, burdens that shamelessly stem from worldwide political neglect of both the health and science of the planet.

You should be disappointed but also challenged. However, a very hopeful characteristic of your generation is that you more often than not see yourselves less as nationalists and more as global citizens. This marks a significant shift from my generation and a hopeful game-changer in the global landscape.

As your volunteerism matures, use whatever bully pulpit you have to expose and change those inequities that you see in the world. The risk is worth it.

I spoke up in Iraq over blatant human rights violations of the Geneva Conventions and was called a "traitor" in the political press. I am most proud I made that choice.

Remember, those who do have the political power to make change frequently do not know what they don't know. Instinctively, all volunteers are also educators and advocates. It comes with the title.

The MOVE [Mobilization of Volunteer Efforts] program, run by the Campus Ministry and the Fire & Rescue Squad, represents realistic "real-world models" that one can neither assume nor get from the classroom alone. I wish I had experienced them myself. These inspiring volunteer initiatives have changed the culture of the college and more broadly and accurately redefined "American exceptionalism."

Harvard, where I teach today, has recently taken a page from the St. Mike's playbook by placing more emphasis on accepting students to college who value caring for the community over individual extracurricular achievements. They claim that "community service" and the ethical concern for the "greater public good" is a more sensitive and true measure of an applicant.

I agree! St. Mike's, emphasizing "service to others," has owned and promoted this belief for many decades.

Aid to the oppressed has never stood still. Volunteerism, in general, is increasingly moving toward prevention, recovery, and rehabilitation. Your role models must be those distinguished recipients of the honorary degrees today. I applaud their selfless commitments to others.

St. Mike's was an unselfish gift to me. My class of 1961 was unique in producing many leaders in science, education, government, law, the military, industry, the social sciences, and medicine and dentistry, to name but a few. They are all great citizens who still argue incessantly over politics. Some things never change—nor should they!

Please promise me that you will see your classmates often. Call them, email them, and return to the reunions. It's a great time to brag and see that everyone is equally aging and putting on weight. I do miss many of my friends and colleagues and also the professors who I tried to model myself on who passed away before I could thank them.

And yes, as a bonus, there is another Harvard study this year that shows that both volunteers and their recipients increase social connections, reduce stress, and live longer lives!

I must close now. As a 31-year Navy and Marine Corps veteran, I wish to leave you with a saying that we, in the service of our country, always thought was strictly a nautical blessing. In point of fact, it is a universal phrase of good luck as one departs on a voyage in life. It reads: "Let me square the yards, while we may, and make a fair wind of it homeward." I wish you all in this audience "Fair Winds and Following Seas." God speed to you and St. Mike's, and thank you for listening.

"Listening to the Heartbeat of Humanity"
by Robert Macpherson

"Dr. Burkle stepped outside the bounds of everyday life and walked into worlds of disaster, violence, and deprivation."

For more than half a century, I have watched Skip Burkle's bravery, courage, and brilliance shine as an inspiration to humankind. Likewise, his compassion serves as a beacon to those who believe in the goodness of people. Dr. Burkle's works are the embodiment of a quote attributed to Andrew Jackson: "One man with courage makes a majority."

I met Skip on April 7, 1969, but I don't remember the meeting because I was unconscious from gunshot and shrapnel wounds from a battle with the North Vietnamese Army [NVA]. I was lying with a group of Marines in a medical triage area at the 3rd Medical Battalion, which served the Marines at Dong Ha, Republic of Vietnam. A military triage has three areas for the wounded. They are staging sites (1) for those who are likely to live, (2) for those for whom immediate care may make a positive difference, and (3) for those unlikely to live, irrespective of their care. I'm told I was in the last group.

After 10 hours of work in the operating room, Dr. Burkle started to make his way to the earthen bunker, which served as his sleeping area. As he walked through the triage area, he heard me moaning. His first instinct was to have a corpsman administer another shot of morphine to relieve the pain and let me die in comfort. However, while checking my wounds, he decided there was a chance I could survive, then contacted the surgeon who agreed, and he moved me to the operating room.

Days later, I was medevacked to a U.S. Naval Hospital in Guam where I remained for seven months before I was well enough to be airlifted back to the United States. While in Guam, I learned the story of how I survived and the name of the surgeon who operated on me. Yet it was a different era without the internet and search engines, and I never located Skip.

Twenty-four years later in February 1993, my workspace was a large tent inside the former U.S. Embassy compound in Mogadishu, Somalia. President George H.W. Bush had ordered U.S. troops to Somalia. Our mission was to end the warlords' violence and assist the UN and humanitarian community with the assets to end the starvation that had already caused the death of nearly 500,000 Somalis.

As I flipped through papers on a small desk, I noticed a tall, slim, white-haired man in civilian clothes walk through the front entrance and speak to a Marine near the tent flap. The Corporal nodded in my direction, and the man approached me. He introduced himself as Dr. Skip Burkle and explained that the Secretary of Defense's Humanitarian Assistance Coordinator for Somalia had sent him to evaluate the American military's support of humanitarian relief efforts.

After a short discussion regarding his assignment, I asked if he was ever stationed at the 3rd Medical Battalion at Dong Ha, Vietnam. He replied he spent 13 months as a battalion surgeon in that expeditionary hospital, which was an earthen compound to protect the facility from NVA shelling. I told him my story and he confirmed the account, adding further details about how close I came to the end of my life that day in April 1969.

In our discussion, we learned we lived less than a mile apart on the island of Oahu. Sitting in that tent, I was amazed. After more than two decades from the day this man saved my life, I meet him in Somalia and discover we live on the same island in the middle of the Pacific Ocean. Over the ensuing years, our friendship grew. When I retired from the Marines and joined the humanitarian organization CARE [Cooperative for Assistance and Relief Everywhere], Dr. Burkle became a mentor as I adjusted to life as an aid worker. His quiet counsel was indispensable as my responsibilities grew within CARE.

Additionally, we often met in complex environments, and I watched him provide medical assistance to vulnerable populations in wars and natural disasters, often in places where others feared to go. He was a force that never accepted the words "too hard," "can't," or "won't." Again, in Sarajevo, Bosnia, during the war, while I was with CARE, I saw him build a system for the International Rescue Committee to support a clinic and house hundreds of children in the city's hospital amid the shelling, snipers, and unending violence. The toddlers and newborns were wounded by snipers, shelling, or dying of pneumonia because there was no medicine. Through his untiring perseverance, he found ways to transport medicine and medical equipment through the Serb blockades.

In 2003, shortly after the surrender of Iraqi military forces, Dr. Burkle was appointed the Interim Minister of Health for Iraq. When I met him in Baghdad while working with CARE, he was troubled because the nation was cascading into a deteriorating social and health care disaster. As sectarian violence increased and medical management collapsed, Dr. Burkle faced a U.S. government administration [President George W. Bush's Administration] that wanted to incur only limited expense for health protection for the Iraqis.

Dr. Burkle counseled that the U.S. was responsible for the Iraqi people under International Humanitarian Law. He was stonewalled. The afternoon of our meeting, he mentioned one recourse, but it would cost him his job. The following day—in front of the international media—he declared a public health emergency throughout Iraq. Dr. Burkle was correct on two counts. First, the media attention forced the Bush Administration to rebuild a health care system to support the Iraqi people. Second, within a week he lost his job.

The words "selfless courage" are a perfect descriptor of Dr. Burkle's work and life for more than half a century. While I have watched others rightfully receive medals and accolades for courageous acts in war, their bravery is remarkable and should be recognized. But there are no parades or stirring speeches for humanitarians like Dr. Burkle. Instead, his achievements may be chronicled in a blog or occasionally as part of a documentary but are quickly forgotten.

However, it is not those momentary acknowledgments that motivate him. He is an unassuming man with a quiet but deep desire to heal, assist, and empower humankind. For more than half a century, Dr. Burkle stepped outside the bounds of everyday life and walked into worlds of disaster, violence, and deprivation. In the chaos, he forged solidarity with others by listening to the heartbeat of humanity. Wading into horrific situations, armed only with his willingness to confront rather than retreat from injustice, there was no deliberation that some people were worth saving while others were not. All lives have value.

Skip Burkle's commitment was not to friend or foe, religion, country, or to a creed. It was from that freedom, when the night was darkest, his light manifested to bring forth the dawn. Dr. Martin Luther King once asked, "Life's most persistent and urgent question is, 'What are you doing for others?'" Dr. Burkle has never had to ponder his answer.

Robert Séamus Macpherson
Charlotte, North Carolina
October 2023

Appendix 2: Four Perspectives on the World's Challenges and Concerns

My long career in humanitarian care and medical disaster assistance took me to distant lands. Decades of practicing global medicine shaped my perspective on critical subjects.

"A Physician in Peril" is a personal account about my friend, Iranian physician Dr. Ahmadreza Djalali, a world-renowned specialist in disaster preparedness. Under false charges of espionage and treason, Ahmadreza has been a victim of hostage diplomacy since 2016. Being imprisoned for more than eight years, he "lives" in solitary confinement at the notorious Evin Prison in Tehran under the daily threat of execution. I don't want Ahmadreza and his courageous story to be forgotten.

"Sowing the Seeds of Global Autocracies" reflects my psychiatric knowledge about how autocrats, past and present, have come into power. Their failure to develop abstract reasoning during adolescence has contributed to narcissistic behavior. And this personality disorder has directly led to their future authoritarian ways. One of the means by which autocratic leaders assert their power is to undermine and downplay public health emergencies.

"Politics and Global Public Health: An Explosive, Tragic Combination" shows how politics has recently interfered with humanitarian and public health emergencies, such as Covid-19. Political intrusion led to thousands of unnecessary Covid-19 deaths in the U.S.

"The Untold Cost of War on Civilians" focuses on the UN's standing today and how Article 43 under the UN Charter's Chapter VII has lost its ability to respond to warring factions. I also discuss the 1949 Geneva Conventions whose articles are ignored or forgotten, thus weakening international humanitarian law.

I hope these additional perspectives will enlighten and give meaning to some of the health-related issues we currently face and will certainly confront in the future.

A Physician in Peril

"The agents forced him to make fabricated confessions dictated by the officers. They threatened to hurt his children, attack his spouse, and arrest his family members if he did not comply and confess what the Ministry of Intelligence requested."

My long career in humanitarian care and medical disaster assistance took me to distant lands. Decades of practicing global medicine shaped my perspective on critical subjects. Countries once admired can easily disappoint, and they can frustrate decades of progress and freedom. Iran is one of them.

"A Physician in Peril" is a personal account of my friend, Iranian physician Dr. Ahmadreza Djalali, a world-renowned specialist in disaster preparedness. Under false charges of espionage and treason, Ahmadreza has been a victim of hostage diplomacy since 2016. Being imprisoned for the past seven years, he "lives" in solitary confinement at the notorious Evin Prison in Tehran under the daily threat of execution. I don't want Ahmadreza and his courageous story to be forgotten.

The Islamic Republic of Iran is no different from other countries in managing prolonged conflict, yet Iran remains unique in systematically using hostages to achieve political goals. Only Iran has gained a level of sophistication in international bargaining by using hostage-taking of foreign nationals, dual citizen nationals, or Iranian citizens as a key foreign policy weapon against its perceived global enemies.

A great fear persisting today is how to end this egregious process before it is routinely adopted by other autocratic régimes around the world. Iran uses hostage-taking for many reasons: initiating prisoner swaps, recovering Iranian assets frozen abroad, exploiting for policy leverage, and obtaining Western money and arms. More recently, the Revolutionary Guard, whose task is to protect the Islamic Revolution (January 1978–February 1979), has taken hostages. The Guard also limits the number of academic scholars from Western countries coming into their country to conduct research with Iranians.

Journalists are not the only ones in the world today being targeted by authoritarian governments or caught up in war. As a physician who has often endured the dangers of war and the actions of repressive régimes, I strongly identify with doctors who have dedicated their lives to global disaster medicine and humanitarian assistance. But these committed physicians have increasingly become targets of terrorist organizations. One of my principal efforts during much of my career was training a new cadre of men and women who would practice this brand of medicine on an international scale when my generation could no longer do so.

I want to relate the as-yet-unfinished account of a resolute young physician, one of my former students, who prepared himself for worldwide humanitarian assistance and disaster medicine. He had just begun making his mark when, unfortunately, his career was cut short by disturbing circumstances no longer deemed "unusual." His cause is my cause. His cause is our cause. And, therefore, the roots of this compelling and highly publicized story begin here about a world-renowned doctor.

A Rising Star

Ahmadreza Djalali, MD, was born in September 1971 in Tabriz, Iran's sixth largest city. He was raised in a family that would be described today as "middle-class" in Iranian society. He was 6 years old when he witnessed the start of the Iranian Revolution in January 1978, and was 9 when the eight-year-long Iran-Iraq War began in 1980. Both events severely affected Iran and its people, particularly the children, who suddenly had to deal with limitations, threats, and fear. Iranians were forbidden to wear colorful clothes and shoes, including foreign brands. And strangely, playing sports was off-limits. A shortage of basic care essentials impacted all children both at home and in school. As a child, Ahmadreza experienced these apprehensions and scarcities.

Despite many social drawbacks, Ahmadreza was a top student by Iran's national standards before studying medicine at Tabriz University of Medical Sciences. He met Vida Mehrannia, who would become his future wife, in Tehran in 2000, having been introduced by mutual friends. It was a friendship for some months before they decided to marry. Two years later, they had a daughter, and after moving to Sweden, they had a son in 2011. Vida has described to me that Ahmadreza is an honest, moral man, maybe a bit idealistic, and a very kind person. He loved to travel with his family to different locations in Sweden or to other European countries. He and his family received Swedish citizenship in February 2018.

Ahmadreza was in Iran from 1997 to 2007. Natural disaster and technological crisis management are his areas of expertise. But while in Iran, he was a researcher, lecturer, and planner. He worked at the Ministry of Health and then moved to the Natural Disasters Research Institute, both located in Tehran. While employed at this Institute, he enjoyed international cooperation with multiple academic and research centers affiliated with both military and civil sectors.

Ahmadreza began studying for his PhD in 2008 at Karolinska Institute in Stockholm. The Institute's academic authorities in the Emergency Medicine Department handled his acceptance and visa issues. He preferred to spend most of his time with his family, especially when they moved to Europe where they had no relatives. He studied hard and worked tirelessly on scientific subjects and projects. Ahmadreza loved to mentor others, which, along with playing with his children and teaching others, always energized him. In one of my email conversations with Vida, she said his dream was to improve the life of people who were in need, admittedly driven by a wish to see Iran free of dictatorship, bigotry, and oppression.

During his doctoral studies, Ahmadreza was occasionally invited back to Iran to give lectures, advise on research projects, and consult on crisis management programs. In Iran once again after receiving his doctorate degree from the Karolinska Institute in 2012, a representative from a military center contacted him. The agent offered a proposal to stay and join a military university in Iran involved in passive defense and counter-terrorism. Passive defense is the régime's plan that would keep the Iranian régime in power even if the country's vital infrastructures were targeted in time of war. Passive defense is the Iranian version of homeland security.[1] But Ahmadreza refused the military's proposition. He wanted to continue his career in the European Union (EU) as a post-doctoral fellow in crisis management at the prestigious Università del Piemonte Orientale's Center for Research and Training in Disaster Medicine, Humanitarian Aid and Global Health (CRIMEDIM), headquartered in Novara, Italy.

Starting in 2012, Ahmadreza was involved in various training and research programs, three of which were funded by the European Commission in Brussels. These undertakings were relevant to health systems within the subjects of crisis management, education, and counterterrorism, as well as chemical, biological, radiological, nuclear, and explosives (CBRNE) weapons in the EU countries. But he still maintained cooperation with Iranian universities and research centers by contributing to crisis management.

I first met Ahmadreza during my affiliation with CRIMEDIM. I also participated as visiting faculty at CRIMEDIM, which allowed me to get to know Ahmadreza and share in his research and the publication of his scientific papers in international medical journals.[2] Worldwide, he was a rising star in crisis management of disasters. Then I learned that he was preparing to arrange study programs for physicians in Iran, a country prone to many natural disasters. He loved Iran and his ongoing goal was to make a positive difference in his native country.

Detained and Tortured

During a trip to Iran in 2014, two people from a military center and the Ministry of Intelligence met Ahmadreza and asked him to cooperate with them in recognizing and gathering information from EU states. The requested "information" would include EU countries' critical infrastructures, counter-terrorism, CBRNE weapons capabilities, and sensitive operational plans. This collaboration would also entail research projects relevant to terrorism and crisis management.

Ahmadreza firmly declined, arguing that he was a scientist, not a spy. He stated that any scientific help to Iran's academic centers stemmed from his commitment to

---

1. "Iran Setting up 'Passive Defense Plan,'" *The Jerusalem Post*, July 4, 2008. Available at https://www.jpost.com/iranian-threat/news/iran-setting-up-passive-defense-plan.
2. Ahmadreza and the author contributed to an article, "Assessment of Disaster Preparedness Among Emergency Departments in Italian Hospitals: A Cautious Warning for Disaster Risk Reduction and Management Capacity," published in the *Scandinavian Journal of Trauma, Resuscitation and Emergency Medicine*, December 2016, 24(1). Available at https://www.researchgate.net/publication/306132158_Assessment_of_disaster_preparedness_among_emergency_departments_in_Italian_hospitals_a_cautious_warning_for_disaster_risk_reduction_and_management_capacity.

Iran. And he further asserted that if asked to spy, he would stop his cooperation with Iran. The intelligence agents, somewhat taken aback, asked him to forget the meeting and the offer. They assured him that he would not have any further problems. The officials asked that he continue his teamwork and teachings at Iran's academic centers.

In the autumn of 2015, the national Passive Defense Organization, which was affiliated with the military system of Iran, invited Ahmadreza to give a speech about health system resiliency against terrorist attacks that use CBRNE weaponry. Additionally, he attended a few meetings about a training program relevant to passive defense and counter-terrorism. Six months after these meetings, he went to Tehran to arrange study programs for Iranian physicians on natural disaster and crisis management. But he was suddenly detained by Ministry of Intelligence officials who, on April 26, 2016, accused him of acting against national security.

Ahmadreza was immediately transferred to solitary confinement in the infamous Evin Prison in Tehran. He was not allowed access to a lawyer or permitted to have any contact with his family. His barren cell, illuminated 24 hours a day, was only 6 feet by 6 feet, and his only "companions" were ants and beetles. He was given three small, dirty blankets to protect himself from the dank chill. To relieve himself, he was limited to knocking on the cell door five times a day to use one of only a few stench-filled bathrooms. Ahmadreza was kept in solitary confinement and routinely tortured for more than three months before he was transferred to a room shared by 18 other prisoners. His torment continued for an additional four months.

The investigators said that Ahmadreza had gathered top-secret data about Iran's critical infrastructure, crisis management, and passive defense systems and projects—classified information, which, they stated, he had shared with Israel. He was charged with having spied for Israel since 2008. The Iranian agents claimed that all his doctorate studies, post-doctoral work, and visa and residency (temporary and permanent) issues in Sweden and Italy had been arranged and offered by Israel in exchange for his espionage services for Israel.

Ahmadreza rejected the charges, declaring that all connections with other countries, as well as relationships with the CRIMEDIM faculty, were legally conducted by the universities. He emphasized that he had never associated or cooperated with any Israeli intelligence services or with any other country. Being put on the defensive, he underscored that he had never traveled to Israel or had any colleagues or friends from Israel. He further pointed out that dozens of professors and researchers in Sweden and Italy were fully informed about his daily activities and his scientific publications from the previous nine years.

Almost four weeks after being held in solitary confinement, the intelligence agents told Ahmadreza that they had decided he was innocent and therefore he would be free to return home. The guards brought him all his clothes and belongings, affirming that he would be free within a few hours. As a condition, however, he had to be interviewed in front of the camera or else he would be left in solitary confinement for a year without any contact with the outside and without further investigation. The officials added that the interview would be used just for the Ministry of Intelligence's training objectives, and his words would never be presented outside the Ministry.

Ahmadreza had to obey the requests of these agents, believing he would be released. The agents dictated what he was to say in front of the camera. During that broadcast, however, he never admitted to espionage and cooperation with a hostile country, such as Israel and the United States. Contrary to the promise, and, as an additional inhumane act, guards escorted him back to solitary confinement.

The investigators from the Ministry of Intelligence were not interested in Ahmadreza's explanations. On December 26, 2016, he was taken to Section 209 of Evin Prison where he was detained once again in a 36-square-foot isolation cell. He immediately began a hunger strike. From that point, his jailors used multiple psychological and physical measures to torture him. They also threatened, humiliated, and deluded him, denying him access to an attorney for seven months. While imprisoned, Ahmadreza was forced to falsely confess to fabricated crimes. His prison file contained lies and groundless accusations, all unsupported by any documentation or reasons for his incarceration.

Living Hourly Under Threat of Execution

After nine months of detention and two hunger strikes, one lasting 42 days and the other for 43 days, Ahmadreza was taken to the Revolutionary Court in mid–February 2017. The presiding judge, Abolghasem Salavati, without any evidence, finally charged him eight months later in October with espionage. He now faced the death penalty for the mystifying crime of "corruption on earth." Although he had legal counsel, his lawyer was not allowed to be present at the hearing and was not authorized to see the case files.

In November 2017, the UN Working Group on Arbitrary Detention launched an inquiry into the reasons for his incarceration. Iran summarily ignored this probe. That same month, under threat of execution and harm to his loved ones, Ahmadreza was presented on Iranian television[3] as a spy with a forced, signed, pre-written text.

Although his health seriously deteriorated since being confined in Evin Prison, Ahmadreza was denied access to adequate medical care despite increasing health complications. He remained in custody under the ever-present threat of execution.

Ahmadreza requested several times to see human rights officials in Iran, but all demands were refused, including his appeal to meet with the Swedish ambassador to Iran. When EU ambassadors visited Evin Prison on July 20, 2017, he was transferred to an isolated cell to prevent any possible meetings with these EU representatives.

---

3. "Iran TV Broadcasts Jailed Doctor 'Confessing to Spying,'" BBC News, December 17, 2017. Available at https://www.bbc.com/news/world-middle-east-42387308.

However, through his attorney, he was able to get out the following message to the world:

"I appreciate all my colleagues, faculties of the universities, human rights organizations, and activists, governments, reporters, media, people … from the whole world that has supported me and helped my family. I ask them to please continue their support and helpful actions until I am released or dead."[4]

That same year, the journal *Nature*[5] addressed the evidence of Ahmadreza's denial of being involved in espionage. Despite all the irrefutable proof as to his innocence, Iran's government and judiciary have rejected all international requests and have not removed the death penalty. The Iranian judiciary and intelligence authorities were known in some circles to accept Ahmadreza's innocence, but none would act to correct this huge travesty of justice by canceling his death sentence and releasing him.

During the next four years, the Ministry of Intelligence repeatedly moved its world-famous political prisoner to various parts of Evin Prison. At the beginning of August 2019, Ahmadreza was taken to an undisclosed location, kept in solitary confinement under psychological torture, and coerced into pleading guilty to new allegations. The agents forced him to make fabricated confessions dictated by the officers. They threatened to hurt his children, attack his spouse, and arrest his family members if he did not comply and confess what the Ministry of Intelligence requested.

Throughout these years, Ahmadreza was the subject of joint appeals sent to the Iranian government by the UN Human Rights Council and other relevant experts. They urged the authorities of the Islamic Republic of Iran to annul the death sentence and release him immediately. Sweden and other EU countries, in particular, Belgium and Italy, strongly acted in his support and have repeatedly pressured Iran's government to free him. Also, the European Parliament adopted four resolutions calling on the Iranian authorities to unconditionally release him. In addition to the actions taken by the European Union and UN, hundreds of academic societies, universities, scholars, scientists, and more than 130 Nobel laureates on multiple occasions have urged Iran to revoke Ahmadreza's death penalty and set him free.

Ahmadreza is not the only innocent victim of the brutality by Iran's intelligence organizations. And he is not the only person with dual nationality who has been taken hostage by Iran's security entities. But he is among only a few political prisoners with dual nationality who have all faced the cruelest and most malicious actions by Iranian officials. In 2020, I published a plea to my emergency medicine and public

---

4. Emily Grant, "'Until I Am Released or Dead': Amadreza Djalali and the Detention of Dual Nationals in Iran," *The Gate*, May 19, 2021. Available at http://uchicagogate.com/articles/2021/5/19/until-i-am-released-or-dead-ahmadreza-djalali-and-detention-dual-nationals-iran/.

5. Michele Cantanzaro, "Iranian Scholar Sentenced to Death," *Nature*, October 23, 2017. Available at https://www.nature.com/articles/nature.2017.22875.

health colleagues in *Prehospital and Disaster Medicine*,[6] the journal of the World Association of Disaster and Emergency Medicine (WADEM). I reminded the readership that the silence on Ahmadreza's case did not indicate that his circumstances had changed. His incarceration without due process and under unspeakable conditions continued unabated. Internationally, his imprisonment represented one of the most recognized and profoundly ruthless acts, a situation that was beyond comprehension by the global health and medical community. I attached to the article an emaciated-looking Ahmadreza photo that had been smuggled out of the prison.

Whatever political advantage Iran thought it might gain by his internment has had the opposite effect. I undertook a campaign on Ahmadreza's behalf. I petitioned by email a proposal that if he died in captivity, academic institutions worldwide should deny acceptance to any more Iranian graduate students. Those universities support more than 70,000 students from the Islamic Republic of Iran. I gave as my reason that those students would suffer a similar fate just as Ahmadreza did when they returned to Iran. Colleagues were reluctant to go that route of protest and the suggestion was voted down.

In my published plea for help, I stressed that Ahmadreza had endured, at that point, more than 1,500 days of imprisonment with increasing mental and physical torture. His health had dramatically worsened. He was now more vulnerable to Iran's Covid-19 surge. Again, I emphasized that physicians, such as Ahmadreza, are neutral, respected, and protected under the Geneva Conventions and International Humanitarian Law. His release and return to his wife and two children in Sweden must occur immediately before he died in prison. He was of no use to Iran as a prisoner.

I pointed out that Iran would benefit greatly in the eyes of the world if its government would immediately let him go on compassionate grounds. His plight was our plight. I asked that members of WADEM and readers of its *Prehospital and Disaster Medicine* journal speak out in any manner possible for Ahmadreza's immediate freedom. But nothing came of my appeal and nothing changed.

At the beginning of the Covid-19 pandemic, I received an email from Ahmadreza's wife, most likely arranged by his lawyer. One of Evin Prison's most prominent inmates had asked for articles on Covid management, which I quickly sent. I talked to several colleagues, and we all hoped that the request might mean a positive move by the Iranian government to use Ahmadreza's talents to help manage their pandemic crisis. But that possible shift in attitude was not the case, and I never heard from his lawyer again. None of my colleagues believed that he could survive the infection if the virus spread throughout the prison. Yet we learned later from his family that all prisoners had been vaccinated. That news suggested that it was in the Iranians' interest to keep him alive.

---

6. Frederick M. Burkle, Jr., "Ahmadreza Djalali, MD, PhD Is Dying," *Prehospital and Disaster Medicine*, 2020, 35(5):1–2. Available at https://www.cambridge.org/core/journals/prehospital-and-disaster-medicine/article/ahmadreza-djalali-md-phd-is-dying/D655A93377D6225ADEFA229E74831644.

Maintaining Dignity in Solitary Confinement

Thousands of hopeless, desperate days have passed since Ahmadreza has been detained by the Iranian régime. He is currently being kept in Evin Prison's ominous general ward. His physical and mental status is fragile, and the authorities continue to deny him access to medical care. In June 2021, his family arranged appointments for surgery and gastrologic visits at an outside hospital, but jail officials ignored that referral. In July 2021, his mother, who resided in Iran, passed away and he was prohibited from calling or seeing her when she was in the hospital. To Ahmadreza, not being able to visit his dying mother created severe mental distress which he had to bear alone in his cell.

I asked Vida, during our many email exchange conversations, how Ahmadreza was managing his isolation. She responded that he decided to survive in prison and maintain his hope, pride, and positive personality.

Vida told me that he spends his days studying available books, journals, and newspapers, trying to improve himself physically, mentally, and morally. While in solitary confinement, Ahmadreza was isolated from the outside world and had no access to reading material. But when he shared space with other prisoners, he was able to access books, journals, and newspapers. Vida went on to state that she had heard from different people, all prisoners and even the prison employees who were very impressed by Ahmadreza's manner of living in the notorious Evin Prison.

Vida muses that her husband's detainment in some ways has made him a much better person, declaring that he is stronger both from spiritual, social, and human aspects. She added in her email that he always talks about Nelson Mandela, who was imprisoned for 27 years. To Ahmadreza, Mandela was a symbol who changed himself and also had a huge effect on the world. Over the phone when he could call her, he always reminded the children about the importance of being a good human being and to enjoy everything about life. In that last communication, Vida said that she manages just by hoping that he will return home. However, since November 2020, his captors have denied Ahmadreza the right to call his family in Sweden.

After five months of solitary confinement from November 2020 to April 2021, Ahmadreza lost several teeth, which is a familiar outcome after hunger strikes. In addition, he suffers from painful gastritis and gallstones, most likely resulting from malnutrition. I have seen these medical conditions before in patients suffering from a poor diet. Along with all the other inmates, he received the first dose of Covid-19 vaccine. The big question is why Iran continues to detain this man.

Iran's Playbook of Hostage Diplomacy

Many in the outside world had hoped that the solution to Ahmadreza's ongoing hostage status would be tied to the fate of an Iranian diplomat being held in Belgium on charges of terrorism. Assadollah Assadi, an Iranian envoy in Vienna, was sentenced by a Belgian court to 20 years in prison for his role in a thwarted 2018 attack on a group that sought to overthrow the Iranian leadership. While attached to the Iranian mission in Austria, he supplied explosives for an attack that was supposed to take place in France during an Iranian opposition rally.[7] Assadi was charged with attempted terrorist murder and participating in the activities of an extremist group.

Ahmadreza Djalali's status is still uncertain. A *Washington Post* article in 2019 by Jason Rezaian titled "Iran's Hostage Factory"[8] describes many such events in which the Iranian government has imprisoned foreign citizens on trumped-up charges, holding them as bargaining chips. Speaking with authority on this subject, Iranian-American journalist Rezaian spent 544 days imprisoned by Iran until his release in January 2016. Rezaian's study claims that the seeds for this tactic began on November 4, 1979, when radical Iranian students stormed the U.S. Embassy in Tehran, taking dozens of personnel as hostages. After 444 days, the mass captivity ended on January 20, 1981. The seizure of the Embassy's junior and senior staff members was considered by the Ayatollah Khomeini government to be a successful model for using hostages as pawns to achieve political goals.

Since the 1980s, such cases have grown in frequency and Ahmadreza was swept up in a highly structured system of hostage-taking, most being hostages with dual citizenship. Rezaian's article is predictably consistent with the following Iranian hostage-taking methodology[9]:

- Iran accuses hostages of fabricated crimes against the state to later gain concessions from their home countries.
- Iran blames hostages for being spies and they are imprisoned for long periods without outside contact.
- Iran uses opaque charges of threatening the country's national security and plotting with foreign governments against the régime.
- Accused hostages are interned in Evin Prison, the same section run by the Revolutionary Guard.
- The hostages remain in solitary confinement and are subjected to long hours of interrogation without legal counsel, and this pattern continues for months.
- The Revolutionary Guard announces the detention and airing of charges through domestic media outlets it controls, sometimes with forced confessions.
- Once internationally known, a closed-door trial is held where hostages are denied due process and adequate legal representation.
- Almost all cases are heard by the same judge, Abolghasem Salavati, who convicts the accused and metes out harsh sentences.

These are procedures the Iranians use in their "standard hostage package" for all political hostages. "Special" prisoners, who potentially will reap more dividends for Iran, are nationals of the United States, Britain, Canada, Australia, and France.

---

7. Steven Erlanger, "Iranian Diplomat Is Convicted in Plot to Bomb Opposition Rally in France," *The New York Times*, February 15, 2021. Available at https://www.nytimes.com/2021/02/04/world/europe/iranian-diplomat-convicted-bomb-plot.html.

8. Jason Rezaian, "Iran's Hostage Factory," *The Washington Post*, November 4, 2019. Available at https://www.washingtonpost.com/opinions/2019/11/04/irans-hostage-factory/.

9. *Ibid.*

These particular internees have added value to Iran. Some are released after paying multimillion-dollar fines, a price for political and diplomatic battles to which they have no connection. Some cases result in a prisoner swap. Other instances are tied to attempts to recover frozen Iranian assets abroad. The Revolutionary Guard, often acting independently of the Iranian government, uses this tactic to deter contact between the outside world and Iranian society. This model has increased during negotiations over Iran's nuclear activities. The number of detained Western academic scholars in Iran has increased.

In return for freeing their captives, Iran has increasingly demanded concessions of all kinds: money, arms, and changes in policy favoring Iran. As of this writing, more than two dozen foreign and dual nationals are still detained in Iranian prisons. *The Washington Post* writer, Jason Rezaian, cautions that this behavior, while unique to Iran, may become an acceptable tool of diplomacy for other countries. The medical community once focused on Ahmadreza as an unusual case that would easily be resolved. Only recently have we learned that his captivity is part of a predictably malignant scheme over which he and his attorney have had no control.

Ahmadreza Djalali is an international tool of the Iranian government, a despotic rule that is abominable in every manner. Will this form of weaponizing hostages as collateral become a blueprint for other repressive sovereignties to wield power with systematic hostage-taking? Not surprisingly, other autocratic régimes, which now dominate our world, have not voiced any objections to this cruel and growing policy of hostage diplomacy.

As of this writing, I don't know what has become of Ahmadreza Djalali. But he and his unconquerable spirit will not be lost in his solitary confinement, will not be lost in torture cells, and will not be lost to history.

Sowing the Seeds of Global Autocracies

"Once in power, a leader with an antisocial personality disorder thrives on continuing discord and never seeks peace."

Throughout the past eight decades, many countries have suffered under the oppression of autocratic regimes. These types of despotic governments were first defined in the 1920s and 1930s, and the rest of the world looked the other way. The singular dictatorial designs of Hitler, Mussolini, Stalin, and Tojo ignited World War II when the Germans invaded Poland in September 1939—less than one year before I was born.

Historical debates, which seem too few in number, have asked the highly essential question: "Why do autocrats emerge and how do they maintain their power?" The end of the Cold War, which is usually considered to be the dissolution of the

Soviet Union in 1991, created the perfect storm of unruly circumstances. This state of affairs either perpetuated those in absolute control or gave birth to unprecedented opportunities for rising authoritarians.

Many of these would-be tyrants showed evidence, in varying degrees, of antisocial behaviors. They took advantage of the power vacuum to seek commanding roles in some of the world's most vulnerable and lawless countries. Incompetent leaders, unlike at any other time in history, were often assured tenure of authority by the easy availability of sophisticated weaponry and ready access to eager followers. Again and again, those massive numbers of supporters were bored, unemployed, disadvantaged, and disaffected youth looking for a cause. They found that cause—and a leader—in that chaotic void.

A repressive rule can be perceived in several forms. A pure autocracy is ruled by one dictator. Oligarchies, which are increasingly popular today, occur when domination is held by members of an elite segment of society, such as in Russia, China, and the Philippines. From 2017 through 2020, the Trump Administration put the United States on that same track with a corporate elite having a greater influence than "the people." Other autocratic models are military dictatorships in which all citizens must adhere to their respective strict military laws, as seen in Thailand, Libya, Pakistan, and, most recently, Burma (Myanmar). An additional type of authoritarianism exists, which can be found in the Northern Triangle of Central America. Gang violence in Honduras, Guatemala, and El Salvador has subverted all existing government authority, leaving people starving for law and order. Because of this pervasive lawlessness, more than 541,000 people fled the region in 2019, heading north for a better life.[10]

An Autocrat's Adolescent Development

In a December 2019 edition of the MSNBC program "Hardball," anchor Chris Matthews, in frustration over yet another one of President Donald Trump's obvious lies, asked, "Why is he like this?" I, too, have asked this same crucial question about all autocrats. The significant response is that the 45th President of the United States was psychologically considered a "narcissist" during his term in office—and out of office. That personality disorder is characterized by an excessive need for admiration, a lack of empathy, an inability to handle criticism, and believing in a deserved sense of entitlement.

A necessary first step in understanding the wide range of despotic, narcissistic leadership comes with knowledge of the basic comprehension of an autocrat's mental and emotional growth from childhood into adulthood. We must recognize the unique role that adolescence plays in ensuring either a stable adulthood or one that

---

10. Diana Roy, "Ten Graphics that Explain the U.S. Struggle with Migrant Flow," Council on Foreign Relations, December 1, 2022. Available at https://www.cfr.org/article/ten-graphics-explain-us-struggle-migrant-flows-2022.

is self-serving and oppressive. In addition, we need to be aware of this process of human development that is universally seen in every culture. The evolution of autocratic leaders in history reveals that many share severe character disorders that are consistently similar across borders and cultures.[11]

In early adolescence—the teenage years, some vanity is demonstrated as "healthy narcissism," which plays a vital role in building a person's emerging but fragile ego. The years between the ages of 10 and 19 are recognized as a critical stage of growth because that time-period is dependent on the unique, age-specific, neurological growth of the brain. That brain development/transitional stage is not biologically available to young people before age 10. On the other hand, if that transition hasn't already occurred for those in their mid–20s to late 20s, then that change most likely won't ever happen.

Individuals either gain reasoning powers by that point through these teenage and young adult learning challenges, or they never will have that analytic capacity. These capabilities of logical thinking are seen as cognitive and emotional qualities of behavior that society accepts as necessary for personality development. The teenager enters adulthood and needs to accept the responsibilities which that role demands. The young person's behavior becomes fixed at this point, although his personality can be further refined and remain so for the rest of his life.

Adolescents are constantly being tested. They are subjected to many social, emotional, and physical challenges, often seeking new and risky situations. For the first time, many feel personal anxiety, doubt, shame, depression, guilt, sorrow, and embarrassment over making mistakes. As young people gain more independence, they learn new avenues of behavior by modeling themselves after more mature adolescents or adults. At this point in their life, they acquire age-appropriate neurologically and socially beneficial developmental skills. Those abilities include learning to share for the common good and finding out how to compromise, namely, not dominating or prevailing over others. Since every child is in love with himself, part of maturation means developing strong feelings for someone else. These are milestones that eventually lead to a sense of accomplishment.

Personality disorder behaviors of this nature should stay in childhood. By the end of young adulthood, society expects the concrete, black-and-white narcissistic thinking, and actions of childhood to have been tamed. If not curbed early, that kind of behavior will run the risk of continuing and overshadowing development into adulthood, becoming a fixed trait reflecting thinking and conduct. These attributes can limit mental growth from concrete thinking to abstract reasoning.

While empathy reveals a deep sense of self-awareness, this ability to understand the feelings of others is a forerunner to the attainment of additional capabilities requiring more conceptual thought. Abstract reasoning is also fundamentally

---

11. F.M. Burkle, Jr., "Character Disorders Among Autocratic World Leaders and the Impact on Health Security, Human Rights, and Humanitarian Care," *Prehospital and Disaster Medicine*, 2019;34(1):2–7. Available at https://pubmed.ncbi.nlm.nih.gov/30642410/.

important because it involves flexible thinking, creativity, judgment, and logical problem-solving skills.

Critical reasoning challenges a person's ability to think outside the box. Abstract thinking also tests the capability to understand the nuances of multiple cultural settings and their all-encompassing global surroundings. This type of abstract consideration is indicative of a higher degree of thought, which is so necessary to grasp the subtleties of democratic concepts for everyone.

Adolescents today have to bear witness to their own individual trials and journeys within their community. To add even more stress during this vulnerable and dynamic thought period, many in this teenage group are now forced to grapple with the earth's planetary health crises and downstream implications for them in their later years.

But the human cognitive timeline for abstract thought has notable chronological limits—a sequential window of opportunity. If critical reasoning is not developed by this point, it cannot be learned later in life. Language, group cooperation, developing networks, and considering and questioning viewpoints, which are all outside our perspective, are essential characteristics. Those traits give meaning to the word "humanity." But the common factor that seems to trigger their progression is abstract thought and reasoning.

To believe that abstract thinking is only for the most educated is absurd. Understanding unique cultures and their social and political behavior defines humanity today, setting the tone for our ability to work together. The U.S. Constitution, even with its flaws, enumerates and defines our freedoms as Americans. A large number of Americans share an understanding of "freedom" no matter what the level of their education. However, our freedoms can easily and underhandedly be taken away by those who are unable to think in-depth, that is, those whose approach is absolute.

The failure to comprehend what makes autocrats tick appears to be universal. I have repeatedly discovered that most negotiators from democratic countries, international humanitarian organizations, and Western militaries have had—and still have to some extent—a blind spot. They were and often are unaware of the overwhelming power, character flaws, and self-serving motives of repressive leaders whose state of mind consists only of those concrete, absolute thought processes. That shortcoming in the negotiators' thinking creates grave diplomatic situations and threatens the health security of endangered populations.

To the point of denial, democratic countries have collectively shied away from exploring the mentality of tyrannical leaders. Self-governing societies have allowed oppressive rulers to secure consummate authority. But democratic social orders don't know how to contain those autocratic leaders' malignant and destructive behaviors.

The prolonged Cold War era provided many examples for the social sciences to study and understand the behavioral nuances of dictatorially driven leaders who would eventually be labeled as "narcissistic" and "sociopathic." These two forms of personality disorders are sometimes used interchangeably, overlap, or appear side by side modifying each other. But the main distinction between these two alarming, troubling, antisocial personality disorders is that a sociopath is more dangerous and more Machiavellian.

Narcissistic sociopaths do not attain this decisive last stage of mental and emotional development, especially abstract thinking, which is necessary for critical analysis. Abstract reasoning allows an individual to consider the broader significance of ideas and information rather than depending on concrete details and impulses alone. Domineering leaders have limited, if any, capacity for empathy, love, guilt, or anxiety, all of which become developmentally permanent and guide their everyday decision-making.

Despite marked differences in their cultures and languages, it is hardly surprising that opportunistic rulers across the globe share the same character traits of these two kinds of antisocial personality disorders: narcissism and sociopathy. Both of these conditions have proven to be predictably common and comparable to other failed leaders throughout history. Once they have achieved dominance, these power holders feel universally threatened and compelled to destroy democratic thought and freedoms. Many people are unable to understand how and why this need to break down the democratic system occurs.

Bullies on a Global Scale

Most people who are in command, good and bad, rose to leadership because earlier wars and internal conflicts had been attributed to multiple unresolved causes. Previous governments and parties in power were no longer trusted or acceptable. Unfortunately, this vacuum of leadership was often filled with heartless, self-serving, vile leaders who frequently would first present themselves as "saviors." They appealed to the masses searching for order after a period of chaos.

After obtaining absolute authority, these self-absorbed men were perceived as despots or common criminals, but still claimed to be "patriots." Collectively, they all share a psychological framework that differs little from those responsible for World War I, World War II, and the conflicts that plagued the Cold War and post–Cold War eras. Even today, what the world is witnessing is a plethora of oligarchic autocracies. In 2018, one-third of the global population lived under outright authoritarian regimes.[12]

These emerging despots are neither mentally ill—by existing clinical criteria—nor are they more inclined to have mental disorders, conditions that may be found in the rest of society. These tyrannical leaders instead represent personality or character disorders dominated across a wide spectrum by various degrees of sociopathy and narcissism. These behaviors result from flaws in their personality or character

---

12. The Economist: Intelligence Unit, "Free Speech Under Attack," Democracy Index 2017. Available at https://www.eiu.com/n/campaigns/democracy-index-2017-free-speech-under-attack/.

development that begins from birth. They do not arise from any defective genetic makeup or any biologically driven illnesses amenable to therapy, such as medication or counseling. Narcissists are fully aware of their self-serving actions, and they do not see themselves as having a mental or personality disorder.

Despite numerous differences in ethnicity, history, and geography, character traits of autocratic leaders in history are consistently similar across borders and cultures. Their shared characteristics can be traced to inappropriate cognitive and emotional development in childhood and early adolescence. The results are fixed, lifelong, concrete thinking patterns. These children and adolescents are first regarded as spoiled children prone to temper tantrums when they don't get their way.

When engaged with society, we call them "bullies." We all grew up with intimidators. They repeatedly exhibit intentional verbal, physical, and antisocial behaviors. This kind of conduct seeks to threaten or marginalize someone perceived as weaker or less powerful. Unfortunately, most societies have their share of these young tormentors and aggressors who grow up to obtain some level of power if they aren't redirected when young.

Common forms of this aggressive and frightening behavior include abusive language and physical harm. This conduct may grow subtler with age as teenage bullies routinely insult and mock their targets. For careers, they typically are drawn to crime, politics, the clergy, the law, and law enforcement. In these occupations that impose outright influence over others, they demonstrate a lack of empathy, remorse, and guilt. For unknown reasons, they do not seem to have a moral compass. They like to continually express grandiosity and overinflated self-worth. They also manipulate and expose their self-serving greed.

Oppressors require adulation and recognition. These authoritarians are also pathological liars. They show no consistency in behavior, and their shallowness, impulsivity, and risk-taking are always in the public eye. They refuse to be held accountable for their actions, revealing a blatant inability to apologize. Harassers are generally promiscuous, may have had multiple marriages, and display a constant daily need to control everything around them—from messaging and texting to diversion. All these offensive behaviors are refined in public by varying degrees of being charismatic, unpredictable, and ruthless. Those who most notice their behaviors and are most critical are in empathetic professions such as medicine. Medical professionals are best equipped to recognize autocrats' bad behavior. Other disparagers of an autocrat's dominance include learned politicians and those in legal circles. As public servants, they become the tyrant's relentless and lifelong targets of abuse through a constant barrage of adolescent-age insults that continue into adulthood. The bully trait has never left them. These highly repugnant characteristics have enabled menacing rulers to get everything they need, including getting elected to the highest office in the land.

This pattern of behavior lies on a continuum from healthy to pathological.

Narcissism turns into a problem when the individual becomes preoccupied with himself. He needs embellished admiration and approval from others, but shows callous disregard for other people's sensitivities. These egotists often portray an image of grandiosity and overconfidence to the world. This self-imposed persona covers up deep feelings of insecurity and a fragile self-esteem that is easily bruised by the slightest criticism. Because of these traits, self-centered individuals find themselves in inconsequential relationships that serve only to satisfy their constant need for attention.

Narcissism on the Rise

When narcissistic traits become so pronounced that they lead to impairment, the presence of a self-absorbed personality disorder is revealed. Persons with such a self-obsessed condition show a pretentious sense of self-importance. They are consumed by fantasies of unlimited success, power, brilliance, beauty, or ideal love, and are extremely sensitive to criticism. Sociopsychological studies show that narcissism is on the rise in Western societies. According to mental health researcher Olivia Remes, these findings hypothesize that this personality disorder, particularly those aspects of "entitlement, exploitation, sense of superiority, and negative evaluation of others,"[13] is not necessarily observed in individuals with high self-esteem.

Even as adults, narcissists mobilize their parents to handle a myriad of difficult social dealings. The parents, as "fixers," deal with their offspring's alarming disorder problems, such as divorces, violations of the law, and debts. Commonalities among narcissists include creating fabrications, exaggerations, and lies about their cultural histories, war records, and education. When challenged, they may rapidly escalate into derogatory and inflated insults meant to frighten their accusers. Once a narcissistic ruler is in authority, willing political, economic, and legal oligarchs assume that protective parental role.

Autocratic behaviors are easily observed in daily antics that worry, frustrate, and anger the population. Those behaviors become even more obvious globally when wars ultimately fulfill the narcissist's desired outcome. His demand for more respect is unstoppable. He will eventually provoke an armed conflict because he fantasizes about sending others into battle. Wanting to be seen as the hero-commander who saves the world, he can then receive those long-desired war medals and adulation. Once in power, a leader with an antisocial personality disorder thrives on continuing discord and never seeks peace.[14]

Every war I've experienced on a personal level has been started or perpetrated by

---

13. Olivia Remes, "Narcissism: The Science Behind the Rise of a Modern Epidemic," *The Conversation*, March 11, 2016. Available at https://www.the-independent.com/news/science/narcissism-the-science-behind-the-rise-of-a-modern-epidemic-a6925606.html.

14. F.M. Burkle, Jr., "Antisocial Personality Disorder and Pathological Narcissism in Prolonged Conflicts and Wars of the 21st Century," *Disaster Medicine and Public Health Preparedness,* February 2016; 10(1):118–128. Available at https://pubmed.ncbi.nlm.nih.gov/26456397/.

narcissistic sociopaths and psychopaths who are even more calculating and manipulating. Saddam Hussein in Iraq, Slobodan Milošević in Serbia, and Mohamed Farrah Aidid in Somalia were driven to pursue war. These autocrats failed as effective leaders in peaceful times. They all thrived on creating and maintaining a state of conflict around them, a tyrannical condition that was part of their psyche. They did not make effective rulers in times of peace because stability was not in their nature. In a strife-free period, they predictably fomented and returned to conflict. This autocratic mentality also applies to Bashar al-Assad in Syria today.

When the Dayton Agreement was signed in 1995,[15] the warring parties of Bosnia, Croatia, and Serbia all came together. Many were aghast that Milošević, an absolute tyrant, was treated as a diplomat who was held in high esteem when, in reality, he was on the contemptible end of the spectrum. The one-time "diplomat" then returned home to Serbia to persecute Kosovo's ethnic Albanians. If the United States and foreign diplomats had listened to non-governmental leaders who distrusted Milošević, then this oppression in Kosovo did not have to occur.

Narcissists are incapable of forming relationships with those having less concrete views, especially if those other people are perceived as having enviable social status that would compete with narcissists' pursuits. On a higher level, egomaniacal leaders' combined admiration and jealousy turn into an obsession over the individual power of other world leaders. Despite their seductive talents and uncanny ability to speak to the universal concerns of every citizen, narcissists never attain mature abstract reasoning. Authoritarians dodge discussions and debates that demand levels of critical thinking, observation, and objectivity. They circumvent issues that do not personally boost their absolute authority and prestige. These autocrats also expend emotional energy to cover up their limitations and turn to childish insults and unrelenting boastful opinions of themselves.

Narcissist-in-Chief

During the 2016 presidential debates, Republican candidate Donald Trump needed to bring attention to himself, other than just responding to questions. About every 90 seconds, he inserted a statement in his answers that gave him credit or brought him back to the forefront of the political discussion. At the debate held on October 9, 2016, Trump closely and menacingly followed Hillary Clinton around the stage, asserting his formidable height behind her to reclaim the limelight—even as she spoke.

On July 3, 2020, President Donald Trump spoke in front of Mount Rushmore, carefully posing for the camera as he positioned his face to appear next to the head of Abraham Lincoln. From the time of his election in 2016, he openly and seriously

---

15. The Dayton Agreement, also known as the "Dayton Accords" or the "General Framework Agreement for Peace in Bosnia and Herzegovina," was negotiated at Wright-Patterson Air Force Base, Dayton, Ohio, in November 1995. The agreement was formally signed in Paris on December 14, 1995, ending the Bosnian War that lasted nearly four years.

mused about having his head chiseled on Mount Rushmore, even going so far as to contact the Republican Governor of South Dakota, Kristi Noem, about how his likeness could be carved on this national memorial. Self-aggrandizers crave visual attention and adoration, especially in granite. The imagery and message weren't lost on his base.

From an early age, narcissists demonstrate unchangeable beliefs and behaviors that are the absolute antithesis of everything a democracy demands of an individual. Their regard for others in power is the extension of an adolescent obsession with more successful bullies. The consistent pattern of praise and envy for other world despots is remarkably consistent. They share similar character traits, such as an absence of conscience and an unquenchable desire for acclamation. Across the personality spectrum, Russian despot Vladimir Putin seems more sociopathic and less demonstrably narcissistic than Donald Trump. But Putin's intimidating and disarming silence provides him with a formidable and convincing self-importance.

In many ways, Trump admires Putin just as Hitler respected Mussolini's early successes. This pathological regard for their dictatorial style assures themselves with the same mentality: "If they can do it, so can I." Putin favoring oligarchs is equivalent to Trump backing politicians and corporate leaders. Both Russian oligarchs, American politicians, and corporate leaders profit greatly from their unbridled loyalty to their respective autocratic leaders.

Donald Trump has served as a model of narcissism before his one-term administration, then during his four years in office, and even following the post–2020 presidential election, which he claimed he won. On every public and tweet occasion, he quickly digressed from the topic at hand just to bring immediate attention to himself. So much of what narcissists do every day is an act, but the adulation and worldly attention, two forms of prestige which the Oval Office affords, are immediately gratifying.

The electorate would naturally assume that intelligence also comes with serving in the White House. But President Trump proudly proclaimed that he does not read books. He prohibited the schools he attended from releasing his grades and test scores—under threat of legal action. Mary L. Trump, the niece of Donald Trump, recounted an incident about his academics in her best-selling book *Too Much and Never Enough: How My Family Created the World's Most Dangerous Man*.[16] She claimed that in 1966, her uncle paid an acquaintance to take the Scholastic Aptitude Test exam under the Donald Trump name in order that Trump could get accepted into the prestigious University of Pennsylvania's Wharton School.

On the world stage, narcissists predictably tend to identify with other authoritarians in times of crises, not to mention cooperating and supporting each other. This admiration can quickly turn malignant if they perceive, in a very concrete, egocentric manner, that they are more deserving of the power.

---

16. Mary L. Trump, *Too Much and Never Enough: How My Family Created the World's Most Dangerous Man* (New York: Simon & Schuster, 2020), p. 72.

Democracy in Retreat

Our world is plagued once more by imperious rulers determined to compromise our struggling democracies. Trump decisively lost the 2020 presidential election. He sought to maintain his presidential authority, however, by vehemently questioning the election's legitimacy. But he also encouraged a "Make America Great Again" mob—his followers—to attack the Capitol, the very symbol of our democracy. The day of this insurrection—in which lives were lost—was seen in real-time around the world. January 6, 2021, will be remembered alongside the "Where were you" dates of Pearl Harbor on December 7, 1941, the Kennedy assassination on November 22, 1963, and the World Trade Center attack on September 11, 2001.

According to the Stockholm-based International Institute for Democracy and Electoral Assistance, a "visible deterioration"[17] was noted in American civil liberties beginning in 2019. In its 2021 report, for the first time, the international think tank added the United States to its annual and growing list of backsliding democracies. The report asserted that "the declines in civil liberties and checks on government indicate that there are serious problems with the fundamentals of democracy...."[18]

The report continued: "A historic turning point came in 2020–2201 when former President Donald Trump questioned the legitimacy of the 2020 election results in the United States."[19] A loss of confidence in this bedrock American rite portended a danger for future state and national elections. This distrust in the election process, as played up by the outgoing President because he didn't win, showed a further weakening of democracy. Until 2020, American elections have been the international democratic gold standard.

Today, the shrinking, democratically elected world is again under the influence of autocratic oligarchies. Putin is hell-bent on restoring the former Soviet Union. Despots in Central America and South America want to maintain corrupt control of El Salvador, Nicaragua, Venezuela, and Peru, all previously democratic countries.

But it is Vladimir Putin, already branded on the world stage as an "autocrat," who has gone beyond that designation of "autocrat." In March 2014, Russia took over Ukraine's Crimean Peninsula. And on February 24, 2022, Russian troops brazenly invaded Ukraine again on many fronts to bring that sovereign nation back into Russian dominance. The Russian aggressors committed multiple atrocities against civilian populations as Russian bombs and missiles reduced many Ukrainian cities to rubble. All this ongoing destruction, pillaging, and other brutalities have transpired despite severe economic sanctions, a united NATO front, and worldwide condemnation.

---

17. "U.S. added to list of 'Backsliding' Democracies for First Time," Agence France-Presse, November 22, 2021. Available at https://www.theguardian.com/us-news/2021/nov/22/us-list-backsliding-democracies-civil-liberties-international.
18. *Ibid.*
19. *Ibid.*

Appendix 2: Four Perspectives on the World's Challenges and Concerns   253

Putin has also been cited as a "war criminal" for perpetrating crimes against humanity. This Russian dictator knows no boundaries as to how much devastation he can inflict on civilians in a democratic Ukraine, and, shockingly, with continued support from Russian citizens. And at the time of this writing, Putin had already laid waste to Ukraine, deliberately bombed civilian populations, and produced an exodus of refugees not seen since World War II, all witnessed by irrefutable evidence and documented carnage.

Two days before the actual 2022 Russian invasion, Trump publicly applauded Putin's initial reason for attacking Ukraine by calling the Russian autocrat "savvy" and a "genius."[20] Trump used these volatile words after the Russian leader blatantly recognized the independence of breakaway eastern Ukraine regions.

Just as Putin galvanized the Russian oligarchs, Trump allowed the empowered economic elites in the U.S. to hijack the economy. As President of the United States, he redefined the U.S. Constitution under a self-serving political and economic autocracy. All despotic world leaders have shared agendas, including newly labeled "war criminal" Putin of Russia, Xi of China, former President Duterte of the Philippines, Kim Jung-Un of North Korea, Nicolás Maduro of Venezuela, and the gangs controlling much of Central America.

Trump also proudly claimed, in a strong, positive, self-confident manner, that he and Kim Jong-Un understood each other. While that questionable relationship may be quite true on an adolescent level, that kind of "rapport" did not translate into mature diplomacy. Even Colin Powell, a longtime Republican serving as Secretary of State under George W. Bush from 2001 to 2005, spoke at the 2020 Democratic National Convention of the importance of having a leader who would "trust in our own intelligence and diplomatic community, not the flattery of dictators and despots."[21]

Joint Russian-Chinese military exercises, which are based on partnerships with like-minded absolute rulers, are stronger than ever. History teaches us about conflicts that have resulted from such flawed leadership. And historians have lacked basic explanations of why these autocratic behaviors continually return to dominate many societies. We have taken democracy for granted, but during Trump's autocratic years in office, the world witnessed the pushback of our republic's values and laws.

Building multidisciplinary capability in societies, much needed to defend existing democracies against despotism, has been tragically weakened. To limit or end such authoritarian dominance, efforts must be two-fold. First, we need to begin with a developmental comprehension of why autocrats exist. Second, we must understand why they persist in externalizing their pathological behaviors on unsuspecting and vulnerable populations.

---

20. Alana Wise, "Trump Praises Putin as 'Savvy' amid New Escalations on Russia-Ukraine Border," NPR, February 22, 2022. Available at https://www.npr.org/2022/02/22/1082478790/trump-praises-putin-as-savvy-amid-new-escalations-on-russia-ukraine-border.

21. "CNN Politics," Transcript: Colin Powell's DNC remarks August 18, 2020. Available at https://www.cnn.com/2020/08/18/politics/colin-powell-speech-transcript/index.html.

Frida Ghitis, a world affairs analyst and writer, contends that "modern-day would-be dictators don't overthrow another government. What they do is take over the system of government."[22] She emphasizes that authoritarians' methods are more gradual because they can gradually wear down democracy to a weak remnant of itself.

Similar to Germany in the 1930s, by the time most people realize what has happened to their democratic state, it's too late to push back. When Xi Jinping took power in 2012, China's once-applauded democratic progression and ownership of private, market-driven advancement, was forced out. The resurgence of the state's role, last seen under Mao Zedong from the 1950s to the 1970s, caused this 180-degree change. This growth increased the Communist Party's impact on private businesses within and outside the country. Dreams of a more democratic leaning China have since disappeared.

A Wired Globe

The world is changing rapidly. Autocratic leaders are gaining confidence and challenging globalization by emphasizing democratic failures throughout an increasingly connected, sophisticated, electronically wired globe. Their actions and behaviors are now instantly reported on the worldwide scene. Oppressive regimes are escalating their efforts to work together. They have adapted and consolidated their strength in claiming historically disputed lands and territories. The ease with which they can manipulate information, as well as generate entire propaganda campaigns, also creates an environment where facts are up for debate. This fusion of power, coupled with climate change, is expected to lead to a projected 143 million fleeing migrants and refugees within a decade.[23]

Despotic rulers view the flight of refugees as an effective weapon against democracy. This tactic has led, especially in the European Union (EU), to a rise in the radical right that has combined populism with anti-immigration and authoritarianism. These leaders have knowingly created a perpetual state of crisis centered on anti-politics, anti-intellectualism, or anti-elite. An autocrat wants to convince his country's populace that he alone is infallible. If various factions within a country are not supportive of Big Brother, then those political groups are automatically considered to be against "the people."

Humanitarians, who serve in an autocratic country, realize that a dictator's sole motivation is to stay in power. They assert that despotic regimes take a cut of UN aid. International financial support may build or improve some vital infrastructure, such as roads, sanitation, and clean water resources, but these indispensable

---

22. Frida Ghitis, "Dictatorship, 21st Century Style," *CNN Opinion*, August 8, 2017. Available at https://www.cnn.com/2017/08/08/opinions/dictator-lessons-opinion-ghitis/index.html.
23. Laura Parker, "143 Million People May Soon Become Climate Migrants," *National Geographic*, March 19, 2018. Available at https://www.nationalgeographic.com/news/2018/03/climate-migrants-report-world-bank-spd/.

systems are rarely maintained. Citizens living in such oppressive environments lack the political rights to protest disastrous public health services. The dictators keep the cash, which is designated for public service aid, and punish those who object to this form of graft. The opposition asserts that if these autocratic regimes continue human rights abuses, then those governments must be threatened by withholding international funding unless democratic measures are put into place.

If humanitarian aid groups or other governments become engaged with despotic rulers, manipulation of assigned assistance funds will ensure that those in need will not receive the aid they require. Pathologically-driven leaders prevent aid to inflict harm, retreat from public responsibility with the emergence of a public health emergency, and/or divert financial resources to further violence or conflict. Authoritarian regimes routinely utilize physical and psychological coercion as their primary method of governance, resulting in predictable health and mental health consequences.

Societies haven't paid enough attention to the unbridled sense of aggrandizement that drives the corrupt mover and shaker. The world has come to accept and excuse the autocrat who personally intimidates those he perceives as obstacles to his authority. When the political party aligns itself with the egomaniac at the head of the government, those party representatives become operationally and mutually narcissistic. They, too, have overblown opinions of themselves and relish staying in office. On December 19, 2019, Nancy Pelosi, Speaker of the House, commented at a press conference in the Capitol Visitor Center: "Our Founders, when they wrote the Constitution, they suspected that there could be a rogue President. I don't think they suspected we could have a rogue President and a rogue Leader [Mitch McConnell] in the Senate at the same time."[24]

Once collective narcissism exists, the head of state can be assured of sustaining his support base. The authoritarian demands total loyalty from his followers who must speak from the same playbook. Yet loyalty between an autocrat and his supporters is only a one-way street: total allegiance to him—and to him alone. On June 12, 2017, five months into Trump's presidency, his cabinet awkwardly paid tribute to him—on camera. Trump listened to each of these so-called accolades and kept nodding in approval.[25]

An autocrat's devotees must be drilled to give daily compliant sound bites. Disloyalty is severely punished by those at the top of the cultish narcissistic pack. The leader's staunch followers have built among themselves a powerful and self-serving political culture. Many in absolute command truly believe in having god-like powers that absolve their faults and other people's judgments. Society is at fault for lavishing praise on an authoritarian and feeding his ego with unfathomable, incomprehensible approval.

---

24. "Transcript of Pelosi Weekly Press Conference Today," December 19, 2019. Available at https://pelosi.house.gov/news/press-releases?page=159.

25. Kevin Liptak, "Cabinet Members Give Trump Unusual Tribute," CNN, June 12, 2017. Available at https://www.cnn.com/2017/06/12/politics/trump-cabinet-tribute/index.html.

In general, democratic communities have, unfortunately, been dismissive of the impact of sociopathy and pathological narcissism on families and society. Power-grabbing is on the rise and also becoming more troubling as previously created democratic advances wear away. The culture of collective narcissism becomes more infectious, and its collaborative power turns out to be more pervasive.

The loyalists, now a political base, see political and economic advantages for themselves, whether or not those rewards would come to fruition. The autocratic country lacks moral direction and many more of its citizens feel they have a new license to express themselves. Destruction of schools, churches, synagogues, and mosques has become commonplace. Bad behavior is ignored, defended, or excused as those benefits accumulate for an authoritarian leader's loyalists.

The 20th century offered two of the most terrifying and oppressive dictators. Mussolini's Fascisti in the 1920s and Hitler's Nazis in the 1930s should have raised early alarms to a war-weary Europe. These two authoritarians took advantage of the devastation created by the Great War of 1914–1918. Having come to power through elections, these brutal dictators eliminated all political opposition through intimidation, violence, and murder. They ignited a global conflagration resulting in 70 to 85 million deaths.[26]

I frequently turn to the writings of Kenneth Roth, who was the Executive Director of the Human Rights Watch (HRW) from 1993 to 2022. The HRW is one of the world's leading watchdog and investigative organizations concerning human rights. Through HRW, Roth explained the contradictions, especially in the former Trump Administration. He stated that autocrats possess an operational agenda that is only as ambiguous as it is effective for authoritarian regimes to keep the status quo and keep themselves in power.

Unlike traditional dictators, Roth also emphasized that, unlike traditional dictators, today's would-be autocrats typically emerge from democratic settings. Most pursue a two-step strategy for undermining their representative form of government. First, they find a scapegoat and demonize vulnerable minorities in order to build popular support. Second, they weaken the checks and balances on government and the authority needed to preserve human rights and the rule of law, such as an independent judiciary, a free media, and vigorous civic groups. Even the world's established democracies, most particularly the United States, have shown themselves vulnerable to this demagoguery and manipulation.[27]

The United States and United Nations at a Tipping Point

The Guardian, a British newspaper, recognized by many as a bastion for the expression of democracy, civility, and truth, has openly questioned the attempts

---

26. "World War II Casualties," Wikipedia. Available at https://en.wikipedia.org/wiki/World_War_II_casualties.

27. Kenneth Roth, "World's Autocrats Face Rising Resistance," *Human Rights Watch: World Report 2019.* Available at https://www.hrw.org/world-report/2019/country-chapters/global.

of the United States to redefine the norms of behavior that guided my generation and the development of the United Nations. John Mulholland, the editor of *Guardian US*, wrote in *The Guardian* on March 6, 2019, during the Trump Administration: "America is at a tipping point, finely balanced between truth and lies, hope and hate civility and nastiness. Many vital aspects of American public life are in play—the Supreme Court, abortion rights, climate policy, wealth inequality, Big Tech, and much more. The stakes could hardly be higher."[28]

The United Nations is also at a very precarious tipping point because these articulated qualities must be reflected and championed in a UN mission statement. That declaration must serve the global community, not the deceivers representing current global power brokers. These false prophets have no more rights than the common man, woman, or child.

In nations already defined as "authoritarian" and earning a "not free" designation from Freedom House, which is another non-governmental overseer organization, regimes have increasingly shed the thin façade of democratic practice established in previous decades. At that time, international incentives and pressure for reform were stronger.[29] More authoritarian leaders, such as Turkish President Recep Tayyip Erdoğan and Hungarian Prime Minister Viktor Orbán, are now banning opposition groups and jailing their leaders, dispensing with term limits, and tightening the screws on any independent media that remain.

Many countries democratized after the end of the Cold War. But these nations have since regressed in the face of rampant corruption, anti-liberal populist movements, and breakdowns in the rule of law. Most disconcerting, even long-standing democracies have been shaken by populist political forces that discriminate against minorities and reject basic principles, such as the separation of powers. Until the Trump era, no American president had ever claimed to be above the three equal branches of government. Donald Trump, as Chief Executive, consistently demonstrated that he was above the Legislative and Judicial branches of the federal government, as well as exceeding those presidential powers delegated by the Constitution.

Causing real alarm are the major democracies that are now becoming less democratic. They seem to be heading in the opposite direction. Witnessing worldwide despotism on the rise is the cause for "a fire bell in the night," to use a Thomas Jefferson phrase that is relevant to so many disturbing political situations. Democracy needs defending. As traditional champions stumble, such as the United States, core democratic norms meant to ensure peace, prosperity, and freedom for all people, are under serious threat around the world.[30] The pandemic of narcissism is killing democracy.

---

28. John Mulholland, "The Gap Between us," February 4, 2020. Available at https://twitter.com/TheGapBetweenU1/status/1224863814526566400 (source no longer accessible).
29. *Freedom in the World: Democracy in Retreat* Annual Report (2019 edition), Washington, D.C: Freedom House, 2019. Available at https://gijn.org/stories/document-of-the-day-freedom-in-the-world-2019/.
30. *Ibid.*

We need to understand how 74 million citizens voted to keep Donald Trump in power in the 2020 election. Did their education and/or upbringing make them identify with Trump's "Make America Great Again" movement? Did a lack of certain important components of their education during adolescence have a major influence on the development of abstract reasoning—or absence of development of abstract reasoning?

Studies have shown that civics knowledge has been at an all-time low. Columbia University sociologist Jonathan R. Cole pointed out that "it is testimony to the failure of the country's education system that a high percentage of the voting-age population is simply ignorant of basic facts—knowledge that is necessary to act reasonably and rationally in the political process."[31] He also noted that "89 percent of those who took a test on civics knowledge in 2009 expressed confidence they could pass it."[32]

But in a 2017 civics knowledge survey, the University of Pennsylvania's Annenberg Public Policy Center found that more than one-third of those questioned could not name any of the rights guaranteed under the First Amendment, and only one-quarter of Americans could name all three branches of the federal government.[33] However, a 2020 Annenberg survey showed a marked increase in knowledge. Just over 51 percent could name all three branches, still not a ringing endorsement of the nation's civics education.[34]

During my adolescence, civics classes were a compulsory part of a high school curriculum, but those courses have since met their demise. Only nine states and the District of Columbia require one year of U.S. government or civics courses, while 30 states require a half year, and the other 11 states have no civics requirement.[35] A 2018 report titled "The State of Civics Education," published by the Center for American Progress (CAP), stated that only 23 percent of eighth-graders performed at or above the proficient level on the National Assessment of Educational Progress civics exam. The report added that achievement levels had virtually stagnated since 1998.[36] One reason for this lack of progress, CAP hypothesized, was the increased emphasis on math and reading in elementary, middle, and high schools, a focus that gave lower priority to other subjects, including civics.[37] For so many teenagers, learning civics

---

31. J.R. Cole, "Ignorance Does Not Lead to Election Bliss," *The Atlantic*, November 8, 2016. Available at https://www.theatlantic.com/education/archive/2016/11/ignorance-does-not-lead-to-election-bliss/506894/.
32. *Ibid.*
33. "Americans Are Poorly Informed about Basic Constitutional Provisions," Annenberg Public Policy Center, September 12, 2017. Available at https://www.annenbergpublicpolicycenter.org/americans-are-poorly-informed-about-basic-constitutional-provisions/.
34. "Amid Pandemic and Protests, Civics Survey Finds Americans Know More of Their Rights," Annenberg Public Policy Center, September 14, 2020. Available at https://www.annenbergpublicpolicycenter.org/pandemic-protests-2020-civics-survey-americans-know-much-more-about-their-rights/.
35. Sarah Shapiro and Catherine Brown, "The State of Civics Education," Center for American Progress, February 21, 2018. Available at https://www.americanprogress.org/issues/education-k-12/reports/2018/02/21/446857/state-civics-education/.
36. *Ibid.*
37. *Ibid.*

in high school may have been the last time their brains were challenged to become proficient in abstract reasoning.

As President, Trump failed to confront many critical issues and make appropriate decisions. Some problems were too complicated for him to comprehend because his sphere of understanding was so narrow and concrete, as expected in an early adolescent. Whenever presented with a quandary that did not fit into a black-and-white dimension of understanding, he simply ignored it or allowed others to make decisions for him—in his name.

Some authoritarians are more violent and abusive than other "Big Brother" leaders, regardless of their title—tyrant, dictator, autocrat, despot, king, oppressor, fascist, or president. But the backgrounds of how these suppressive heads of state came to power, as well as understanding their developmental gaps through childhood and adolescence, are all too similar. Their narcissism and sociopathy form the common strategy of coercion and fear with identical tactics: They abuse human rights and they disregard, overtly or covertly, the laws of their country.

Beware the narcissists who use religion to acquire more influence and dominance as though God is talking directly to them. Religions see their role as enlightening the multitudes, as well as being an important element of consolidating and informing the community and controlling community behaviors. Autocratic leaders, who are usually non-religious, will pursue special relationships with religious leaders. These despots may claim that God speaks through them. They may also profess they have a special connection with God, which makes them superior to the masses.

* * * *

Narcissistic sociopathy presents a more virulent threat to peace and justice than at any other time since the end of the Cold War. Democracy is the arch enemy of every concrete thinking, pathologically narcissistic sociopath. The concept and functioning of a representative government are abstractions that autocrats can neither define nor comprehend. The momentum toward democracy, which swept the globe as I grew up and which advanced in my career, reversed course from January 20, 2017, to January 20, 2021. The Narcissist-in-Chief for those four years was Donald Trump. Ever optimistic, the years ahead may bring about winds of change for the better: Democracy will triumph over autocracy.

Politics and Public Health: An Explosive Combination

"Political meddling in public health is as perilous domestically as it is globally. We continue to see how the decades-old international legal framework is easily overwhelmed by political inaction and interference."

My life's work in public health was captured in my 2017 article titled "The Politics of Global Public Health in Fragile States and Ungoverned Territories." This perspective article reflects the essence of that 2017 *Currents Disasters* journal piece.[38] My colleagues and I have always tried to stay the course to practice and advance the just cause of global public health—and to steer clear of politics.

In 2004, I was interviewed for *The Lancet* medical journal's Lifeline Series. I had left my disastrous short tenure as the Interim Minister of Health in Iraq in 2003 following the Iraq War. Secretary of State Colin Powell had given me the following instructions: Mitigate the destruction of vital public health infrastructure and protections. Powell knew that U.S. forces were now designated as "occupiers." Under two articles of the 1949 Geneva Conventions, Articles 55 and 56, the U.S. was now required to ensure and maintain the medical services, public health, and hygiene of the occupied territory, in this case, Iraq.

Predictably, the loss of critical public health protections in food, water, sanitation, shelter, health, and energy leads to illness and loss of life. Mortality statistics, which accrue from a lack of public health safeguards, exceed death and injury from war weaponry by 50 to 70 percent—or perhaps a higher percentage. The George W. Bush Administration immediately squelched the plan we had already developed for Iraq when Secretary of Defense Rumsfeld unexpectedly transferred these post-war humanitarian responsibilities from the Department of State to the Department of Defense.

Donald Rumsfeld claimed that U.S. forces were not "occupiers" but "liberators." This decision promptly reversed any previously planned public health recovery and rehabilitation. The State Department's seasoned nation-building specialists, including myself, were summarily replaced. But before leaving Iraq, I had the last word by publicly declaring Baghdad a "public health emergency." My pronouncement fell on deaf ears.

Many in Iraq see that decision as the most egregious policy enacted after the Coalition invasion in which women, children, the elderly, and the disabled suffered the most. While the "liberator" claim was debunked and reversed 18 months later, it was too late. Reliable public health data and surveillance systems were also thwarted in the war's aftermath. American politicians were largely protected from further scrutiny. Two decades later, Iraq is still considered a public health emergency.

The Lifeline Series interviewer from *The Lancet* asked me in 2004, "What do you believe is the most exciting field of science?"

Without hesitation, I replied, "Public health. It has the most potential and the least support."

The interviewer, somewhat surprised, stated that to date no one had ever mentioned public health. And when he asked what I believed was the greatest political danger to the medical profession, I answered unequivocally, "Political interference in public health."

---

38. Frederick M. Burkle, Jr., "The Politics of Global Public Health in Fragile States and Ungoverned Territories," *PLOS* [Public Library of Science] *Currents Disasters*, January 9, 2017, 9. Edition 1. Available at https://www.ncbi.nlm.nih.gov/pmc/articles/PMC5300740/.

My response from 2004 would be the same answer I'd give today. Political meddling in public health is as perilous domestically as it is globally. We continue to see how the decades-old international legal framework is easily overwhelmed by political inaction and interference. Moreover, we can still perceive struggles for relevance given today's modern challenges. The reasons for humanitarian crises—and how the world responds to these catastrophes—have dramatically changed every decade. The 1945 United Nations Charter, International Humanitarian Law, and the 1949 Geneva Conventions were designed to protect humanitarian aid in cross-border wars.

Although the language remains relevant, attempts have been made to adapt twentieth-century language to modern-day civil wars. But many warring factions and signatory governments do not respect public health protections, or they choose to blatantly disregard them. In instances of civil war, therefore, public health officials can no longer guarantee the continued safety of citizens, out-of-combat military casualties, vital public health infrastructure, and humanitarian personnel.

As armed conflict erupts, essential public health infrastructure rapidly disappears and populations flee. Disasters define public health and expose its vulnerabilities. The global community must emphasize prevention and preparedness. The world community also needs to re-legitimize prevention and preparedness under international law to ensure protection in fragile states before they weaken to the point of no return.

Lessons Not Learned for Public Health Emergencies

More than a decade after the Iraq War, a broader brand of global health engagement has emerged, yet public health's role remains in limbo, ignored, or ill-defined. What interventions exist under international law to protect public health before conditions deteriorate? Working from up-to-date laws of war, the International Committee of the Red Cross (ICRC) has been influenced by the consequences of Iraq, Syria, Ethiopia, Burma (Myanmar), and Afghanistan.

The ICRC acknowledges the overwhelming and dramatic cumulative impact brought about by urban system breakdown. What invariably transpires from that collapse is the loss of interconnected infrastructure that health systems cannot keep pace with. At present, we painstakingly try to verify the deaths of health personnel in war. But no means exist to document the deaths of indispensable public health recovery personnel, especially those specialized personnel whose skills are required to restore water and sanitation.

Despite the desperate call for a renewed emphasis on disaster risk reduction in 2015's Hyogo Framework for Action,[39] the fledgling global community is fixated on

---

39. The Hyogo Framework for Action (HFA) was the international proposal for disaster risk reduction efforts between 2005 and 2015. The HFA's goal was to decrease by 2015 the following disaster losses: lives and damages in the social, economic, and environmental assets of communities and countries. The HFA was adopted at the World Conference Disaster Reduction in 2005 in Kobe, Hyogo, Japan. Available at https://climate-adapt.eea.europa.eu/en/metadata/publications/hyogo-framework-for-action-2005-2015-building-the-resilience-of-nations-and-communities-to-disasters.

interventions that still favor response over preparedness and prevention for natural disasters. But what if the consequences of a natural disaster, including that of climate change or global pandemics, inextricably lead to conflict or war?

Today's domestic and regional crises are increasingly influenced by climate change, biodiversity loss, rapid and unsustainable urbanization, and water, food, and energy scarcity. These catastrophes have become more severe, affecting massive populations across many borders. Some limited and often primitive public health protections have remained. But those protections have been ineffectual, dangerously managed, and selectively denied to the most vulnerable. Those in power have persistently ignored solutions offered by the scientific community.

While some standard indicators already exist, the most perceptive signs are often multidisciplinary and transdisciplinary. The rate of dengue fever, for instance, which escalates when trash collection is inadequate, is a subtle indicator of both poor governance and urban decay. The humanitarian community is far from solving this problem. We do not know, for example, how to operate effectively in dense, rapidly urbanized settlements, a most likely site for both future conflicts and pandemics.

Unless measures are taken to develop the means to include indirect mortality and morbidity, political scientists, humanitarians, and military analysts will be unable to calculate the human cost of public health decline. Their calculations will remain an inexact process of estimation. The capacity to access vital information concerning the location, function, and extent of destroyed necessary infrastructure is currently not possible. The lives at risk and those lost will remain unseen, uncounted, and unnoticed. We have not learned the lessons for effective prevention and protection.

More than ever, we need strong international humanitarian laws, accountability, and recourse for those who fail to respect the laws that are already in place. Why wait for conflicts to occur when we have a clear, evidence-based global mandate to lessen the public health consequences? With so many examples of public health infrastructure and protections, which have been obliterated, overwhelmed, unmaintainable, or population-denied, we have a massive global health emergency.

While we have had "laws of war" for centuries in an increasingly globalized world plagued by public health emergencies, now is the time for "laws of prevention." Public health protections are a human right. An emerging global society has the tools to wage war—but a global society cannot prevent them.

The Politics of a Pandemic

War, conflict, drought, crop destruction, famine, and climate change are not the only events affecting global health. Diseases and pandemics, such as Covid-19, have had an earth-shattering impact. The worst health crisis I have seen in my lifetime is the pandemic from late 2019 to the present day. How nations, including our own, have handled the pandemic has been incomprehensible. The deadly virus has illustrated why politics and public health are an explosive combination.

Appendix 2: Four Perspectives on the World's Challenges and Concerns

As Covid-19 engulfed the planet, sickening and killing millions, we first witnessed the denial of its danger and then an unending conflict over what works or does not work in controlling the pandemic. Controversies erupted over the wearing of preventive masks, the use of questionable and untested therapies, and, most importantly, the refusal of getting life-saving vaccines. In the United States, a world leader in medicine, science took a back seat as did scientists and public health experts. For the first time, a global disease became political.

In autocratic regimes, public health science has been discounted. I emphasized this fact early in the pandemic in my study titled, "Declining Public Health Protections within Autocratic Regimes: Impact on Global Public Health Security, Infectious Disease Outbreaks, Epidemics, and Pandemics."[40] Autocrats cannot challenge science and so they forcefully ignore it or try to alter its message. Political loyalists run their health departments or ministries, but they differ greatly in capability, capacity, and assessments regarding containment. These decisions define public health, along with strict economic and political imperatives that are dangerously similar in all autocratic countries. These régimes have failed across the board to prepare for a pandemic by denying for decades any investments in public health infrastructure, education, and prevention. They fail to keep pace with population growth and densities upon which the spread of infectious disease is dependent.

In my 2020 article, "Declining Public Health Protections within Autocratic Regimes," I focused on the predictable manner in which these self-serving régimes failed to identify, alert, and manage health crises. Autocrats and their respective populations placed the rest of the world at increasing risk. China, lauded for its economic advances, was the first authoritarian government to be judged. Unfortunately, China failed miserably by ignoring World Health Organization (WHO) agreements to which it was a signatory. Even more distressing was China's move to stifle and then arrest physicians whose early Covid-19 alerts to the rest of the world were systematically disregarded.

But when I witnessed similar disturbing behaviors in the United States, I realized we were doing no better in not being able to control the pandemic. Also in 2020, I co-authored another article titled "50 States or 50 Countries: What Did We Miss and What Do We Do Now?"[41] Some states supported public health officials and epidemiologists both locally and nationally to make the necessary public health, population-based decisions to contain the spread. Yet other states, often sharing adjacent borders, became mired in both political and economic competition and pressures. To date, more than 200 public health experts have been fired, replaced multiple times, or resigned early.

---

40. Frederick M. Burkle, Jr., "Declining Public Health Protections within Autocratic Regimes: Impact on Global Public Health Security, Infectious Disease Outbreaks, Epidemics, and Pandemics," *Prehospital and Disaster Medicine*, April 2, 2020, 1–10. Available at https://www.ncbi.nlm.nih.gov/pmc/articles/PMC7156578/.

41. Frederick M. Burkle, Jr., and Asha V. Devereaux, "50 States or 50 Countries: What Did We Miss and What Do We Do Now?" *Prehospital and Disaster Medicine*, May 22, 2020, 1–5. Available at https://www.ncbi.nlm.nih.gov/pmc/articles/PMC7261962/.

This inconsistency in judgments resulted in discernible differences in disease transmission from state to state. Their borders, which were only lines on a map, were easily crossed, making it impossible for national health authorities to respond effectively. So the question then arises: Is the United States made up of 50 states or 50 countries? Despite attempts at the federal level to place response control of Covid-19 under a single organizational umbrella, the management of the pandemic markedly differed because each of the states went its own way.

From the outset of the pandemic, either the public health leaders were unprepared or had their decisions challenged by state politicians, most often governors. And to make managing this virus worse, many public health officials across the United States were shunned, ignored outright, or fired. Nationwide, political pressure accounted for hundreds of health care workers' confirmed resignations, firings, leaving voluntarily, or taking early retirement.

One key to success in conquering Covid-19 and other pandemics is a reliance on public health professionals. These experts normally work every day behind the scenes in prevention, preparedness, administering vaccines, and controlling infectious and environmental diseases. They often think of themselves as being the invisible health authorities, yet they are largely responsible for the majority of improvements in global life expectancy. During the Covid-19 pandemic, public health specialists silently assumed leadership roles in multiple countries and within the United States, as they do with all epidemics and pandemics.

The functional and population-based approaches are complementary ways of understanding a complex problem. Both methods must be considered in preparedness and response to pandemics to assess the health status and health needs of a target population. But hospitals and clinics are managed by clinicians trained primarily in individual care—and the patient is right in front of them at the time. Population-based care and management have shifted emphasis to population-based decisions. These clinicians are trained to recognize limited or absent resources to ensure the best possible outcome for society as a whole. Overall, nations with a competent state apparatus—a government that citizens trust and listen to—have shown that effective public health leaders perform well.

A Fear of Future Pandemics

The greatest fear that global health practitioners have is that recovery from Covid-19 will not advance major change in how the world prepares for and responds to future epidemics and pandemics. Denial is possibly the strongest of human defenses. We recognize that worldwide public health crises will continue unless we have full acceptance of the multiple global calamities that contribute to infectious disease events. Also, the global public health community cannot tolerate the increasing political interference that authoritarian governments, as well as local, state, and federal politicians in our own country and other Western democracies, have displayed.

Appendix 2: Four Perspectives on the World's Challenges and Concerns

The coronavirus ravaged the United States. In its early stages, the Trump Administration formally moved to withdraw our nation from the World Health Organization, accusing WHO of being under China's control in the wake of the Covid-19 pandemic. This purely political action, an effort to divert attention from the administration's disastrous handling of the pandemic, weakened the international response and isolated the United States. President Trump stated in July 2020 that he was pulling the U.S. out of WHO, a withdrawal to go into effect in July 2021. But President Biden, on his first day in office in January 2021, fortunately reversed that decision.

The World Health Organization's international health regulations need serious restructuring. And to that end, two other colleagues and I published a two-part article[42] proposing how WHO could undertake this challenge. Unlike other pandemics, Covid-19 management has led public health experts to conclude that the poor response and outcomes were predictable and preventable. With the onset of this pandemic, WHO officials voiced that no country would be going back to "normal." Public health decisions would mean the difference between life and death. These warnings by an internationally recognized organization, WHO's role was minimized by international politics. Our study pointed out that global public health information and management deficits have led to very unfortunate outcomes.

Two major factors are necessary for making over the World Health Organization. The first component would have WHO-sanctioned, population-based management teams serve the world's entire population through WHO regional centers. These sites would support "centers for disease control" to be established in every nation. These centers would be staffed by trained, population-based health care managers and scientists with a major grasp of the nuances of global public health and global crises.

The second element would require worldwide population-based management teams to be universally linked with updated population and public health information. These facts and figures would be readily accessible on a global public health database,[43] which is essential to make population-based decisions. Such a database has been glaringly absent during Covid-19, leading to few vital public health decisions being made in a timely fashion.

The World Health Organization, as an operational structure supported by a

---

42. Frederick M. Burkle, Jr., David A. Bradt, and Benjamin J. Ryan, "Global Public Health Database Support to Population-based Management of Pandemics and Global Public Health Crises, Part I: The Concept," *Prehospital and Disaster Medicine*, 36(1), 95–104. Available at https://www.cambridge.org/core/services/aop-cambridge-core/content/view/87458FB265E23D2FF8BD9A5FAD7CEB45/S1049023X20001351a.pdf/global-public-health-database-support-to-population-based-management-of-pandemics-and-global-public-health-crises-part-i-the-concept.pdf.

43. Frederick M. Burkle, Jr., David A. Bradt, and Benjamin J. Ryan, "Global Public Health Database Support to Population-Based Management of Pandemics and Global Public Health Crises, Part II: The Database," *Prehospital and Disaster Medicine*, 36(1), 105–110. Available at https://www.cambridge.org/core/journals/prehospital-and-disaster-medicine/article/global-public-health-database-support-to-populationbased-management-of-pandemics-and-global-public-health-crises-part-ii-the-database/2C-F1F9CA713E055AE91080668F6ECC1F.

global public health information database, needs to be revamped. The overhaul of WHO must exist as a UN treaty-based body funded by the United Nations and all its members—that is, *all* members. This international health agency cannot be dependent on outside financial assistance to conduct its work. We can no longer tolerate an ineffectual and passive international response system. Equally important, we cannot accept the self-serving political interference that authoritarian régimes have exercised over WHO and its crucial global role.

Practitioners and health decision-makers must break their silence and strongly encourage a return of WHO's singular global authority, and these specialists must support professional, coordinated, population-based management. In the early 1900s, Sir William Osler, a pioneer in the study of zoonotic[44] diseases, promoted his "one medicine, one health" concept. Even more than a century ago, that concept defined what global public health should be striving for today.[45]

* * * *

In a highly globalized world, WHO has the potential to become one of the most effective mechanisms for crisis response and worldwide risk reduction. The world's health practitioners, especially public health administrators, must advocate for a return of WHO's singular global authority that is so well coordinated, multidisciplinary, and science-based. The Covid-19 pandemic tells us that we can no longer wait to develop a non-political global public health system. When it comes to health, every country in the world is entitled to be treated on an equal basis. We have no other choice. Time has run out.

The Untold Cost of War on Civilians

> *"When protective thresholds in public health are absent, destroyed, or inundated with war casualties, both direct and indirect dire consequences affect the health of a population."*

Even before World War II had ended, the outcry around the world was the same: "Never again!" On April 25, 1945, representatives from 50 nation-states met in San Francisco and began drafting the United Nations (UN) Charter. The world had just witnessed unimaginable levels of evil and devaluing of human life. Countries across the war-ravaged globe were committed to never allowing those crimes against

---

44. Zoonotic infectious diseases are transmitted from animals to humans or from humans to animals; for example, rabies, Lyme disease, plague, and possibly COVID-19.
45. Frederick M. Burkle, Jr., "Political Intrusions into the International Health Regulations Treaty and Its Impact on Management of Rapidly Emerging Zoonotic Pandemics: What History Tells Us," *Prehospital and Disaster Medicine*, 35(4), 426–430. Available at https://www.ncbi.nlm.nih.gov/pmc/articles/PMC7167298/.

Appendix 2: Four Perspectives on the World's Challenges and Concerns 267

humanity to happen again. The UN Charter was signed on June 26, which formally established the United Nations. The Charter took effect on October 24, 1945. On that historic day, the new international peacekeeping organization became a reality. The UN member states promoted the fledgling institution as nations combining "to save succeeding generations from the scourge of war."[46]

I was born before the United States entered World War II. I remember post-war school classes in which the UN flag stood proudly alongside the American flag. Studying the geography and cultures of new UN member nations was an expected part of the curriculum. As a hobby, we exchanged our prized collection of country flags. My classmates and I fell silent as our teachers, some having fought in the war, offered our first lesson in "humanitarianism." In the elementary school classroom setting in the late 1940s and then in junior and senior high school in the 1950s, we learned the plight of those left destitute, hungry, and sick by the prolonged war. But having the UN in place, those post-war years were seen as an encouraging time that guaranteed an end to all wars.

Regrettably, within just a year of the signing of the Charter, the idealistic expectations of the UN's one-world view were shattered. East-West antagonisms, rivalries between the growing list of new UN members, and the communist status of those nations all played into the slow demise of an optimistically united world. The high anticipation in 1945, however, was that war would be relegated to the history books. But the debates, which flourished with the conclusion of the Second World War, focused on a new struggle tied to the competing ideologies of the United States and the Soviet Union. The emergence of tension-filled, overt hostility came to be called the "Cold War." And those apprehensions were undeniably very cold and very dangerous.

The potential for the UN and its Charter, though, remained a dominant subject in schools and communities well into the 1950s. The focus of attention was on the UN Charter's promises to protect member states, as stated through Chapter VII titled "Action with Respect to the Threats of Peace, Breaches of the Peace, and Acts of Aggression."[47] The UN Charter spelled out the original system of collective security, which was outlined in two of the Charter's chapters. Chapter VI covered the voluntary settlement of disputes, and Chapter VII dealt with enforcement action. Chapter VII's Article 39 first authorized the Security Council to determine, according to its chapter title, "the existence of any threat to the peace, breach of the peace, or act of aggression."[48] Chapter VII's Article 42 was designed to take such action by "air, sea, or land forces as may be necessary."[49]

---

46. The Preamble to the United Nations Charter. Available at https://www.un.org/en/about-us/un-charter/preamble.
47. Chapter VII of the UN Charter. Available at https://www.un.org/en/about-us/un-charter/chapter-7.
48. *Ibid.*
49. *Ibid.*

Worldwide Indifference to the UN Charter's Article 43

Article 43 committed all UN member states "to make available to the Security Council, on its call, armed forces, assistance, facilities, including rights of passage necessary for maintaining international peace and security."[50] Under Article 43, UN enforcement actions would be ordered and directed by the Security Council and its Military Staff Committee. In essence, this agency was to be a military source of strength available to the UN to save democracy—whenever, wherever, and however the need might arise. Hope for the future was placed in Article 43, but sadly, with two exceptions,[51] the UN's instrument of force was never applied. All that was available was the empowerment of the General Assembly to restore peace if aggressive situations developed.[52]

Today's generation is not aware of the original existence and intent of Article 43. Over the decades, some half-hearted Article 43 suggestions were proposed to alleviate flare-ups between countries. But the UN drafters had granted veto control to the five permanent members of the Security Council: the United States, the United Kingdom, France, the Soviet Union, and the Republic of China (Taiwan).[53] Any one of these five members could unilaterally terminate a Security Council resolution.

During the Cold War, the Security Council was often deadlocked by a veto, which prevented Article 43 from being employed. Had Article 43 been implemented as designed, I believe that authorization of military force could have led to the global maintenance of international harmony and security. Instead, the Security Council veto control established a wedge between nations that rose out of the ashes of World War II. This veto power pitted countries against each other: Those nations that wanted a governing democratic base against those countries whose despotic leaders intended to have a governing autocratic base. The division of powers between the Security Council and the General Assembly has never found a functional, satisfactory equilibrium to prevent clashes and war.

This deliberate attempt to avoid UN enforcement was a concerted plan on the part of those in authority to severely limit the activities of the UN. For years, Article 43's language has been purposely ignored as an option. But the General Assembly has the influence to intervene to avoid conflicts and restore peace when the need occurs. This authority has given license to many UN programs to mitigate and reestablish full accord, but those options have been short of employing a military force.

The consequences of the UN's limitations have become painfully clear in recent decades. The most unforgettable example of this failure was seen in Rwanda in 1994.

---

50. *Ibid.*

51. The UN committed forces in September 1950 to serve with the Army of the Republic of Korea in the Korean War. Ten years later, the UN also sent troops to the Republic of the Congo in July 1960.

52. Frederick M. Burkle, Jr., "United Nations Charter, Chapter VII, Article 43: Now or Never," *Disaster Medicine and Public Health Preparedness* 2019, August 13(4), 655–662. Available at https://www.researchgate.net/publication/320943680_United_Nations_Charter_Chapter_VII_Article_43_Now_or_Never.

53. On October 25, 1971, the People's Republic of China (mainland China) took over the Security Council seat belonging to the Republic of China (Taiwan).

In a matter of weeks, the UN peacekeeping soldiers in that country were unable to stop the slaughter of more than 800,000 Tutsi, an ethnic group comprising 14 percent of the population. With several Belgian peacekeepers killed at the beginning of the genocide, the political will to strengthen the UN undertaking quickly waned. Consequently, the peacekeeping mission ended abruptly, resulting in distrust and bitterness from the Rwandan people toward the UN—resentment that lingers today. Kofi Annan, Secretary-General from 1997 to 2006, even acknowledged the systematic failure of the UN during that time.[54]

During the past decades, I have made an effort several times to explain the figurative disappearance of the once omnipresent Article 43, as being critical to failings in the UN consciousness. Since the end of the Korean War in 1953, we have rarely heard a debate that confirms the legitimate integration of global peace and security by Article 43. Nothing has prevented existing autocracies from taking increased advantage of the most vulnerable of nations, placing European Union (EU) countries once again the most at risk.

Members of the UN fully recognize today that both the scope and complexity of violent conflicts have surpassed the global community's capacity and capability to address and manage current and future crises. Even for foreign and domestic health care workers attempting to maintain the population's health welfare, their day-to-day living and working conditions have become unsafe. At one time, physicians, nurses, and other medical personnel garnered the greatest respect, even under wartime circumstances. However, we now see an annual rise in attacks and confrontations against these aid workers. International humanitarian law, which is codified in the Geneva Conventions, as well as international human rights law, prohibits attacks on health facilities and health workers.

Nevertheless, such aggressive acts continue to escalate, often due to unstable governments that cannot or will not provide protection. In 2018, at least 973 reported brutal acts took place against health workers, medical facilities, and patients across 23 countries in conflict.[55] This surge in assaults is up from 701 attacks in 2017. These statistics are most likely very much underreported because of the challenge of data collection. A lack of governmental protection has likely been a leading cause of the rapid decline in hope for humanitarian relief in recent years.

I believe the only structure that would work in this instance is the implementation of Article 43 with a ready reaction force capability. This armed strength could respond rapidly to regional, national, and global crises. United Nations troops could be deployed before the fighting has advanced to the point that the essential public health infrastructure and protections are destroyed. For its survival, the UN requires many long, overdue reforms for organizational structure and governance

---

54. Nicole Winfield, "UN Failed Rwanda," Global Policy Forum, December 16, 1999. Available at https://www.globalpolicy.org/component/content/article/201-rwanda/39240.html.

55. "2018: A Year of Dangerous Attacks on Health Workers, Facilities: Hundreds of Attacks in 23 Countries Documented," Press Release for Physicians for Human Rights, May 15, 2019. Available at https://phr.org/news/2018-a-year-of-dangerous-attacks-on-health-workers-facilities/.

power, including a robust UN standing task force to be put into effect under Article 43.

Disregard of the 1949 Geneva Conventions

I am a committed student of the Geneva Conventions and international humanitarian law, both protections that are likely unknown to most Americans. But despite their obscurity, the Geneva Conventions have the United States as a signatory, ratifying the protections that this series of treaties calls for in time of war. And the U.S. wasn't the only nation to sign these treaties; 196 other member states added their signatures in 1949 to set up these rules. The provisions of international humanitarian law under the Geneva Conventions' Articles 55 and 56 have been recognized by the humanitarian and public health communities for decades. Nevertheless, they are rarely appreciated by the current generation of political decision-makers, who are inhibited by the outlay of time, personnel, and funds required to restore such infrastructure.

The United States is often quick to criticize other countries' violations of these provisions while it has risen to the position of world police enforcer. Yet frequently and ironically, America has not complied with the rules and regulations. The United States time and again chooses to interpret adherence to the Geneva Conventions in a way that best suits its needs, which does not come as a surprise to anyone outside the country. Avoidance of our duties as a signatory to the Geneva Conventions included two prime offenses. The U.S.-led Coalition forces tortured and abused Iraqi prisoners at Abu Ghraib prison 20 miles west of Baghdad. The U.S. also incarcerated Iraqi prisoners and suspected terrorists at Guantanamo Bay Detention Camp in southeast Cuba, many of whom were not convicted of any crimes.

After I returned from Iraq in 2003, the Iraq War had severely escalated and many quickly realized this conflict was not going to be short-term. A physician at Walter Reed Army Medical Center in Washington requested that I give a presentation to physicians and nurses who were then being rushed to Iraq. At the outset of my address in a cafeteria filled with eager medical staff, I assured them my discussion would answer their concerns. I requested that the attendees refrain from asking questions until I ended my talk. Despite this appeal, within minutes a woman began waving a piece of paper causing a major distraction. I stopped and allowed her to speak.

She stood up and angrily stated that she was clutching the schedule listing the training that the military had been giving to them for the past two weeks. The course's military director had, unfortunately, decided that these nurses and staff physicians could skip the scheduled lectures on international humanitarian law and the Geneva Conventions and instead have a last-day party. She added that she had specifically come to my talk because she and others were unaware of these international laws. The class applauded in affirmation. With an increasingly attentive audience, I got down to facts to tell them what they needed to know operationally about these mechanisms. I was given a standing ovation. Unfortunately, that war resulted in seven international humanitarian law violations against the United States, three of them medically related.

The George W. Bush Administration also considered "reinterpreting" Common Article 3 of the Geneva Conventions to protect interrogators from being labeled as "war criminals."[56] The Bush Administration wanted to continue business as usual in the interest of the United States with little regard for human rights or international law. Fast forward to the beginning of the 2020 decade, and the same international humanitarian law protections were again being ignored in Syria.

To some degree, previous wars may have seemed more "civilized" than conflicts today, and they were fought with a "set of rules," if that phrase can legitimately be said about any war. As uniformed U.S. military health care providers, those personnel had explicit obligations and were allowed specific protections that civilian health care workers did not enjoy. As military health professionals, the Geneva Conventions gave military health care workers, if captured, the status of "military detainees," not "prisoners of war" (POWs). As military detainees, physicians, dentists, nurses, medics, and corpsmen were still allowed to practice the art of medicine. These personnel were supposed to be given supplies to do their jobs and protect their prisoner-patients. But even though these rules of war are spelled out in the Geneva Conventions, they are now being increasingly disregarded.

Statistics from German prisoner-of-war camps in Europe are revealing. The death rate during World War II for Allied POWs—Americans, British, and Canadians—was approximately 3.6 percent. For Russian POWs held by the Germans, the death rate was about 57 percent.[57] The Germans pointed out that the Russians were not signatories to the 1929 Geneva Convention, therefore the Germans were not obligated to treat the Russian POWs according to the Geneva Convention's rules. Not abiding by those international rules made a difference in whether or not a POW survived.

I firmly believe that adherence to the 1929 Geneva Convention and 1949 Geneva Conventions historically mattered. Observing those humanitarian rules would still make a vital difference today. Operationally, they were first applied to cross-border wars. But with the disappearance of that type of warfare,[58] applying these same rules to internal wars has become much more difficult. That complexity is easily seen in the unending Syrian civil war, an incredible departure from the norm. Making the Geneva Conventions relevant to contemporary, non-cross-border conflicts is an

---

56. Lionel Beehner, "The United States and the Geneva Conventions: Backgrounder: U.S. Debate over Treatment of Detainees Hinges on Interpretation of the Geneva Conventions," Council on Foreign Relations, September 20, 2006. Available at https://www.cfr.org/backgrounder/united-states-and-geneva-conventions.
57. "German Mistreatment of Soviet Prisoners of War," Military Wiki. Available at https://military.wikia.org/wiki/German_mistreatment_of_Soviet_prisoners_of_war.
58. The Russo-Ukrainian war, the largest conflict in Europe since World War II, is a notable exception.

ongoing struggle that I've tried to comprehend and articulate in recent decades. The nature of a country's humanitarian obligations is a profound international legal issue.

Manufactured Fears

The post–Cold War era has seen many protracted internal tensions and wars that have lasted for decades, carrying with them both chronic nation-state and regional instability that we still witness today, some even perpetrated by the United States. The responsibility for many of these clashes has been attributed to repressive governments that are no longer trusted or acceptable. With the recent rise and dominance of authoritarian régimes, globalization has almost become a nonentity. The concept has disappeared under a very coordinated false narrative campaign by autocrats.

The Democracy Index[59] report annually ranks countries as having either a "full democracy," "flawed democracy," "hybrid régimes," or an "authoritarian régime." The 2019 report's analysis placed less than half the world's population in a democracy. The percentage of those living in a "full democracy" has fallen by almost 5 percent. According to the 2019 Democracy Index, the United States was ranked 25th and labeled as a "flawed democracy" because of a serious decline and erosion of confidence in our democratic institutions.[60] And that 25th-ranked designation was before the insurrection at the U.S. Capitol on January 6, 2021.

We have seen the rise of neo-fascism during the last several years across a broad range of geography and nations. Madeleine Albright, in her book *Fascism: A Warning* (2018), reminds us that while these disreputable leaders all "claim to speak for a whole nation or group," they are "utterly unconcerned with the rights of others, and willing to use violence and whatever other means necessary to achieve the goals he or she might have."[61]

Although this trend has clear implications for world order, the gradual but critical influences on the mental and physical health of populations may be less obvious. Dictatorship in the Central Asian nation of Turkmenistan, for example, has had documented negative effects on population health. The regime's strategy was to keep statistical data secret and also intentionally neglect to report health indicators to the international community. The authorities' policy of concealment was especially true for infectious diseases considered ripe for epidemic outbreaks, such as avian influenza, tuberculosis, HIV/AIDS, and plague. The Turkmenistan government's state of denial saw the solution to health care problems as suppression rather than

---

59. The Democracy Index is an index compiled by the UK's Economist Intelligence Unit (EIU). Available at https://en.wikipedia.org/wiki/The_Economist_Democracy_Index.
60. Andrea Germanos, "United States Doesn't Even Make Top 20 on Global Democracy Index: Nation Classified 'Flawed Democracy,'" Common Dreams, January 11, 2019. Available at https://www.commondreams.org/news/2019/01/11/united-states-doesnt-even-make-top-20-global-democracy-index..
61. Madeleine Albright, *Fascism: A Warning* (New York: HarperCollins, 2018), 11.

prevention. Moreover, its leaders found it more expedient to enable the trafficking of drugs from Afghanistan than to confront the nation's failing health care system.

Caught in the Crosshairs of War

Looking back, I believe the most common public health challenge for the 20th century, as well as the first decades of the 21st century, was trying to improve the health status of populations trapped in this vicious cycle of war. In many developing countries, war creates intimidation, hunger, desperation, migration, and death. It is difficult for a country to function optimally for all citizens if it doesn't have essential public health infrastructure. But that country must also have the ability to maintain that structure for the entire population. When protective thresholds in public health are absent, destroyed, or inundated with war casualties, both direct and indirect dire consequences affect the health of a population. Appalling outcomes are amplified when public health resources are not recovered or maintained, or these agencies are simply denied to populations due to the many disasters that have already infiltrated their lives.[62]

Since the end of World War II in 1945, disasters and worldwide responses to them have changed about every 10 to 15 years, sometimes more frequently. Desperate situations, including economic, environmental, ecological, and health-related circumstances, vary greatly across regions.[63] These conditions are progressively marked by widely integrated global changes and forces. Those impacts may often seem as moving too slowly, but they are increasingly severe and massive because they affect larger populations across many borders. Nevertheless, subtle crises are powerful and encompassing, magnified even more within public health frameworks and essential health protections that have become overwhelmed through the years.

Even though society today possesses some of the most advanced technological innovations and achievements, we ironically face the greatest number of people worldwide who lack access to clean water, food, shelter, and basic health care.[64] Unfortunately, these kinds of conditions hold true in even more "developed" wealthy countries. Losses are not often even measured, which means they go unnoticed or disregarded by those in authority, while millions suffer from the cascading effects of war. Civilians around the world, who are unlucky enough to be caught in the wrong place or speak the wrong language, are often subject to war's horrors.

The tragedies and misfortunes of conflict are not new. But war's disproportion-

---

62. Frederick M. Burkle, Jr., and P. Gregg Greenough, "Impact of Public Health Emergencies on Modern Disaster Taxonomy, Planning, and Response," *Disaster Medicine and Public Health Preparedness* 2008 October; 2(3), 192–199. Available at https://pubmed.ncbi.nlm.nih.gov/18562943/.

63. Elin A. Gursky et al., "The Changing Face of Crises and Aid in the Asia-Pacific," *Biosecurity and Bioterrorism* 2014, November–December; 12(6), 310–317. Available at https://pubmed.ncbi.nlm.nih.gov/25268048/.

64. "The Contribution of the Water for Life 2005–2015 Decade," United Nations Office to Support the International Decade for Action, February 22, 2014, 64–83. Available at https://www.un.org/waterforlifedecade/pdf/WaterforLifeENG.pdf.

ately devastating effect on civilians is a recent measure of calculating casualty figures because noncombatant deaths have previously been ignored as a necessary "cost of war." The Center for Systemic Peace, an organization that monitors and quantifies political violence around the world, clearly states that those not fighting are by far the ones losing their lives in modern wars. Both military and civilian medical personnel, who treated Vietnamese civilians during the 20-plus-year conflict, witnessed this wide-ranging consequence of war every day. It was not just the horrendous wounds suffered by civilians, especially children, but also the indirect effects of severe malnutrition and epidemics of infectious diseases. The bubonic plague I encountered in Vietnam was considered the worst outbreak in the 20th century.

Although statistics of military wounded and dead from the Vietnam War are well documented, disputes remain over civilian deaths, with estimates ranging from 1.3 million to more than 4 million people. The arrival of military casualties by helicopter at Delta Med, the Marine Forward Casualty Receiving Facility where I served, were treated within minutes of injury. But civilian casualties, if cared for at all, took hours or days. The local villagers, who were caught in the crosshairs of ongoing warfare, had to wait their turn to be seen by a doctor. While this "cost of war" has been hidden from the public eye for decades, we need to pay more attention to war's impact on civilians. We must publicly demand transparency that can lead to an honest civilian casualty assessment.

We recognize the absence of the fundamental needs of life for many, but we also have to acknowledge the incredible advancement that has been forged in recent decades to reduce the number of people living in poverty. Major gains have also been made in preventing and treating infectious diseases to decrease child mortality. Yet the frequency and intensity of extreme events are escalating and threaten much of this progress. With the parallel explosion of population growth in megacities across the globe, as well as autocratic leaders caring little for their respective societies, the number of people affected by these disasters is also expected to continue rising.

We used to maintain a distinction between natural and manmade disasters, but these two kinds of calamities are now becoming so interrelated that it is difficult to know where to attribute proper blame. The rise of "mega-catastrophes" is a call to arms not only for global public health leaders, but also a motivation for all of society to act on them. If we are to truly address the massive changes in humanitarian crises happening before our very eyes, a multidisciplinary, cooperative effort on a global scale will be required.

Unpredictable Forces

As political oppression and armed conflict erupt in countries around the world, as a never-ending arcade game of whack-a-mole, public health infrastructure disappears, populations flee, and anarchy reigns. Now in the third decade of the 21st century, such active illustrations of failing frameworks already exist in Yemen, Syria,

Somalia, Ethiopia, the Democratic Republic of the Congo, and Venezuela. Many more nations are also just on the verge of a structural breakdown. What invariably transpires from this collapse is the loss of interconnected infrastructure, increased demand, and supply chain disruptions that health systems cannot keep pace with—and this breakdown occurred even before the Covid-19 pandemic began in late 2019.

Early in my medical career in the 1960s, about 50 million refugees could be counted, but that number has now risen to more than 70 million. Even more disturbing, the 2018 World Bank Group reported that people fleeing climate change's various impacts on the land may number more than 140 million by 2050.[65] At the highly anticipated 2019 UN General Assembly meeting, Secretary-General António Guterres called upon world leaders, the private sector, and society at large to address the climate emergency with the urgency it demands. Even in November 2021, more ideas were discussed at the 26th UN Climate Change Conference of the Parties in Glasgow. But the world is still waiting for direct and widespread action.

Many crises receive international attention only when they result in conflict. The Syrian civil war is a case in point. From 2011 to 2016, 60 percent of Syria's agricultural northeast and south suffered its worst drought, water shortage, and crop failure, compounded by the breakdowns in Bashar al-Assad's governance and mismanagement.[66] With previous droughts, the Syrian government provided relief despite the population's religious differences. But with oil prices dropping, the Assad regime claimed it was unable to respond as it had in the past. Poverty accelerated the exodus of farmers, herders, and rural families to cities in the western part of Syria, fueling the beginning of today's major sectarian war.

In retrospect, multiple public health interventions were available in Syria, which could have stopped or mitigated the population exodus and human rights tragedies. But Assad did nothing as the crisis worsened and the world has remained silent. Similar lost opportunities for preventive engagement occurred in Sudan, Somalia, Ethiopia, and Eritrea. Internally displaced persons (DPs) or refugees,[67] who are escaping from a public health collapse, will exceed those casualty figures from warfare alone. The increasing number of refugees will further exacerbate the fragile public health protections in host countries, such as Jordan, Lebanon, Turkey, and Greece.

The humanitarian community strongly adheres to the global political commitment of "responsibility to protect," as endorsed by all member states of the United

---

65. Alex Kirby, "Climate Refugees May Reach Many Millions by 2050," *Climate News Network*, March 20, 2018. Available at https://climate-diplomacy.org/magazine/environment/climate-refugees-may-reach-many-millions-2050.

66. Scott Greenwood, "Water Insecurity, Climate Change, and Governance in the Arab World," *Middle East Policy*, 2014; 11, 140–156. Available at https://onlinelibrary.wiley.com/doi/abs/10.1111/mepo.12077.

67. "Refugees" flee across international borders to escape ongoing war, oppression, or natural disasters in their homeland. "Displaced Persons" or "Internally Displaced Persons—IDPs" have been forced out of their homes due to being caught between opposing militant factions, but they decide to remain in their respective country.

Nations. The UN recognizes that migrants have an equal right to live and thrive in the country and culture in which they were raised. Not surprisingly, many immigrants to EU nations have openly declared their dream to return to their native country. Despots, primarily in the Middle East, can passively assist or engineer the fleeing of massive numbers of their citizens mostly to EU nations. In many of those EU countries, the perceived refugee crisis has contributed to what might be seen as a "populist uprising," referring to anti-immigrant sentiment.

The convergence of all these issues is alarming. The progressively more destructive catastrophes, triggered by climate change and disappearing biodiversity, have caused desperate and vulnerable populations to take flight from grave and untenable circumstances. At the same time, narcissistic leaders are taking control of countries all over the world. Each autocrat has an eye only for military might and ignores the true power that lies in diplomacy. American foreign policy long held the vision of the "three-legged stool" concept: development, diplomacy, and defense. Keeping those three legs balanced was responsible for many of the global achievements of the 20th century. But in recent years that three-legged stool stands on only one leg, and therefore has lost its critical stability.

Current models of expansion, which created both great wealth and rising inequities in emerging economies, put the health and survival of the people and the planet in peril. For autocrats, "global health" is an inspirational expectation of their economic promises. These leaders, often describing themselves as "patriots," have hijacked global health as "economic health." Unwisely, the realm of public health yielded. A minority has grown rich from the unsustainable use and large-scale exploitation of land resources, beginning with colonization in the 19th century, and resulting in conflicts intensifying in many countries. We have reached a point where we must reconcile these differences. We must rethink how we plan, use, and manage the land—for the sake of all our futures.[68]

Restoring the Global Authority of WHO and the UN

The UN also needs to regain its voice, the one of assurance and assertion that I heard in the early post–World War II years. Several articles have questioned if the political climate in the near future would be appropriate for the UN to invoke Article 43. If not at this time, we then have to ask if the UN exists only to monitor the consequences of violence without intervening, as seen in the failures in the 1990s. Rethinking Article 43 would require making a major change in the structure of the Security Council. Shielding susceptible populations, as well as preventing aggression and brutality against the vulnerable, increasingly defines regional needs. But strong, unbending leadership is required for justice and human rights. While these rights were never previously questioned, they often seem to be conditional today.

---

68. "Global Land Outlook: Key Messages," United Nations Convention to Combat Desertification, October 31, 2017. Available at http://www2.unccd.int/sites/default/files/documents/2017-10/GLO%20KEY_ESUM-%20finalweb.pdf.

This new kind of threatening environment, created by the confluence of climate change, despotic leaders, war, and humanitarian crises, has become ominous for the citizens living in such countries as Yemen, the Philippines, Syria, Sudan, Nigeria, Somalia, and Ethiopia. But other nations are also caught up in the turbulence created by these multifaceted humanitarian emergencies. Yet despite the cascading negative effects that politics, war, and narcissistic leaders have inflicted on the world stage today, I have noted tremendous achievements to celebrate. In my own time as a humanitarian professional, great progress has been made in terms of infant and child mortality, gender equality, and literacy rates, as well as exciting innovations led by those within their communities.

* * * *

Positive advancements have been made thanks to the extraordinary contributions of researchers, doctors, nurses, anthropologists, and others around the world who have devoted their careers to providing better lives for mankind. I have been privileged to work with many of these passionate men and women through the years, and have found great hope in the next generation of young people. They often see themselves as global citizens not bound by arbitrary country lines. While our humanitarian work is not finished—and never will be, I am emboldened in my retirement by recognizing that so many people are still committed to these deep and sincere causes.

Index

Numbers in **_bold italics_** indicate pages with illustrations

academic positions *see* CDC (Centers for Disease Control and Prevention); Harvard Humanitarian Initiative; Johns Hopkins Bloomberg School of Public Health; Manoa School of Medicine (University of Hawaii); National Academy of Medicine; Woodrow Wilson International Center for Scholars
admirals *see* Prueher, Adm. Joseph W.; Smith, Vice Adm. Leighton
adolescent medicine 64; *see also* pediatrics
Africa *see* Ethiopia; Kenya; Liberian civil war; Libya; Nigeria; Rwanda; Somalian civil war
Agency for International Development (USAID) *see* USAID (U.S. Agency for International Development)
Agent Orange 218, 218*n*8
Aidid, Mohamed Farrah 135, 137, 138
Air Force *see* U.S. Air Force
Akamai Telemedicine Program 152–153, 158–164; *see also* Tripler Army Medical Center
Al Khanjar Navy-Marine Corps Trauma Center 105–118, ***106***, ***110***, ***115***, 121, 133; *see also* Persian Gulf War
Alpha Med 36, 57, 108; *see also* Vietnam War
ambassadors *see* Bodine, Amb. Barbara; Bremer, Amb. L. Paul, III; Chamberlin, Amb. Wendy; Lyman, Amb. Princeton; Prueher, Adm. Joseph W.
American Red Cross 6, 65, 121, 123, 152; *see also* International Committee of the Red Cross

(ICRC); Red Cross and Red Crescent Societies
Apollo (space program) 53, 221
Army *see* U.S. Army
Asia *see* China; Japan; North Vietnam; Pakistan; South Vietnam; Thailand
Asia-Pacific countries 152–156
Audrey and Theodor Geisel School of Medicine *see* Dartmouth Medical School
Australia 210–212
autocratic leaders 6, 64, 137, 143, 165, 216
awards and honors 1–6, 18–19, 22, 155, 210

Ba'ath Party 125, ***125***, 170*n*3, 171, 180–181; *see also* Hussein, Saddam; Iraq War
Babangida, Ibrahim 94–95; *see also* Nigeria
Baby Boy M 24, 25, 26
Baghdad, Iraq 124, 129, 166, 171–179, ***172***, ***173***, 179–183
Balkan Peninsula *see* Bosnian War; Yugoslavia (former)
Barzani, Masoud 120, 121, 129, 130
Beijing, China 97, 100
Berkeley, California 2, 65, 80–81, 88, 97
Bloomberg School of Public Health *see* Johns Hopkins Bloomberg School of Public Health
Bodine, Amb. Barbara 179
Bond, Doug 155–156
Bosnian War 5, 134–149, ***144***, ***146***, ***147***; *see also* Yugoslavia (former)
Boston, Massachusetts 64
Bremer, Amb. L. Paul, III 179, 181
Brown, Commander William (Bill) 108, 109

bubonic plague 40–47, 44*n*7, ***45***, 201; *see also* illnesses
Buchanan, Liberia 188, 189, 190, ***191***; *see also* Liberian civil war
Burke, Mary (mother) 2, 12–15, 34, 62
Burkle, Christopher (son) 19–20, 23–24, ***28***, 62, 215
Burkle, Dr. Frederick Martin, Jr. (Skip): board certifications (*see* adolescent medicine; emergency medicine; pediatrics; psychiatry; public health); cities lived in (*see* Berkeley, California; Boston, Massachusetts; Burlington, Vermont; Colchester, Vermont; Hanover, New Hampshire; Hawaiian Islands; New Haven, Connecticut; Newport, Rhode Island; Old Saybrook, Connecticut; San Diego, California; Tacoma, Washington); deployments (*see* Disaster Assistance Response Team (DART); Iraq War; Liberian civil war; Operation Restore Hope (Somalian civil war); Persian Gulf War; Vietnam War); family members (*see* Burke, Mary [mother]; Burkle, Christopher [son]; Burkle, Frederick, Sr. [father]; Burkle, Heidi [daughter]; Burkle, Jennifer [daughter]; Burkle, Joan [sister]; Burkle, Phyllis [wife, née Dinnean]; Burkle, Richard [brother]; Burkle, Robert [uncle]; Dinnean family [in-laws]); higher education (*see* Dartmouth Medical School; Harvard Medical School; Saint Michael's

Index

College; UC Berkeley School of Public Health; University of Geneva; University of Vermont Medical School; Yale-New Haven Hospital; humanitarian positions (*see* American Red Cross; International Rescue Committee [IRC]; Operation Provide Comfort [Kurdish refugee crisis]; Operation Restore Hope [Somalian civil war]; WHO [World Health Organization]); international travels (*see* China; Ethiopia; Geneva, Switzerland; Iraq; Japan; Kenya; Liberian civil war; Micronesia; Nigeria; Saudi Arabia; Somalian civil war; South Vietnam; Turkey; Yugoslavia [former]); leadership roles (*see* Al Khanjar Navy-Marine Corps Trauma Center; Center of Excellence [COE]; Defense Threat Reduction Agency; Disaster Assistance Response Team [DART]; Emergency Medical Services [Hawaii]; Interim Minister of Health [Iraq]; International Development Global Health program; International Rescue Committee [IRC]; Maui Memorial Hospital); medical positions (*see* Division of Emergency Medicine [University of Hawaii]); Kapiolani Medical Center for Women and Children; Madigan Army Medical Center; Mary Hitchcock Memorial Hospital; Maui Memorial Hospital; Naval Health Clinic New England; Yale-New Haven Hospital; tributes to (*see* "Listening to the Heartbeat of Humanity" [Appendix 1]; "Senator Leahy's Tribute" [Appendix 1]; U.S. Air Force service *see* ROTC [Reserve Officers' Training Corps]; U.S. Army service (*see* Madigan Army Medical Center); U.S. Marines service (*see* Naval Health Clinic New England; Navy-Marine Medical Company [Persian Gulf]; 3rd Marine Division [Vietnam]; U.S. Navy service (*see* Delta Med [Vietnam War]; Naval Health Clinic New England; Navy-Marine Medical Company [Persian Gulf]; U.S. Navy Captain; U.S. Navy Reserves *see* Operation Provide Comfort [Kurdish refugee crisis]; Operation Restore Hope [Somalian civil war]); upbringing (*see* childhood and youth; family life; Notre Dame [Catholic high school]; Saint Raphael Hospital [volunteer work])

Burkle, Frederick, Sr. (father) 2, 5, 9–18, 24, 29, 34

Burkle, Heidi (daughter) 28, **28**, 62

Burkle, Jennifer (daughter) 21–23, **28**, **35**, 62

Burkle, Joan (sister) 9–10

Burkle, Phyllis (wife, née Dinnean): as advisor and companion 23, 72, 91, 154, 162–165, 200, 215–220; career 18–20, 22, 28, 65; courtship 19–21, 26–27; home relocations 64–65, 86, 92, 162, 183; as military spouse 6, 60–63, 67–70, 79–81, 118, 202, 208; as mother 20–24, 28, **28**, 65; parents 16–17, 63, 219; pictured with husband **28**, **87**, **219**; reunions or separations 34–35, 57–58, 90–91, 103–104, 148–149, 214–218; as student 16–20, **18**; travels 48, 66n1, 108

Burkle, Richard (brother) 9–10

Burkle, Robert (uncle) 62

Burlington, Vermont 17–22, 48

Burma *see* Myanmar (Burma)

Bush, Pres. George H.W. 103, 119, 119n1, 135

Bush, Pres. George W. 166–168, 180–181

Cambodia 68–69, 80; *see also* Vietnam War

casualties of war 49–51, 113, 199–201, 207, 216; civilian 6, 40–42, 121, 135, 167–169, 216, 233; *see also* war injuries; war zones

CDC (Centers for Disease Control and Prevention) 152, 154–156, 162–163

Center for Humanitarian Civil-Military Cooperation *see* Center of Excellence (COE); Pan-American Health Organization (PAHO); WHO (World Health Organization)

Center for Humanitarian Health *see* Johns Hopkins Bloomberg School of Public Health

Center of Excellence (COE) 150–165, 150n1, 216; *see also* Manoa School of Medicine (University of Hawaii); Tripler Army Medical Center

Centers for Disease Control and Prevention *see* CDC (Centers for Disease Control and Prevention)

"Challenging the Next Generation: Service to Others" *see* Appendix 2

Chamberlin, Ambassador Wendy 2, 167–168, 167n1

chemical warfare 107, 111n6, 113, 117, 121

Cheney, Vice President Dick 180–181

child soldiers 188–191, 188n4, **191**; *see also* Liberian civil war

childhood and youth 5–18; abuse or bullying during 2, 12–16, 18, 24, 29; creativity 5, **10**, 10–14, 173; disabilities 3, 5, 13–15, 18; education 13–15, 18, **18**; father 5, 9–18, 24, 29, 34; mother 2, 12–15, 34, 62; portraits during **10**, **12**; role models during 2, 5, 14; *see also* family life; Notre Dame (Catholic high school); Saint Raphael Hospital (volunteer work)

children: African 96, 186; Cambodian 80; orphaned 2, 5, 66–71, 66n1, 80; psychology 10–11, 14; rights 96; as soldiers 180–181, 188–191, 188n4, **191**; Vietnamese 66n1, 69, 77–78; worldwide 95; *see also* children's hospitals; pediatrics

children's hospitals 39, 56, 67–68

China 69, 97–101, 202, 212, 222; Forbidden City 97–101, **98**, **99**; Tiananmen Square 97–101, **100**

Civil-Military Operations Center (CMOC) 135–136

civil wars *see* Liberian civil war; Somalian civil war

civilian–military cooperation 122–123, 130–136, 151–160, 180–182, 216–217

Clark Air Base 67–69, 77, 79

climate change 212–213, 217, 221

Coalition Forces (Iraq War) 109, 110n5, 118, **125**, 127, 167–174, 180; *see also* Iraq War

Index 281

Colchester, Vermont 17–18
combat medicine *see*
  emergency medicine; war
  injuries; war zones
Combined Humanitarian
  Assistance Response
  Training (CHART) 161
conflict zones *see* global
  crises; war zones
Congressional Federal Program
  of the Year 155
COVID-19 pandemic 233
Crawford, Alvin 93–96
critical care *see* disaster
  medicine; emergency
  medicine; urgent care
  medicine
Croatia *see* Yugoslavia
  (former)
cross-cultural awareness 39,
  45–46, 53–60, 77–78, 93–94,
  123–134
Crown Prince of Jordon 123–
  124, 130

Da Nang, South Vietnam
  35–38, *47*, 50, 59–60, 68, 109
Daly, Ed 68, 79
Dartmouth Medical School
  86–88, 86n1, 94n3
David (CBS cameraman) 73–74
Davos, Switzerland 206
death threats 2, 59, 90–93, 177
Defense Department *see*
  Department of Defense
  (DOD)
Defense Threat Reduction
  Agency 162–163
Delta Med (Vietnam War) 33–
  67, 85, 105–109, 199–200, 210,
  218–221; medical treatments
  40, 45, 55; triage bunker *41*
Department of Defense (DOD)
  135, 152, 168–170, 178–182,
  203–205
Department of State *see* State
  Department
Department of Veterans Affairs
  (VA) 203–204
deployments: homecomings
  from 59–62, 118; of medical
  professionals 104–105, 151,
  210, 216–217; readjustment
  after 62–63, 200, 209, 219
Dinnean family (in-laws) 16–17,
  63, 219
diplomacy: in Africa 92–93,
  96, 137, 184, 195; in Middle
  East 123; vs. military force
  166; post–World War II 131;
  psychology 137, 165, 190–191;
  skills in 134 , 137, 195
disabilities: childhood 3–5,

13–15, 18, 23; cognitive 5,
13–15, 18, 199, 204; dyslexia
13, 18; fugue states 85–86;
hearing-related 50, 201–203,
202n2, 214; psychological
60, 85–86, 206–208; seizures
202–203; stuttering 2, 13,
16, 18; visible vs. invisible
199–203, 207–208; vision-
related 95; *see also* illnesses;
war injuries
Disaster Assistance Response
  Team (DART) 2, 169–178; *see
  also* Persian Gulf War
disaster medicine 92, 97–102,
  116, 142, 150–157, 186,
  209–219
Disaster Medicine (textbook)
  212
Division of Emergency
  Medicine (University of
  Hawaii) 92, 150–151, 162–163
Djalali, Dr. Ahmadreza
  see "Physician in Peril"
  (Appendix 2)
DMZ (demilitarized zone) *see*
  Vietnam War
Doctors Without Borders *see*
  Médecins Sans Frontières
  (MSF)
Dong Ha village (Vietnam) 36,
  41–42, 46–47, 54–56, 61; *see
  also* South Vietnam; Vietnam
  War
Dooley, Dr. Tom 5, 15, 23, 28

education *see* Dartmouth
  Medical School; Harvard
  Medical School; Notre Dame
  (Catholic high school);
  Saint Michael's College; UC
  Berkeley School of Public
  Health; University of Geneva;
  University of Vermont
  Medical School; Yale-New
  Haven Hospital
Emergency Medical Services
  (Hawaii) 91–92
emergency medicine 27, 42, 64,
  88–96, 142, 182–194, 209–217;
  in Balkan Peninsula 145–148;
  in China 97–98, 100; field
  89, 97–100, 157, 188, 210–212;
  in Nigeria 15–16, 92, 95–96;
  teaching of or training in 64,
  85, 92, 100–102, 150–151, 162–
  163, 210; triage management
  33–38, *41*, 49–57, 105–112, 146,
  200–201; vs. urgent care 97n6;
  wartime 109, 111
Ethiopia 5, 135–138, 184, 202
ethnic conflicts 132, 139–149;
  see also Bosnian War;

Kurdish refugee crisis;
  Myanmar (Burma); Rwanda;
  Somalian civil war
EUCOM (European Command)
  130, 159

family life: financial hardship
  17–21, 23; with in-laws 16–17,
  63; with parents 2, 5, 9–24, 29,
  34, 62; with wife and children
  19–20, *28, 35*, 58–65, 86–88,
  87, 200; work-life balance
  20–28, 48, 57–63, 88, 104–105,
  147, 200, 219
field hospitals *see* Al Khanjar
  Navy-Marine Corps Trauma
  Center; Delta Med (Vietnam
  War)
1st Marine Expeditionary Force
  (Persian Gulf) 104–107,
  106n4; *see also* Al Khanjar
  Navy-Marine Corps Trauma
  Center; Navy-Marine
  Medical Company (Persian
  Gulf); Persian Gulf War
Flying Tigers 68–71, 68n2, 73
Forbidden City 97–101, *98, 99*;
  see also China
Fourteenth of July Bridge (Iraq)
  173, 173n4, *177*; *see also* Iraq;
  Iraq War

Garner, General Jay 2, 168,
  178–179
Geisel, Theodor Seuss (Dr.
  Seuss) 86, 86n1
generals *see* Garner, Gen. Jay;
  Krulak, Brig. Gen. Charles;
  Krulak, Gen. Victor (Brute)
Geneva, Switzerland 156–159,
  169–170, 183, 194–195
Geneva Conventions 36n4, 51–
  52, 156–157, 170–175, 175n5,
  180–181, 233
global crises 6, 132–139, 200,
  209–212, 217–218
global public health *see* public
  health

Hamden, Connecticut *see* New
  Haven, Connecticut
Hanover, New Hampshire
  86–88
Harvard Humanitarian
  Initiative 6, 210
Harvard Medical School 64
Hawaiian Islands 48, 81,
  89–92, 131, 213; Honolulu
  92; Kapiolani 91–93; Kula
  88–92; Maui 88–92; Oahu
  48, 149, 183; *see also* Center
  of Excellence (COE);
  Kapiolani Medical Center for

Women and Children; Maui Memorial Hospital
health care *see* illnesses; medical professionals; patient care; public health
Health Emergencies in Large Populations (HELP) program 156–161; *see also* International Committee of the Red Cross (ICRC)
health issues: asthma 2, 12–13, 18–19, 23, 116; cancer 218; food poisoning 130; hearing-related 50, 201–203, 202n2, 214; heart-related 213–215; seizures 202; self-diagnosed 202; syphilis exposure 26; vision-related 50, 203
HELP program *see* Health Emergencies in Large Populations (HELP) program
Ho Chi Minh City (Saigon) 36, 54, 66–72, 66n1, 74n4, 78–80, 80n6; *see also* Operation Babylift (Fall of Saigon); Vietnam War
Honolulu, Hawaii 81, 213; *see also* Hawaiian Islands
human rights 51–52, 121, 139, 145, 185n2; *see also* Geneva Conventions; war crimes
humanitarian aid: Christian 46, 158, 192–193; community 67, 95–96, 123, 130–169, 186, 195; international 122, 133–145, 166, 195; security concerns and 131, 178, 189; *see also* NGOs (non-governmental organizations)
humanitarian medicine 38–40, 56–67, 92–97, 116–129, 156–159, 167–175, 192–210; advocacy 181, 186, 215–217; coordination 123, 216; NIH lecture 210; power dynamics 2–3, 130, 167–171, 211; teaching or training 97, 148–150, 209–211; *see also* Médecins Sans Frontières (MSF); WHO (World Health Organization)
humanitarian positions *see* American Red Cross; International Rescue Committee (IRC); Operation Babylift (Fall of Saigon); Operation Provide Comfort (Kurdish refugee crisis); Operation Restore Hope (Somalian civil war); WHO (World Health Organization)
Hussein, Saddam 102–103, 111–129, **125**, **126**, 137, 170–181

ICRC *see* International Committee of the Red Cross (ICRC)
illnesses: bacterial 46–47, 64–65, 213; brain-related 202–208; bubonic plague 40–47, 44n7, 201; chronic 186, 199; contagious 48, 189, 212; dehydration 69, 78, 148, 148n11, 212; diarrheal 77–78, 186–189, 202; epidemics or pandemics 42–45, 65, 97, 142, 186–189, 194–196, 217–218; heart-related 59; Lyme disease 64; malarial 140, 186–189; malnourishment **78**, 97, 135, **136**, 148, 186–189, 212; meningitis 27, 58; mental health 14, 85–88, 137, 144, 165, 210, 218; parasitic 96, 189; respiratory 58, 116, 189; syphilis 26–27; tuberculosis 47; viral 42, 46, 196, 196n5; *see also* disabilities; war injuries
Imperial Palace 97–101, **98**, **99**; *see also* China
Inouye, Sen. Daniel 152–161
Interim Minister of Health (Iraq) 6, 96, 166–179, 183
internally displaced persons (IDPs) *see* refugees
International Children's Emergency Fund *see* UNICEF (UN International Children's Emergency Fund)
International Committee of the Red Cross (ICRC) 36, 121, 131, 142, 151–177, 192; *see also* American Red Cross; Health Emergencies in Large Populations (HELP); Red Cross and Red Crescent Societies
International Development Global Health program 163–169
International Humanitarian Law (IHL) 121, 131, 156–157, 170–175, 175n5
International Rescue Committee (IRC) 139–149
Iran 103, 111, 121, 127, 206–207; *see also* Kurdish refugee crisis
Iraq: antiquity 118; armed forces 110–119, 119n1, 124–130, 181; Baghdad 124, 129, 166, 171–183, **172**, **173**; Fourteenth of July Bridge 173, 173n4, **177**; Future of Iraq Task Force (USAID) 169–170; government 124–127, 130, 170, 179–180; Iran war 111, 121; medical crisis 166–174, 179–183; missile attacks 113–114, 113n8, 206; no-fly zone 120, **120**, 126–127; oil fires 116, **117**; ransacking 181; Red Crescent Society 124–126, 129; Tigris River 173–175, **177**; travels 127–131; UN peacekeeping forces 121–122, 130; *see also* Interim Minister of Health (Iraq); Iraq War; Kurdish refugee crisis
Iraq War 124, 166–182, **172**, **173**, **177**, 199, 206–209; *see also* Disaster Assistance Response Team (DART); Iraq; Persian Gulf War
Israel 111, 113n8, 217

Japan 202, 212–213
Johns Hopkins Bloomberg School of Public Health 157–163, 167, 183, 210
Johnson, Maj. Alan 206–208
Jordan 123–124, 130, 213

Kapiolani Medical Center for Women and Children 91–93; *see also* Hawaiian Islands
Karenni 139–140, 139n6; *see also* Myanmar (Burma); refugee camps
Kellermann, Dr. Arthur L. 1–3
Keltz, Army Sgt. Kimo 206–208
Kennedy, Pres. John F. 168
Kenya 5, 135, 184, 202
Kosovo *see* Yugoslavia (former)
Kowell, Jerry 190, 196; *see also* Liberian civil war
Krulak, Brig. Gen. Charles 105–109, 113, 133
Krulak, Gen. Victor (Brute) 108–109
Kurdish refugee crisis 119–138, **122**, **123**, **125**, **126**, 150–151, 166–168, 216; *see also* Kurds
Kurds: diverse religions of 120; Kurdish Democratic Party (KDP) 120–121, 129–130; Kurdistan Region 127–131; Kurdistan Workers' Party (PKK) 120, 132; Patriotic Union of Kurdistan (PUK) 120, 129–130; People's Protection Units (YPG) 132; statelessness of 119–121, 119n2, 131, 132n6; violence against 111, 120–121
Kuwait 2, 102–105, 111–118, 171, 178; *see also* Iraq; Persian Gulf War

Index

Lagos, Nigeria 15–16, 42–45, 92–96; *see also* Nigeria
leadership roles *see* Al Khanjar Navy-Marine Corps Trauma Center; Center of Excellence (COE); Defense Threat Reduction Agency; Disaster Assistance Response Team (DART); Emergency Medical Services (Hawaii); Interim Minister of Health (Iraq); International Development Global Health program; International Rescue Committee (IRC); Maui Memorial Hospital
Leahy, Sen. Patrick J. 18n1, 223; *see also* "Senator Leahy's Tribute" (Appendix 1)
Li, Dr. Zonghao 97–98
Liberian civil war 121, 125, 183–196, **185**, **191**, 202, 209
Libya 121, 125
"Listening to the Heartbeat of Humanity" *see* Appendix 1
Lofa Bridge (Liberia) 188–189; *see also* Liberian civil war
Long Island Sound 9–12
lunar exploration 53–54, 211–212
Lyman, Amb. Princeton 89, 92, 96

Mabus, Ray (Secretary of the Navy) 205–206
Macpherson, Robert Séamus (Bob) 135, 143, 223; *see also* "Listening to the Heartbeat of Humanity" (Appendix 1)
Madigan Army Medical Center 89
malaria 140–142, 186–189; *see also* illnesses
malnourishment **78**, 97, 135, **136**, 148, 186–189, 212; *see also* poverty
Manoa School of Medicine (University of Hawaii) 91, 150–153, 190
Marine Corps Forward Casualty Field Hospital *see* Delta Med (Vietnam War)
Mary Hitchcock Memorial Hospital 86–88, 86n2
mass violence 111n6, 144, 216–217
Maui, Hawaii 88–92
Maui Memorial Hospital 88–89, 90–91
Mayo Clinic 114, 202, 215
McConnell, Bernd (Bear) 167–168
McDonald, Bob 61–62

Médecins Sans Frontières (MSF) 129, 136, 141–142, 156, 192
Medical Center for Women and Children *see* Kapiolani Medical Center for Women and Children
Medical Corps *see* Medical Service Corps (MSC)
medical lectures 63, 92–97, 142, 151, 210–215; *see also* publications
medical-military cooperation *see* civilian-military cooperation
medical positions *see* Division of Emergency Medicine (University of Hawaii); Kapiolani Medical Center for Women and Children; Madigan Army Medical Center; Mary Hitchcock Memorial Hospital; Maui Memorial Hospital; Naval Health Clinic New England; pediatric practice; psychiatric practice; Yale-New Haven Hospital
medical procedures: antibiotics 26–28, 42, 213; defibrillation 43; immunization 95, 167, 189; rehabilitation 146; resuscitation 24–28, 34, 48, 54, 87, 94, 111, 201; surgeries 23, 28, **40**, 43, **55**, 111–112, **115**; tracheotomies 34, 38; transfusions 26, 54, 56, 110; vaccinations 48, 217
medical professionals: deployments 104–105, 151, 160, 210, 216–217; nurses 47, 59, 85, 88, 210–211; paramedics 38, 49, **80**, **81**, 186–189, 211; *see also* "Physician in Peril" (Appendix 2)
Medical Service Corps (MSC) 64–66, 104–109, 133
medical training 22–28, 34, 86–89, 101; *see also* Dartmouth Medical School; Harvard Medical School; Saint Michael's College; UC Berkeley School of Public Health; University of Vermont Medical School; Yale-New Haven Hospital
mental health 85–88, 112, 144, 199, 210, 218
Micronesia 103
Middle East *see* Iran; Iraq; Iraq War; Kurdish refugee crisis; Pakistan; Persian Gulf War; Syria; Turkey

military-civilian cooperation *see* civilian-military cooperation
military service: U.S. Air Force (*see* ROTC [Reserve Officers' Training Corps]; U.S. Army (*see* Madigan Army Medical Center); U.S. Marines (*see* Naval Health Clinic New England; Navy-Marine Medical Company [Persian Gulf]; 3rd Marine Division [Vietnam]); U.S. Navy (*see* Delta Med [Vietnam War]; Naval Health Clinic New England; Navy-Marine Medical Company [Persian Gulf]; U.S. Navy Captain); U.S. Navy Reserves (*see* Operation Provide Comfort [Kurdish refugee crisis]; Operation Restore Hope [Somalian civil war])
Mogadishu, Somalia 135–139; *see also* Somalian civil war
Monrovia, Liberia 184–194; *see also* Liberian civil war
the moon 53, 104, 112, 221–222; exploration 221–222
mortality and morbidity: in African continent 186; during Bosnian War 144, **144**; of children in war zones 144–148, 186, 216; of civilians in war zones 121, **136**, 167, 213–216; infant and maternal 25, 97; during Vietnam War 48–49, 74; *see also* casualties of war
MSC *see* Medical Service Corps (MSC)
MSF *see* Médecins Sans Frontières (MSF)
Muslims: Bosnian 143–145, 147; Shia 115–127, 170n3, 171, 179; Sunni 115, 119, 170, 170n3, 179
Myanmar (Burma) 134, 139–141, 139n5, 139n6

NASA 53, 221
National Academy of Medicine 3, 6
National Resident Matching Program (NRMP) 20–21, 20n2
NATO (North Atlantic Treaty Organization) 132, 145, 149
Natsios, Andrew 166–167
Naval Health Clinic New England 63–64
naval hospitals 38, 63–65, 109–113

Navy-Marine Medical Company (Persian Gulf) 104–107, **106, 110, 115**, 133; *see also* Al Khanjar Navy-Marine Corps Trauma Center; Persian Gulf War
Navy Reserves Captain 63–66, 89, 93–107, 131–133, 156, 169, 190–191, 202
New Haven, Connecticut 9, 14, 21–28, 60
Newport, Rhode Island 63–64
NGOs (non-governmental organizations) 59, 66–68, 121–139, 145–161, 184–193, 209; *see also* humanitarian aid
Nguyen Van Thieu *see* Thieu, Pres. Nguyen Van
Nierle, Jim 205–206
Nigeria 88, 94–96, 184, 188, 202
9/11 terrorist attacks 166, 181
non-governmental organizations *see* NGOs (non-governmental organizations)
North Atlantic Treaty Organization *see* NATO (North Atlantic Treaty Organization)
North Vietnam 36–42, 51, 66–73, 80; government 53n1; healthcare in 5–16; North Vietnamese Army 46, 51; Viet Cong 46, 51, 59, 80; *see also* South Vietnam; Vietnam War
Notre Dame (Catholic high school) 14–18

Oahu, Hawaii 48, 149, 183
Obama, Pres. Barack 1, 132
Old Saybrook, Connecticut 64–65
Operation Babylift (Fall of Saigon) 66–81, **69, 78, 79, 80, 81**, 106, 114; *see also* South Vietnam; Vietnam War
Operation Iraqi Freedom *see* Iraq War
Operation Provide Comfort (Kurdish refugee crisis) 119–135, **122, 123, 125**, 168; *see also* Kurds
Operation Restore Hope (Somalian civil war) 88, 130–139, **136**, 150, 184, 202
Operations Desert Sheild and Desert Storm *see* Persian Gulf War

PACOM *see* U.S. Pacific Command (PACOM)
PAHO/WHO Collaborating Center for Humanitarian Civil-Military Cooperation *see* Center of Excellence (COE); Pan-American Health Organization (PAHO); WHO (World Health Organization)
Pakistan 167n1, 217
Pan-American Health Organization (PAHO) 157
patient care 47n8, 211, 214; diagnoses 60, 88, 141, 192, 204–210; power dynamics 214, 218; unique cases 24–28, 45–47, 55, 87–88
peacekeeping forces 121–122, 130, 145, 160
pediatric practice 64–65
pediatric residency 23–28, 34, 42, 101
pediatrics 24–26, 40, 58–64, 85, 93–95; adolescent 64, 85, 101; hospitals 39, 56, 67–68; neonatal 127; obstetric 24, 39; orthopedic 93; and psychology 10–11, 14; surgeries **40, 55**; young adult 64, 85, 101
Perrin, Dr. Pierre 157–159
Persian Gulf War 102–119, 125, 133, 202, 209; *see also* Al Khanjar Navy-Marine Corps Trauma Center; Iraq; Iraq War
photography 79, 99–101, 116–118, 127–128, 191; humanitarian 130–131, **187**; medical **45**, 45–46, **78, 81, 187**; photojournalism 14, 69, 73, 79–80; of Saddam Hussein 127–128
"Physician in Peril" *see* Appendix 2
policy writings *see* publications
"Politics and Global Public Health: An Explosive, Tragic Combination" *see* Appendix 2
post-traumatic stress disorder *see* PTSD (post-traumatic stress disorder)
poverty 36, 44, 66, 71–79, 95–97, 195; *see also* malnourishment
Powell, Colin (Secretary of State) 167–168
POWs (prisoners of war): Iraqi 110–116, **115**; Vietnamese 51–52
Prehospital and Disaster Medicine (textbook) 212
professorships *see* Johns Hopkins Bloomberg School of Public Health; Manoa School of Medicine (University of Hawaii)
Prueher, Adm. Joseph W. 151, 156–160
psychiatric practice 91
psychiatric residency 85–86, 86n1, 88, 94n3
psychiatry 10–11, 85–91, 190, 218, 233
PTSD (post-traumatic stress disorder) 60, 85–86, 200, 206–208
public health 38, 65, 85–86, 142–144, 167, 180–184, 212–218; advocacy 85–89, 181–186, 209–210, 215–217; crises 129, 134, 217; economics 97, 217; global approaches 64–65, 88–92, 101–102, 132–134, 215–218; NIH lecture 210; politicization 90, 130, 169–170, 207n14; protections 169, 175, 182–186, 192, 217; *see also* "Politics and Global Public Health: An Explosive, Tragic Combination" (Appendix 2)
public medicine: 6, 89, 101, 149, 211–217; advancements 94, 94n3, 146, 211; advocacy 181, 186, 215–217; coordination 123, 216; NIH lecture 210; power dynamics 2–3, 130, 167–171, 211; teaching or training 97, 148–150, 209–211
publications: biographical 199–200; medical 40, 199–200, 212, 218; policy writings 209–210, 215; scholarly 40, 212, 218; *see also* medical lectures
Purple Heart 205, 207n14
Putin, Vladimir 216

Quang Tri (Vietnam) 36–38, 36n2, 56; *see also* South Vietnam; Vietnam War

Red Cross and Red Crescent Societies: European 121; Iraqi 123n4, 124–126, 129–130; Jordanian 123–124, 123n4; Liberian 192; in Vietnam 36, 65; *see also* American Red Cross; International Committee of the Red Cross (ICRC)
refugee camps: in Balkan Peninsula 134–149, 159; Iraqi 121–123, **122, 123**, 129–130; Jordanian 124; malaria 142; psychology 86–88; Somalian 88; Thai-Burmese 134, 139–

142, 139n6; *see also* Kurdish refugee crisis; refugees
refugees 6, 151, 169; climate change and 212–213; family separation 59–67, 72, 95, 122, 146, *187*, 188–189; Kuwaiti 114; Liberian *187*, 188–190; Nigerian 88, 95; Vietnamese 40, 46, 71, 80, 201; Vietnamese infants *69*, 69–81, *78*, *79*, *80*, *81*; *see also* Kurdish refugee crisis; refugee camps
residencies *see* pediatric residency; psychiatric residency
Rice, Dr. Matthew *100*, 100–101
ROTC (Reserve Officers' Training Corps) 89–90
Rowe, Dr. Bob 43, 59
Rumsfeld, Donald (Secretary of Defense) 168–170, 175–182
Rwanda 139–140

Sadr, Muqtada al- 2, 177–179
Saigon *see* Ho Chi Minh City (Saigon)
Saint Michael's College 17–18, 18n1, 89; *see also* "Challenging the Next Generation: Service to Others" (Appendix 2)
Saint Raphael Hospital (volunteer work) 17–18, 22, 22n4
San Diego, California 34–36
Sarajevo, Bosnia-Herzegovina *see* Yugoslavia (former)
Saudi Arabia 103–107, *106*, 113, 113n8; *see also* 1st Marine Expeditionary Force (Persian Gulf); Navy-Marine Medical Company (Persian Gulf)
scholarly collaboration 97, 149–158, 209–212, 217; *see also* medical lectures; publications
School of Public Health (Johns Hopkins) *see* Johns Hopkins Bloomberg School of Public Health
School of Public Health (UC Berkeley) *see* UC Berkeley School of Public Health
Schweitzer, Dr. Albert 2, 5, 14, *15*
2nd Force Service Support Group (Persian Gulf) 105–108, *106*
2nd Medical Battalion (Persian Gulf) 104–105, 133; *see also* Al Khanjar Navy-Marine Corps Trauma Center; Navy-Marine Medical Company (Persian Gulf); Persian Gulf War
Second World War *see* World War II
Serbia *see* Yugoslavia (former)
Shia Muslims *see* Muslims
Smith, Vice Adm. Leighton 130–133
snakes 50, 60, 141, 201
Somalian civil war 88, 130–139, *136*, 150, 184, 202
South Vietnam 15–16, 41–57, 66–67, 202; children 5, *57*, 60–72, 80; culture 36–57, 67, 72, 221–222; Dong Ha village 36, 41–42, 46–47, 54–56, 61; 1989 visit to 66n1; *see also* North Vietnam; Vietnam War
Southeast Asia *see* Cambodia; Myanmar (Burma); North Vietnam; Pakistan; South Vietnam; Thailand; Vietnam War
Soviet Union *see* USSR (the former Union of Soviet Socialist Republics)
spirituality 53–54, 221
State Department 79, 149, 168–170, 179
Stinnett, Robert *69*, *78*, 79, *79*, 79n5, *80*, *81*
Stop the Bleed® campaign 216, 216n6
stuttering 2, 13, 16, 18; *see also* disabilities
suicide 86, 144, 218–219; *see also* mental health
Sunni Muslims *see* Muslims
supply-chain logistics 42–43, 55, 104–105, 111–113, 137
Syria 119n2, 120, 127, 131–132

Tacoma, Washington 89
Talabani, Jalal 120–121, 129
Taylor, Charles 185–188, 185n2, 188n4; *see also* Liberian civil war
TBIs (traumatic brain injuries) 51, 199–208; *see also* war injuries
teaching 86–94, 111, 149–151, 160–161, 210–213; *see also* Combined Humanitarian Assistance Response Training (CHART); Health Emergencies in Large Populations (HELP) program; medical lectures; publications
teaching hospitals 20, 20n2, 86–87; *see also* Madigan Army Medical Center; Mary Hitchcock Memorial Hospital; Yale-New Haven Hospital
terrorism 181, 216–217
Thailand 139–140, 139n6, 202
Thieu, Pres. Nguyen Van 67, 71; *see also* South Vietnam; Vietnam War
3rd Marine Division (Vietnam) 34–35
Thoreau, Henry David 5, 6
Tiananmen Square 97–101, *100*; *see also* China
Tigris River (Iraq) 173–175, *177*; *see also* Iraq; Iraq War
Tito, Josip Broz (Marshal) 1, 143–145
traditional medicine *45*, 45–46, 57, 61
traumatic brain injuries *see* TBIs (traumatic brain injuries)
travels *see* Australia; China; Ethiopia; Europe; Geneva, Switzerland; Ho Chi Minh City; Japan; Kenya; Liberian civil war; Micronesia; Nigeria; Saudia Arabia; Somalian civil war; South Vietnam
Tripler Army Medical Center 150–161, 164; *see also* Akamai Telemedicine Program; Center of Excellence (COE); Manoa School of Medicine (University of Hawaii)
Trump, Pres. Donald 132, 206
Tubmanburg, Liberia 188–189; *see also* Liberian civil war
Turkey 119–123, 127–132; *see also* Kurdish refugee crisis

UC Berkeley School of Public Health 65–66, 79–81, 85–88, 97
UNICEF (UN International Children's Emergency Fund) 140, 169–170, 182
United Nations (UN) 96, 124–130, 137, 156–159, 188–194; civilian protections 96, 121, 135, 183–184, 233; Emergency System 184; humanitarian efforts 135–138, 169, 183; peacekeeping forces 121–122, 130, 160, 183; training programs 161, 164; UNICEF (International Children's Emergency Fund) 140, 169–170, 182; *see also* UNICEF (UN International Children's Emergency Fund)

Index

United States (US) see Department of Defense (DOD); Department of Veterans Affairs (VA); State Department; U.S. Air Force; U.S. Army; U.S. Foreign Service; U.S. Marines; U.S. Navy; U.S. Pacific Command (PACOM); USAID (U.S. Agency for International Development)
U.S. Air Force: in Europe 130; in Persian Gulf 114; ROTC program 89–90; transports 35–36, 64–66, 74–80, 105, 114, 118; in Vietnam 73–77, 74n4; see also Flying Tigers
U.S. Army 42–43, 89, 109, 116–118, 154–164, 179
U.S. Foreign Service 137, 179
U.S. Marines: in Iraq or Persian Gulf 104–118, 127–133, 171–179, *172*, *173*; in Somalia 135–136; training camp 34–36; in Vietnam 33–64, 85–86, 89; see also Delta Med (Vietnam War)
U.S. Navy: hospital ships 34, 38, 113; medals 205–206; in Persian Gulf 2, 102–107, 131, 181; scholarships 1, 19, 23; veterans 79n5, 93, 108; in Vietnam 33–34, 38, 48, 54–63; see also Medical Service Corps (MSC); naval hospitals
U.S. Navy Captain 63–66, 89, 93–107, 131–133, 156, 169, 190–191, 202
U.S. Pacific Command (PACOM) 151–162
University of California, Berkeley see UC Berkeley School of Public Health
University of Geneva 156–157; see also Geneva Conventions; International Humanitarian Law (IHL)
University of Hawaii see Center of Excellence (COE); Manoa School of Medicine (University of Hawaii)
University of Vermont Medical School 17–18, 20–21
"The Untold Cost of War on Civilians" see Appendix 2
urgent care medicine 92, 97; see also disaster medicine; emergency medicine
USAID (U.S. Agency for International Development) 163–170, 183

USSR (the former Union of Soviet Socialist Republics) 113n8, 132

Vietnam War 15, 23–38, 51–89, 104–118, 167, 192, 199–218; demilitarized zone (DMZ) 2, 36–38, 36n4, *47*; draft 1–2, 34; fatalities 41; Operation Babylift 66–81, *69*, *78*, *79*, *80*, *81*, 106, 114; Quang Tri 36–38, 36n2, 56; Route 1 36, 36n3, 59; 17th Parallel 36n4, 51; veterans 58–61; see also North Vietnam; Operation Babylift (Fall of Saigon); South Vietnam

war crimes 51–52, 111–115, 139–157, 170–186
war injuries: from Agent Orange 218, 218n8; amputations 40–43, *115*, 146–147, *147*; blast wounds 50, 69–70, 199–207, 216–217; and family members 199, 207–208; psychological 60, 85–86, 200, 206–208; PTSD (post-traumatic stress disorder) 60, 85–86, 200–208; TBIs (traumatic brain injuries) 50–51, 199–208; tinnitus 50, 201–202, 206; see also casualties of war
war zones: children *57*, *136*, 144–148; civilians 96, 121, 135, 167–174, 192–195, 216, 233; environmental conditions 116, *117*, 218, 218n8; family displacement *57*, 79, 95, *144*, 188–190, 213; Iraqi *172*, *173*; Kuwait 104, *106*, *110*, 113–118, *117*; medical facility looting 171–174, 178–179; psychology 85–86; sexual violence 188n4, 191; Somalian 137, *185*; Vietnamese 201, 209; see also "The Untold Cost of War on Civilians" (Appendix 2)
warlords see Aidid, Mohamed Farrah; Hussein, Saddam; Putin, Vladimir; Taylor, Charles
wars: camaraderie during 58–59; destructiveness 54, 126, *144*, 167, *185*, 195, 209; ground 40, 107–109; homesickness 44, 57; nameless 134; reverberations 9; shared experience 59; 21st-century 217; in urban areas 212; see also Bosnian War; Iraq War; Liberian civil war; Persian Gulf War; Somalian civil war; Vietnam War; World War I; World War II
weapons: automatic weapons 36, 44–51, 73, 124, 176, 188–189, *191*; bombs 50, 75–76, 80, 195, 217; IEDs (improvised explosive devices) 199; machetes 189–192, *191*; rocket launchers 127; Scud ballistic missiles 113, 113n8, 206–207, 207n14; surface-to-air missiles (SAMs) 70, 119n1; trafficking 124
Whiteman, Lt. Comm. Jamie 114–116
WHO (World Health Organization) 65, 92, 121, 129, 140, 151–170, 183–195
WHO-AFRO (WHO Regional Office for Africa) 184, 192–195
women's rights 13, 138, 191
Woodrow Wilson International Center for Scholars 6
World Airways 67–68, 70–71, 77, 79; see also Operation Babylift (Fall of Saigon)
World Health Organization see WHO (World Health Organization)
World War I 11, 131–132, 207–208
World War II 9–14, 42, 105–108, 147, 208

Xiaoping, Deng 99–100

Yale-New Haven Hospital 20–29, 34, 42, 48, 55, 64
Yarmouk Hospital (Baghdad) 171–172, 178–179
young adult medicine see pediatrics
Yugoslavia (former): Bosnia-Herzegovina 136–147, *144*; Bosnian Muslims 143–147; Croatia 139, 143–148, *147*; Kosovo 149, 149n12, 159; Sarajevo siege 143–144, *144*; Serbia 139, 143–145, *146*, 149, 149n12

Zagreb, Croatia 146–147, 147n10; see also Bosnian War; Yugoslavia (former)

www.ingramcontent.com/pod-product-compliance
Ingram Content Group UK Ltd.
Pitfield, Milton Keynes, MK11 3LW, UK
UKHW050541150426
5217IPUK00026B/2020